Practical Alternatives to the Psychiatric Model of Mental Illness

Beyond DSM and ICD Diagnosing

Edited by

Arnoldo Cantú, Eric Maisel, and Chuck Ruby

Practical Alternatives to the Psychiatric Model of Mental Illness is the fifth Volume of the Ethics International Press *Critical Psychology and Critical Psychiatry Series.*

Practical Alternatives to the Psychiatric Model of Mental Illness: Beyond DSM and ICD Diagnosing

Edited by Arnoldo Cantú, Eric Maisel, and Chuck Ruby

This book first published 2024

Ethics International Press Ltd, UK

British Library Cataloguing in Publication Data

A catalogue record for this book is available from the British Library

Print Book ISBN: 978-1-80441-286-2

eBook ISBN: 978-1-80441-287-9

To Dara, my loving and unwavering rock,

who has helped keep me sane in an insane world.

-AC

Contents

Editor's Introduction

Arnoldo Cantú

"Get it out of me!" This was how a bright 17-year-old male I saw for therapy described his response to be as he recounted the moment during which he, as a child, was told he had "ADHD" by his pediatrician. That story has stuck with me—the panic and fatalism he reported feeling. And in my time working as a clinician helping children, families, and adults share their stories while I, simultaneously, dictated it for them through the act of affixing a psychiatric diagnosis (primarily for billing and insurance purposes, at least here in the US), the cognitive dissonance has only amplified.

The philosopher Kwame Anthony Appiah wrote a provocative book entitled *The Lies That Bind: Rethinking Identity* in which he argued that certain notions of identity, such as those predicated on race and nationality, are built on inconsistent, unstable, and disjointed ideas.[1] I contend that "mental disorder" is additional contemporary example of a lie that binds humanity given their intractable and questionable, at best, epistemological foundations—and the longstanding universality of human suffering they erroneously continue to mislabel.

Therefore, this volume is an attempt at helping the reader learn of and understand different ways of supporting people experiencing difficulties— conceptualizations that an individual would ordinarily be described as suffering from a "mental disorder" or "mental illness." This book recognizes and appreciates standing on the shoulders of giants; that is, those who have contributed to the abundance of literature critiquing the biomedical model of mental health and practice of psychiatric diagnosing. As such, this an attempt to move *past* that rhetoric and discourse—and,

---

[1] Appiah, K. A. (2018). *The lies that bind: Rethinking identity*. Liveright Publishing Corporation.

instead, envision *practical* and *implementable* alternatives to psychiatric diagnosing.

In short, the aim of this volume is to help people walk away with ideas and novel thinking for alternative yet practical ways of working with people without having to resort to medicalizing and pathologizing their experiences—to sidestep and resist the pull of the traditional and predominant biomedical model's ritual of affixing questionable psychiatric diagnoses onto vulnerable individuals as a way to "explain" and "treat" their suffering and difficulties—lest we perpetuate the deception and oppression.

When I told the 17-year-old male that not only is "ADHD" and its concomitant menu of mental disorders controversial, but that there are other ways to help (provisionally) make sense of—and address—his difficulties, a noticeable look of relief and hopefulness appeared on his face. As I have argued elsewhere, "[T]he default setting of the human experience is to consist of challenges and suffering. Dysfunction is normal and having problems is to be expected throughout a lifetime. As such, when struggling we deserve to enter systems of care that will lift us up, rather than tell us what, at our existential core, is wrong or 'disordered' with us while we are already suffering."[2] It is my hope that this volume can provide the reader with a refreshing, newfound set of tools for going about doing that.

Disclaimer: *If you or anyone you know is taking a prescriptive psychiatric medication for any reason deemed appropriate by the prescribing physician, alteration or discontinuation of the drug(s) is not recommended by any of the information provided by the reading material found in this volume, Similarly, the content in this book should not be interpreted, directly or indirectly, as suggestions for any other current support (e.g., psychotherapy, counseling) to be abruptly discontinued without discussion with your healthcare provider.*

---

[2] Cantú, A. (2023). Toward a descriptive problem-based taxonomy for mental health: A nonmedicalized way out of the biomedical model. *Journal of Humanistic Psychology*, 1–24. https://doi.org/10.1177/00221678231167612, p. 17.

Setting the Stage

The Myth of Psychiatric Diagnosis

Wayne Ramsay

Abstract: *Psychiatric diagnosis can determine who is hired for a job, who can be licensed to practice law or medicine, or pilot an airplane, or legally possess a firearm, or have custody of their children. The stigma of a psychiatric diagnosis can ruin or end careers. People who have never committed a crime are involuntarily committed to institutions for days, weeks, years, or a lifetime because of psychiatric diagnosis. People who have committed crimes are excused from responsibility as not guilty by reason of insanity because of psychiatric diagnosis. In this chapter, the author shows psychiatric diagnosis is unscientific, arbitrary, and unreliable and should never be the reason for a decision.*

In a telephone conversation with a state legislator who at the time was Speaker of her state's House of Representatives, and who had been quoted in a newspaper saying she was proud to have sponsored legislation requiring health insurance policies to pay for psychiatric treatment, I referred to people being "accused of mental illness." She disagreed with or corrected me, saying "It's not an accusation. It's a diagnosis."

People who disagree with the concept of mental illness and with the associated idea of psychiatric diagnosis call psychiatric diagnoses "labels." Such critics allege psychiatric "diagnoses" or labels are no more scientifically valid than pejorative nonscientific insults. As psychologist Jeffrey Schaler said in 2006:

> Think of how when people get angry with one another, they inevitably resort to some kind of diagnosis. They say, "You're crazy! You're mentally ill! You're paranoid!" Can you imagine somebody

getting angry with someone and saying, "You have diabetes! You have Parkinson's Disease!"[1]

Accusing someone of mental illness is an insult. Accusing someone of having diabetes or Parkinson's Disease or any other physical illness is not. Because we do not live our lives in isolation but in a society of other people, and because a psychiatric "diagnosis" can change how other people treat a person, a psychiatric "diagnosis" can deprive a person of many of life's most important opportunities and can harm or ruin a person's life. The childhood taunt, "Sticks and stones can break my bones, but words can never hurt me" is simply not true if the words are a psychiatric "diagnosis." As was said by psychiatry professor Thomas Szasz, M.D.,

> The problem with psychiatric diagnoses is not that they are meaningless, but that they may be, and often are, swung as semantic blackjacks: cracking the subject's dignity and respectability destroys him just as effectively as cracking his skull. The difference is that the man who wields a blackjack is recognized by everyone as a thug, but the one who wields a psychiatric diagnoses is not.[2]

Psychiatric "diagnosis" can result in a person who seems normal to the average person, and who is law-abiding, spending his or her whole life imprisoned in a mental institution rather than living in freedom. Psychiatric "diagnosis" can defeat the proper functioning of the system of justice, examples being a person being found not guilty by reason of insanity and avoiding punishment for a serious crime, or a good parent losing custody of his or her child. In an interview on February 11, 2012, psychologist Paula Caplan, Ph.D. said:

> [P]sychiatric diagnosis is the fundamental building block of everything else bad that happens in the mental health system. If you don't get a label, you can't get put on drugs that might help you but are more likely to hurt you. If you don't get a label, then you can't lose your job or custody of your kids or your legal rights because of

---

[1] "Jeffrey A. Schaler, Ph.D., Professor of Psychology",
https://www.youtube.com/watch?v=_-iYngr6N60 at 4:05
[2] Thomas S. Szasz, M.D., *The Second Sin*, Anchor Press, 1973, p. 71

having a label…When you hear somebody say "I lost custody of my children because I had a label that I thought was pretty mild, but you know what—it 'proved' that I'm mentally ill, and they took my children away from me."…You can't hear these stories…year after year…and not try to do something about it. People's lives have been destroyed by getting a psychiatric label.[3]

In his book *Saving Normal: An Insider's Revolt Against Out-of-Control Psychiatric Diagnosis, DSM-5, Big Pharma, and the Medicalization of Ordinary Life* (2013), psychiatrist Allen Frances, M.D. says this:

I led the Task Force that developed *DSM-IV* [American Psychiatric Association's *Diagnostic and Statistical Manual of Mental Disorders*, fourth edition] and also chaired the department of psychiatry at Duke [University], treated many patients … *DSM* has gained a huge societal significance and determines all sorts of important things that have an enormous impact on people's lives—like…who gets to be hired for a job, can adopt a child, or pilot a plane, or qualifies for life insurance … Done poorly, psychiatric diagnosis can be an un-mitigated disaster leading to aggressive treatments with horrible complications and life-shattering impact…Psychiatric diagnosis is a serious business with major and often lifelong consequences."[4]

In Chapter 3 of *Saving Normal*, "Diagnostic Inflation," Dr. Frances includes a section quite appropriately titled "The Power to Label Is the Power to Destroy."[5] Because of the damaging, even life-ruining power of psychiatric diagnosis (or of psychiatric "labels"), the validity, accuracy, reliability, and predictability of psychiatric diagnosis is important. Investigations repeatedly reveal psychiatric diagnosis has *no* reliability or validity.

---

[3] MindFreedom Live Free Web Radio: "Paula Caplan v. Psychiatric Labeling!", https://www.blogtalkradio.com/davidwoaks/2010/03/13/ mindfreedom-mad-pride-live-free-web-radio

[4] Allen Frances, M.D., *Saving Normal: An Insider's Revolt Against Out-of-Control Psychiatric Diagnosis, DSM-5, Big Pharma, and the Medicalization of Ordinary Life,* Harper Collins, 2013, pp. xi, xii, 277

[5] *Id.,* p. 109

In 1887, Nellie Bly (1867-1922), a newspaper reporter, feigned insanity to gain admission to New York's Blackwell's Island insane asylum. She described how she did it and what she saw at the asylum in a book titled *Ten Days in a Mad House*. "I had little belief in my ability to deceive the insanity experts," she wrote in Chapter 1, and in Chapter 2, "to be examined by a number of learned physicians who make insanity a specialty, and who daily come in contact with insane people! How could I hope to pass these doctors and convince them that I was crazy?" In Chapter 6 while at Bellevue Hospital, after it was apparent she had succeeded before her transfer to Blackwell's Island, she wrote:

> And so I passed my second medical expert. After this I began to have a smaller regard for the ability of doctors than I ever had before, and a greater one for myself. I felt sure now that no doctor could tell whether people were insane or not.

In chapter 7, listening to Tillie Mayard, a fellow patient at Bellevue Hospital who had just found out she was in an insane asylum after being told she was going to a "convalescent ward to be treated for nervous debility," Nellie Bly heard Ms. Mayard say to a doctor, "If you know anything at all you should be able to tell that I am perfectly sane. Why don't you test me?" Bly said the doctor "left the poor girl condemned to an insane asylum, probably for life, without giving her one feeble chance to prove her sanity." In Chapter 8, Bly describes this same Tillie Mayard pleading with a doctor after arriving at Blackwell's Island insane asylum:

> I could hear her gently but firmly pleading her case. All her remarks were as rational as any I ever heard, and I thought no good physician could help but be impressed with her story...She begged that they try all their tests for insanity, if they had any, and give her justice. Poor girl, how my heart ached for her! I determined then and there that I would try by every means to make my mission of benefit to my suffering sisters; that I would show how they are committed without ample trial.

Of herself, Bly wrote in Chapter 1:

From the moment I entered the insane ward on the Island, I made no attempt to keep up the assumed *role* of insanity. I talked and acted just as I do in ordinary life. Yet strange to say, the more sanely I talked and acted, the crazier I was thought to be by all except one physician, whose kindness and gentle ways I shall not soon forget.

Of her own departure from Blackwell's Island, after intervention by her editor, she said:

I left the insane ward with pleasure and regret—pleasure that I was once more able to enjoy the free breath of heaven; regret that I could not have brought with me some of the unfortunate women who lived and suffered with me, and who, I am convinced, are just as sane as I was and am now myself.

A similar experiment was done in the 1970s by Stanford University psychology professor David Rosenhan and his colleagues that was published in 1973 in *Science* magazine.[6] Dr. Rosenhan and seven of his colleagues who had no history of or evidence of mental illness (called "pseudopatients" in the study) went to 12 different psychiatric hospitals on the East and West coasts of the U.S.A. as inpatients where they remained as long as 52 days. They found that no matter how normally they behaved they were not recognized as normal by the psychiatrists and other mental health professionals they came in contact with.

Despite being normal, all were prescribed psychiatric drugs: "All told, the [eight] pseudopatients were administered nearly 2100 pills, including Elavil, Stelazine, Compazine, and Thorazine," which undermines the commonly held belief psychiatric drugs are given only to people who need them. (A more important question is whether *anybody* needs psychiatric drugs: see Peter R. Breggin, M.D., *Psychiatric Drugs: Hazards to the Brain* [1983], *Brain Disabling Treatments in Psychiatry, Second Edition* [2008], or

---

[6] *Science* magazine, "On Being Sane in Insane Places", Vol. 179 (January 19, 1973), pp. 250-258; available online at
https://www.canonsociaalwerk.eu/1971_stigma/1973%20Rosenhan%20Being%20sane%20in%20insane%20places%20OCR.pdf

Joanna Moncrieff, M.D., *The Myth of the Chemical Cure: A Critique of Psychiatric Drug Treatment* [2009]).

When the results of this experiment were revealed to the psychiatrists and other staff members of another psychiatric hospital, they "doubted that such an error could occur at their hospital." Dr. Rosenhan said "The staff was informed that at some time during the following 3 months, one or more pseudopatients would attempt to be admitted into the psychiatric hospital." During that time the hospital staff identified "Forty-one patients...with high confidence, to be pseudopatients...Twenty-three were considered suspect by at least one psychiatrist. ... Actually," said Dr. Rosenhan, "no genuine pseudopatient (at least not from my group) presented himself during this period."

Dr. Rosenhan concluded that the inability of psychiatrists and other mental health professionals to distinguish normal persons, such as himself and his colleagues, from true mental patients is "frightening." He said:

> How many people, one wonders, are sane but not recognized as such in our psychiatric institutions? How many have been needlessly stripped of their privileges of citizenship, from the right to vote and drive to that of handling their own accounts? How many have feigned insanity in order to avoid the criminal consequences of their behavior, and conversely, how many would rather stand trial than live interminably in a psychiatric hospital — but are wrongly thought to be mentally ill? How many have been stigmatized by well-intentioned, but nevertheless erroneous, diagnoses?[7]

In his book *Psychiatry: The Science of Lies*, psychiatry professor Thomas Szasz, M.D. says:

> The assertion rests on an erroneous premise, namely, that the doctors were interested in distinguishing insane inmates properly committed from sane inmates falsely detained. The whole history of psychiatry belies this assumption...each time experience was

---

[7] *Id.*, canonsociaalwerk.eu, p. 184

consulted, it showed that the experts were unable to distinguish the sane from the insane.[8]

A study titled "Suggestion Effects in Psychiatric Diagnosis" by psychologist Maurice K. Temerlin, Ph.D. published in 1968 explored "interpersonal influences which might affect psychiatric diagnosis" by having "psychiatrists, clinical psychologists and graduate students in clinical psychology" diagnose a "sound-recorded interview with a normal, healthy man."

When they heard the tape-recorded interview after introductory remarks by "a professional person of high prestige" saying the interview was with a perfectly healthy man, the "psychologists, psychiatrists, and graduate students agreed unanimously." When the tape-recording was heard by a group after introductory remarks by "a professional person of high prestige" saying the recorded interview was with a man who "looked neurotic but actually was quite psychotic...diagnoses of psychosis were made by 60 per cent of the psychiatrists, 28 per cent of the clinical psychologists, and 11 per cent of the graduate students," even though they had listened to the same tape-recording.[9] This study like others shows psychiatric diagnosis has *no* reliability and no validity.

Psychiatrist Allen Frances criticizes the lack of science and the pathologizing of normality in both his own and the current *DSM* in articles, lectures, and his book, *Saving Normal.* Lecturing at the University of Toronto on May 6, 2012, he said "We're giving too much treatment to people who don't need it."[10] In his book *Saving Normal,* Dr. Frances says overly broad psychiatric diagnostic criteria have caused "false epidemics of autistic, attention deficit, and adult bipolar disorder, and ... of several other disorders."[11] In an article on November 8, 2011 he said, "Since the DSM 5 suggestions will all broaden the definition of mental disorder, why

---

[8] Thomas S. Szasz, M.D., *Psychiatry: The Science of Lies,* Syracuse University Press, 2008, pp. 67-68

[9] Maurice K. Temerlin, *The Journal of Nervous and Mental Disease* Vol. 147, No. 4, pp. 349-353

[10] "Allen J. Frances on the overdiagnosis of mental illness", https://www.youtube.com/channel/UCHCmjknv18tgygUD7d38lkQ at 29:30

[11] *Saving Normal* (see note 4, above), p. 75.

should we not worry about diagnostic inflation and the massive mislabeling of normal people as mentally ill?"[12]

Bona-fide diagnosis reveals the *cause* of a problem. A psychiatric "diagnosis" does not do that. A psychiatric "diagnosis" is merely a *description* of disliked behavior.

In his book *Psychiatry: The Science of Lies*, psychiatry professor Thomas Szasz, M.D. says "Modern psychiatry—with its *Diagnostic and Statistical Manuals* of nonexisting diseases and their coercive cures—is a monument to quackery on a scale undreamed of in the annals of medicine."[13]

According to U.S. National Institute of Mental Health (NIMH) director Thomas Insel, M.D., in an article published on the NIMH web site on April 29, 2013, "The strength of each of the editions of DSM has been 'reliability'—each edition has ensured that clinicians use the same terms in the same ways. The weakness is its lack of validity." (Validity means *truth*.) For this reason, Dr. Insel says, the "NIMH will be re-orienting its research away from DSM categories."[14] No less than America's preeminent mental health government agency has rejected American Psychiatric Association's *DSM* "diagnosis."

Dr. Insel seeks to substitute an equally invalid approach. In the same article he says "Mental disorders are biological disorders involving brain circuits" and that the NIMH will seek to create "a new nosology" that is more scientific than that of the *DSM*, one based on biological factors.[15] Because the defining characteristic of a mental "illness" or "disorder" is merely *disapproval*, and biology is no more the cause of mental illnesses or disorders

---

[12] Allen Frances, M.D., "APA Responds Lamely to the Petition to Reform DSM-5", November 8, 2011, https://www.psychologytoday.com/us/blog/dsm5-in-distress/201111/apa-responds-lamely-to-the-petition-to-reform-dsm-5
[13] Thomas S. Szasz, M.D., *Psychiatry: The Science of Lies*, Syracuse University Press, 2008, pp. 18-19
[14] Thomas Insel, M.D., "Director's Blog: Transforming Diagnosis", April 29, 2013, https://web.archive.org/web/20130527220058/ http://www.nimh.nih.gov:80/about/director/index.shtml
[15] *Id.*

than electronics are the cause of bad television programs, this NIMH effort is doomed to failure.

Contrary to Dr. Insel's observation, the *DSM-5* interrater reliability results were actually poor, at least in the opinion of *DSM-IV* and *DSM-IV-TR* Task Force chairperson Allen Frances, M.D. In his book *Saving Normal*, Dr. Frances says this:

> APA [American Psychiatric Association] flunked — instead of admitting that its reliability results were unacceptable and seeking the necessary corrections that might meet historical standards, the goalposts were moved. Declaring by fiat that previous expectations were too high, *DSM-5* announced it would accept agreements among raters that were sometimes barely better than two monkeys throwing darts at a diagnostic board.[16]

In an article titled "A Response to 'How Reliable Is Reliable Enough?'" on January 18, 2012, Dr. Frances said:

> In the past, "acceptable" meant kappas of 0.6 or above…For DSM-5, "acceptable" reliability has been reduced to a startling 0.2-0.4. This barely exceeds the level of agreement you might expect to get by pure chance. … Can "accepting" unacceptably poor agreement uphold the integrity of psychiatric diagnosis?[17]

So, actually, psychiatric diagnosis not only has no validity (truth), but also no "reliability" (agreement among observers).

Because psychiatric diagnosis has neither validity nor reliability, nor general acceptance even within psychiatry, it does not meet legal criteria for acceptance as scientific or expert evidence in courts of law under either of the standards applied by courts in the U.S.A., namely, the *"sufficiently established and accepted"*[18] standard of *Frye v. U.S.*, 293 F. 1013 (D.C. Cir. 1923)

---

[16] *Saving Normal* (see above, note 4), p. 175
[17] Allen Frances, M.D., "A Response to 'How Reliable Is Reliable Enough?'", January 18, 2012, https://www.psychiatrictimes.com/view/response-how-reliable-reliable-enough
[18] As interpreted in *Diaz v. Secretary*, 2:14-cv-91-JES-MRM (M.D. Fla. Sep. 27, 2021), footnote 8, https://casetext.com/case/diaz-v-secy-doc-1

that is used in some states, nor the *scientific validity* standard of *Daubert v. Merrell Dow Pharmaceuticals*, 509 U.S. 579 (1993) that applies in federal courts and other states of the U.S.A.[19]

Courts should recognize this and stop accepting psychiatric testimony. Involuntary commitment law typically requires commitments be based on "competent psychiatric testimony." For example, Texas Constitution Article 1, Sec. 15-a provides that "No person shall be committed as a person of unsound mind except on competent medical or psychiatric testimony." However, there is no such thing as "competent psychiatric testimony" any more than there is, for example, "competent astrology testimony" or "competent palm reader testimony."

In her book *Whores of the Court: The Fraud of Psychiatric Testimony and the Rape of American Justice*, Boston University psychology professor Margaret Hagen, Ph.D., laments the fact that "we buy the accreditation of psychiatry at medical schools as if it were on the same standing as any other medical specialty" when it is not. She says, "Judges and juries, the people alone, must decide questions of insanity, competence, rehabilitation, custody, injury, and disability without the help of psychological experts and their fraudulent skills." She adds that by accepting psychiatrists and psychologists as expert witnesses in court, "Society has created its own monster".[20]

How much of a monster we have created by recognizing psychiatric and psychological diagnosis as valid (when it is not) is illustrated by Robyn M. Dawes, Ph.D., a psychology professor at Carnegie-Mellon University, former head of the psychology department at the University of Oregon, and former president of the Oregon Psychological Association, in his book *House of Cards: Psychology and Psychotherapy Built on Myth*. He tells a true story of a young woman who was determined to need involuntary commitment to a state mental hospital because of her interpretation of a single inkblot in what is known as the Rorschach inkblot test.

---

[19] "Frye Standard", https://en.wikipedia.org/wiki/Frye_standard
[20] Margaret Hagen, Ph.D., *Whores of the Court: The Fraud of Psychiatric Testimony and the Rape of American Justice*, Harper Collins, 1997, pp. 303, 313 & 310

He says on the basis of her interpretation of a single inkblot (she thought it looked like a bear), the young woman was "diagnosed" as schizophrenic and (italics are Dr. Dawes'): *"The staff—over my objection—further agreed that if her parents were ever to bring her back, she should be sent directly to the nearby state hospital...*she may well have been condemned to serve time in that snake pit on the basis of a single Rorschach response."[21] Dr. Dawes says psychiatrists and psychologists lack expertise and "should be thrown out of court."[22]

The bottom line is this: Psychiatric diagnosis is nonsense and should be ignored by all. Psychiatric diagnosis serving as the basis of state and federal laws and judgments of courts is the triumph of pseudoscience over justice.

---

[21] Robyn M. Dawes, Ph.D., *House of Cards: Psychology and Psychotherapy Built on Myth,* Free Press, 1994, p. 153-154
[22] *Id.,* p. 25.

The Alternatives

Restoring the Humanity in Human Services: Pathways Vermont's Relationship-First Practice

J River Helms

Abstract: *In this chapter, the author outlines the principles of Pathways Vermont's Relationship-First Practice: humanity, authenticity, collaboration, humility, curiosity, and hope. Readers will gain insight into the efficacy and sustainability of a practice that centers lived experience as expertise and conceptualizes discomfort and challenges in relationships as opportunities for growth, learning, and transformation. Our Relationship-First Practice is rooted in the disability justice, mad pride, and psychiatric survivor movements—and is inspired by various frameworks including harm reduction, the social model of disability, trauma-informed care, and person-centered care. This practice offers a practical alternative to the way services are provided under the medical model of mental illness, which has long fostered disconnection, inauthenticity, fear, coercion, and control in human services systems. Through the principles of our Relationship-First Practice, service providers and service participants co-create collaborative relationships that inspire and welcome change: roles aren't always static; experiences aren't only ever regarded as chronic or permanent; and beliefs about self, relationships, and the world shift. Utilizing this practice allows service providers to establish and build relationships that are more sustainable long-term as well as participate in transformation that extends beyond the relationship into social and systems change.*

Pathways Vermont is a social justice organization that seeks to build community, increase connection, and support autonomy, choice, and self-determination by providing housing services and innovative mental health alternatives across the state of Vermont. Many Pathways staff come to this work with their own lived experiences including psychiatric diagnoses, thoughts of suicide, extreme states, hearing voices, self-harm, substance use challenges, homelessness, institutionalization, and incarceration.

In our experience working within the human services system (as well as receiving services ourselves), we've observed that service providers are often taught to distance themselves from service participants in various ways: they're discouraged from talking about their lives outside of their work (though life and work overlap for most, if not all, of us); they're discouraged from talking about their own relevant lived experience; or they're discouraged from showing up authentically or connecting with service participants on a human-to-human level. These conditions are, in part, byproducts of the psychiatric model of mental illness.

At base, the psychiatric model asserts a "normal" or "acceptable" range of human emotion and behavior; experiences outside of this range are pathologized as mental disorders or illnesses that require treatment (nay, *correction*) with interventions such as psychiatric drugs, institutionalization, and therapy. Throughout the history of this model, its assertions of "normal" or "acceptable" have been rooted in various oppressive systems and ideologies including white supremacy, colonialism, capitalism, patriarchy, heteronormativity, cisnormativity, and ableism.

Rather than diagnose a society and its systems as oppressive and unjust, the approach has been to pathologize individual people for their identities, emotions, actions, and desires as well as their resistance to oppression, injustice, and inequity. The model has decontextualized the complex, nuanced experiences of human beings and framed a person's response to their circumstances as the problem.

We want to be clear: we do not seek to begrudge, judge, or shame individual people who find meaning in personally identifying with a mental illness or psychiatric label. We know that some feel validated by a diagnosis—that a psychiatric label can feel like an answer to a question that's previously been painfully unanswerable. We value choice, autonomy, and self-determination—and this means that we support people to make meaning in ways that work for them individually.

We also seek an alternative to the psychiatric model of mental illness which has, by and large, located social problems within individual people— precisely because we value choice, autonomy, and self-determination. The psychiatric model of mental illness has created a process of othering that's been used to justify coercion, force, restraint, isolation, abuse, sterilization, and genocide. There is no use in downplaying or tiptoeing around this history and context.

Our work at Pathways Vermont is driven by our commitment to disability justice. We are particularly informed by the social model of disability. In this model, disability is not regarded as a "problem" located within an individual person in need of "fixing" or "correcting." Instead, our focus must be on addressing and dismantling social barriers that are disabling. We're all impacted by social barriers, our nuanced experiences of the world, and the things that have happened to us, though many of us have been taught to decontextualize the suffering of others—to practice sympathy rather than empathy, to "fix" rather than to understand—and, in turn, to decontextualize our own suffering.

To do this is inherently protective, of course: to truly be with and understand someone in their suffering is hard, to truly be with and understand our own suffering is hard. If I'm disconnected from the suffering of others as well as my own suffering, then I don't have to acknowledge the ways that each of us are impacted by grief, loss, disempowerment, inaccessibility, discrimination, inequity, and injustice. This disconnect robs us from doing the profound, meaningful work of exploring possibilities, creating change, and inviting growth and transformation. The social model of disability suggests that, in order for anything to truly change, we all have to work towards change together.

Since our inception in 2010, Pathways Vermont has been trying to do something different—to put the human back in human services and create change through our Relationship-First Practice. We recognize providing services is not about an "us versus them" (service providers versus service participants) dynamic. Service providers are not "whole" and service participants are not "broken"—we believe that we are all part of the human experience, that service providers and service participants are linked together in community.

Our Relationship-First Practice necessitates that service providers reconnect with their humanity, tune into their own emotions, and show up authentically in their relationships. We recognize that there are social barriers and systems of oppression that seek to disconnect us from ourselves and each other because disconnection and disempowerment go hand in hand. Our Relationship-First Practice is meant, in part, to be an antidote to disconnection and disempowerment.

This practice also asks (nay, *requires*) service providers to tolerate and even embrace discomfort in their relationships with service participants. Discomfort is, after all, frequently a precursor to learning, growth, and transformation. And we've seen the harm that can be done when people in positions of power struggle to tolerate discomfort in relationships—discomfort becomes fear, fear leads to seeking control.

Our Relationship-First Practice serves as a reminder that even when we're afraid, even when nothing makes sense or everything feels hard or impossible in a relationship with a service participant, we're in a relationship *first*, so we always have a starting place. To illustrate our Relationship-First Practice, here's a bit about my relationship with a Pathways service participant who consented to having this story about his self-harming experience shared:

When I was a service coordinator in our Housing First program, I supported a service participant who sometimes self-harmed, cutting in particular. One afternoon we were on a hike (we often went for walks during our time together, Vermont weather permitting) and he told me he'd recently cut using an X-Acto knife. We talked about how he used self-harm as a strategy when his distress became overwhelming (in this case, his feelings about an anniversary related to a significant traumatic experience).

He reflected that the cutting was a tool he used to make his distress feel more manageable. I validated his experience and conveyed my appreciation that he had a tool that worked for him. I spoke about my own history of getting tattoos during times of intense distress—how the process of being tattooed reminded me that pain and distress can be transformative.

He noted that the wound from the cut was long and somewhat deep. My authentic response at that moment was concern that his wound may become infected if not cared for properly; I asked if I could share my concerns with him and he consented. He said that he did not want to have an infected wound. I asked if I could look at the wound with him (he was wearing long sleeves that day and his forearm, where he'd cut, was covered). He consented and lifted his sleeve to show me his wound which, as he'd described, was long and somewhat deep.

Together we talked about options for wound care and bandaging. I offered that we could stop by the store for wound care supplies on the way back to his house, though he said he didn't need that support. We continued our hike and conversation for another hour or so during which we explored the meaning of the distress he was experiencing and talked about various other unrelated topics.

I believe this experience highlights the principles of our Relationship-First Practice: *Humanity. Authenticity. Collaboration. Humility. Curiosity. Hope.* I trusted this service participant as the expert of his own experience. I acknowledged and validated that he used self-harm as a survival strategy. I shared some about my own experiences with navigating distress. With his consent, I voiced my own concerns about wound care and together we had a mutual conversation wherein I offered support that he declined. I did not try to problem solve nor change or control his experience.

My approach was to show up authentically, center our relationship, remain curious, and, above all, trust him and his capacity to know and meet his own needs. This experience changed my life. My relationship with this service participant changed my life. Together we practiced vulnerability and connected about some of our deepest pains. We talked about our needs, we made meaning together, we trusted each other, and we co-created a relationship that became a transformative space. This was all possible because we tolerated discomfort together, focused on the relationship first, and built something truly authentic and collaborative.

How do we build relationships rooted in authentic human connection?

First and foremost, we trust service participants as experts of their own experiences. At Pathways Vermont, we do not train staff to show up to relationships thinking they need to have all the answers or solve all the problems a person might be experiencing.

We train staff to show up with humility, curiosity, and a willingness to learn alongside the folks they're paid to support. We prioritize autonomy, choice, self-determination, and mutual responsibility. We understand that it's an honor to be part of someone's journey and we treat it as such, even on tough days (and sometimes there are some really tough days!).

We talk about the relationship, how things are going, what's working well, what feels challenging or difficult, and how we might try something different. We understand that relationships change over time because people change over time. We aspire to be flexible and to remember that each interaction is new—an intense disconnect last week doesn't mean that today's visit won't go well.

We utilize this practice across our programs: permanent supportive housing and rapid rehousing, a peer support warmline, a community center, and our Soteria House (a therapeutic residential program for folks experiencing extreme states often referred to as "psychosis"). We've found that this practice works well for everyone involved—service participants and service providers alike, regardless of their background and lived experience—because the focus is on collaboration and building meaningful, authentic relationships.

In our practice, traditional helper-helpee dynamics and clinical notions of expertise are left behind and relationships become co-creative spaces. Each person is understood to have valuable wisdom, insight, and knowledge. Power imbalances are directly addressed, and power is shared in relationships. When collaboration is the focus, service providers and service participants can explore opportunities for meaning-making and figure out together how to build a sustainable relationship dynamic. This practice minimizes coercion and centers the transformative power of building authentic and collaborative relationships.

Through collaborative relationships, each person has the opportunity to learn and grow because there's shared understanding and agreement about what the relationship means, how it works, each person's needs and expectations, and each person's capacity to contribute—all of which may be continuously negotiated throughout the relationship. As such, collaborative relationships inspire and welcome change: roles aren't always static, experiences aren't only ever regarded as chronic, and beliefs about self, relationships, and the world can shift.

Collaborative service relationships are rooted in the belief that all people, including service participants, have the capacity for self-defined and self-determined change and growth, that each person can build a different life for themselves if they so desire. We know a service relationship works when each person communicates openly and honestly, talks about their needs and boundaries, and gives feedback (not just positive!) to let the other person know what is/isn't working for them. We co-create service relationships via the following principles:

Humanity

We encourage service providers to show up as their **whole, human selves** in service relationships. This requires intentional ongoing self-reflection: *Who am I? What pieces of myself do I want to bring to my service relationships? How do I make meaning? How do I move through my own fear and discomfort? What dynamics do I fall into? Are there dynamics that I want to change?* This self-reflection inspires curiosity and flexibility. Relationships work well when they're dynamic and flexible (not static and rigid) because humans are dynamic.

We invite service participants to show up as their whole selves, too—to reflect on how they've made meaning out of their experiences and to share with us what they feel comfortable sharing. This practice is trauma-informed and person-centered. Trauma is fundamentally about a loss of power and identity. When a service participant is able to show up as their whole self and experience empathetic support without judgment or coercion, they're able to (re)claim their power within relationships and be authentic. When a service provider is able to show up as their whole self, they're able to build authentic, sustainable relationships.

There is much value in hiring staff with various backgrounds and lived experiences, including folks who've experienced homelessness, folks who've received psychiatric diagnoses, folks who've experienced extreme states, folks who've considered and/or attempted suicide, folks who've experienced challenges with substance use, and folks who've been institutionalized or incarcerated. Lived experience is an asset to service relationships.

Service providers can share pieces of their experiences in ways that are mutual, meaningful, and intentional in their relationships with service participants. Mutuality and intentionality are key here: service providers aren't encouraged to utilize their relationships with service participants for therapeutic benefit, though mutual relationships can certainly be therapeutic and healing! Service providers are encouraged to recognize that connecting about shared or similar experiences can be powerful and meaningful.

An example: a trans service provider who has navigated legally changing their name may offer support to a trans service participant who is navigating the name change process—this service provider is not expected to share their experience, though they're also not expected to act as if they don't have their own experience or feel like it's "crossing boundaries" or an "ethical" issue to share intentionally about their experiences.

We've found that service relationships work well when service providers don't feel pressured to fit some predetermined mold of detached expertise or hide experiences they may have in common with service participants. This principle is not about creating an us (service providers) and them (service participants) dynamic—it's about recognizing that we're all in community together. Empathy is more possible when each person shows up as their whole self and is not disconnected from their emotions and experiences.

Authenticity

We encourage service providers to be **authentic** and treat service participants as community members (because they are community members!). What does this mean? Be honest about your needs, boundaries, and limitations. Be upfront about expectations. Embrace difficult conversations—share your authentic response when a disconnect or conflict happens with a service participant and invite them to do the same.

Don't fall back on "program rules" to avoid having an uncomfortable conversation. Have honest conversations about natural consequences. Don't treat participants as if they're fragile or try to protect them from having difficult experiences.

If you're having a rough day, it's okay to say so! Service providers don't need to "turn off" their emotions and experiences at work. If a service participant or fellow service provider says or does something that stirs up some emotion for you, it's okay to acknowledge it. Moments of disconnect and conflict often take up space and energy within the relationship, so it makes sense for service providers to talk about these moments (when they're able) because the focus is on the relationship that's being co-created. When a conflict or challenge arises, each person has an opportunity to reflect on their own beliefs and needs, talk about their experience of relationship dynamics, and figure out how to move forward together.

It's important to acknowledge that the service provider-service participant relationship has an inherent power imbalance because one person is paid to provide services and one person is receiving services. It's imperative that service providers share their emotions and experiences in ways that are authentic as well as thoughtful, intentional, and mutual.

An example: you're meeting with a service participant who's feeling frustrated and yelling at you. Rather than talking about what's "appropriate" or using language that blames or shames, we suggest using "I" statements to convey your personal observations, feelings, and needs: "It seems like you're feeling strongly about this. I want to hear about what's going on for you, though it's difficult for me to stay connected when you're yelling. What if we take a five-minute break and come back to this?"

Collaboration

Our practice is **collaborative**. Each person is regarded as their own expert, shows up as themselves, and talks about their nuanced needs and experiences. Through a collaborative relationship, service participants and service providers decide together what support and services will look like. This allows service providers to be more invested in the relationship than the outcome, to bear witness to someone's journey, and offer support that's agreed upon, not coercive.

A collaborative model assumes the service participant knows themself best, that each service participant is a unique individual with nuanced needs and wants. Thus, a service provider's role is to support a service participant in their journey in ways that are mutual and non-coercive. While a service provider may have expertise and knowledge in their particular field—be it mental health, internal medicine, speech-language pathology—they are not an expert on the individual folks they are paid to support.

This collaborative model is often a paradigm shift for folks who've worked in traditional social services: many service providers have been trained to understand themselves as experts, helpers, and problem-solvers in their relationships with service participants. In our relationship-first practice, service providers humbly learn alongside the service participants they support with the goal of creating collaborative relationships.

We know that service providers may have some insight or knowledge they want to share with service participants: ways of making meaning or reframing; strategies for navigating distress or managing experiences; solutions to tangible problems. Our practice asks service providers to slow down, be curious and open, and seek to truly understand what kind of support a service participant is actually looking for. Through this collaboration, there is room for consensual problem-solving, advice, and offering of insight and knowledge.

A collaborative relationship also necessitates shared understanding about what the relationship means, how it works, each person's needs and expectations, and each person's capacity to contribute (which is often negotiated interaction to interaction). This means that a relationship is working well when it's working for both parties. In a collaborative relationship, service providers and service participants share responsibility and steer the relationship together; both risk vulnerability, both are open to learning and growing together. Thus, it's key that service providers practice humility in their relationships, which bring us to our next principle:

Humility

If you're a service provider, it's imperative that you let go of the idea that you have all the answers, that you know what's best for the service participant, that the work is inherently about problem-solving, fixing, or correcting. Our relationship-first practice prioritizes **autonomy, choice, and self-determination**.

Service participants have choice and control and are able to determine what kind of support does and doesn't work for them. If a relationship isn't working for both people, we acknowledge that it's not working, negotiate needs and boundaries, and explore possibilities. Here are ways to practice humility in service relationships:

- Honor that we are all human beings navigating a world with our respective wisdom, insight, strengths, and challenges.
- Share power and decision-making as much as possible.
- Center the voice and autonomy of the service participant.
- Co-create relationships wherein each person talks about their experiences, needs, boundaries, and limits.
- Acknowledge that there is a power imbalance inherent in service provider/service participant relationships—it would be disingenuous and a disservice to everyone in the relationship to not acknowledge the imbalance—and avoid leaning into this power.
- Acknowledge limits of relationships in general. There is only so much any one person can do for another. One relationship cannot be the only source of support. It's not the job of any one person to "save" anyone else.
- Be open and upfront about any obligations such as mandated reporting and duty to warn.

We understand that practicing humility can be challenging, particularly for folks who've been trained to understand themselves as experts. We have also observed that assertions of expertise in service relationships often result in denial of autonomy, choice, and self-determination—that a service provider's desire to "help" based on their preconceived notions of what "help" means can actually cause harm and disconnect in their relationships with individual service participants.

By practicing humility, we aim to share power because sharing power in our individual relationships can lead to systemic transformation—we've seen this in action. We've also seen humility beget curiosity and, in turn, hope.

Curiosity and Hope

We believe in **the possibility of people**, what they can be, and what they can do: this is the true heart of our practice. We encourage service providers to believe in themselves, believe in service participants, and believe in the transformative power of being in authentic, collaborative relationships.

We encourage service providers to practice from a place of curiosity and hope, even and especially when things get difficult and when things feel scary: to be curious about how a service participant is making meaning, to be aware of their own biases and beliefs, to investigate their own discomfort, to seek connection and understanding rather than control.

This practice embodies harm reduction: the non-judgmental and non-coercive approach, fundamental beliefs, and tools used to provide services that reduce potential harm and risk. Harm reduction can be used when supporting folks having a variety of experiences because this practice:

- supports people to use their self-identified survival tools and understands there is often value in the survival tools
- meets people where they are
- prioritizes self-defined and self-determined health and wellness options
- acknowledges and refuses to perpetuate stigma and cultural norms that have left people isolated, alone, and ashamed

- acknowledges and accepts that life is inherently risky—many activities and experiences involve the potential for risk *and* benefit

It's imperative that we support service participants in ways that center their expertise and human rights, even and especially when they're self-harming, using substances, considering suicide, doing sex work, deciding to discontinue psychiatric drugs—all experiences that involve risks *and* benefits.

Self-determination and the dignity of risk are integral to our practice. If a service provider, out of fear, seeks to remove all risk for a service participant, they're impeding upon that individual's capacity to utilize their self-identified survival skills, make and learn from their own decisions, experience natural consequences, and build and sustain their own self-confidence.

It's essential that service providers honor that a service participant (like any other human) will make mistakes, learn from those mistakes, and change and grow in their own time as they see fit for themselves. This is where the hope comes in: we trust that each of us is able to learn and grow, that no experience is necessarily permanent, and that authentic and collaborative relationships make it possible to explore opportunities for transformation together.

Pathways Vermont's Relationship-First Practice: A Social Justice Framework

Our Relationship-First Practice is, at its core, liberatory: we believe in people's capacity to change and transform themselves, their relationships, their communities, and the world around them. Through our practice, we want to decrease shame, dismantle systems that aren't working, and increase authentic connection. We understand shame impedes growth, change, and transformation: shame reduces individual people to their mistakes and harmful choices, and robs them of context, nuance, complexity, and the capacity to learn and be different.

We want to build a better, more accessible, and more livable world for all of us. And we believe this work starts with relationships: fundamentally and intentionally shifting how we show up for ourselves and each other. The way forward is embracing humanity, authenticity, and true collaboration. The way forward is humility, curiosity, and hope. The way forward is together.

Clinical Case Formulation and Intervention Using a Shame-Informed Model

Harper West

Abstract: *As a pro-social emotion, shame is a positive influence on intra-personal emotional wellbeing and inter-personal behaviors because it promotes healthy guilt and accountability. However, hypersensitivity to shame can cause emotional distress and dysfunctional behavior by provoking feelings of low self-worth and fears of social exclusion. It can disrupt feelings of love and attachment, and even drive us away from loving ourselves, which is why it provokes levels of painful self-loathing labeled as mental illness. Shame is a trans-diagnostic influence on mood disorders, personality disorders, psychosis, and child behavioral disorders. Therefore, a model that considers mental health diagnoses as originating from poor shame tolerance would be more accurate and clinically useful than the biomedical model. Unlike the DSM, a shame-informed model directly and logically links etiology, assessment, case formulation, treatment planning, and interventions. Clinicians can easily identify indicators of negative self-image and unworthiness by assessing for acute and chronic trauma, attachment history, relational patterns, view of self, view of other, and affect. Compassion-focused therapy provides evidence-based interventions that teach mindfulness and soothing skills, decreases social threat responding, strengthens self-worth, and builds earned secure attachment patterns.*

Introduction

An increasing number of mental health professionals and those harmed by the profession are speaking out against the *Diagnostic and Statistical Manual of Mental Disorders* (*DSM-5-TR*) (American Psychiatric Association [APA], 2022). Numerous authors have documented the many faults of the "medical model," such as its lack of scientific rigor, poor reliability and validity, disregard for psychosocial and cultural influences, and overly cozy relationship with pharmaceutical companies (see Deacon, 2013; Kinderman, 2014; Vanheule, 2014; Whitaker, 2010; Whitaker, 2019; Whitaker & Cosgrove, 2015).

Consumer activists also assert that the *DSM* stigmatizes sufferers, leads to preferences for medication as a treatment option, and harms far more than it helps. Research has failed to find any significant functional, genetic, or biochemical causes of problems of thinking, feeling, and behaving. Notably, a meta-analysis of 107,000 studies failed to find a biological marker for any psychological issues (Kapur, 2012). If the biological disease paradigm remains unproven, it makes sense to consider that emotional distress is caused by certain emotions.

Specifically, the emotion of shame is widely known to be a major influence on psychological well-being. Research has linked self-criticism and inner shame to many forms of psychological difficulty including: mood disorders, social anxiety, anger and aggression, suicide, self-harm, alcoholism, post-traumatic stress disorder, hearing voices, affect regulation and personality disorders, and interpersonal difficulties (Gilbert, 2008). Hypersensitivity to shame exacerbates fears of rejection, driving us away from love and a sense of attachment to others. It also drives us away from loving ourselves, resulting in self-loathing, loneliness, and anxiety that are often mislabeled as "mental illness."

Benefits of a Shame-Informed Model

An innovative model based on the impact of shame as a trans-diagnostic cause of emotional distress offers many benefits. For clinicians, it provides one simple, integrated conceptual framework. Rather than merely listing symptoms, a shame-informed model describes causes of behavior based on scientific findings. It corrects a long-standing complaint about the *DSM* by describing a healthy, emotionally functional person—one with self-acceptance who can tolerate shame in non-reactive ways. By normalizing behaviors as adaptive responses to external factors, it reduces stigma for clients and improves agency and autonomy.

A shame-informed model leads logically and coherently from assessment and case conceptualization to treatment planning and intervention. Because compassion is the antidote to shame, compassion-focused therapy provides evidence-based interventions based on actual causes of emotional distress, not false assumptions such as biochemical imbalances. Interventions are not temporary solutions or harmful as are psychoactive medication but can lead to permanent changes in emotional health.

Five Factors Exacerbating Shame Sensitivity

According to a shame-informed model, five factors interact to exacerbate shame sensitivity:

> Factor 1 - Threat Response
> Factor 2 - Fear of Social Exclusion
> Factor 3 - Shame as an Attempt to Prevent Social Exclusion
> Factor 4 - Acute Trauma
> Factor 5 - Attachment Status or Chronic/Developmental Trauma

The first three factors are naturally occurring while factors 4 and 5 reflect life experiences. Exposure to acute and attachment traumas heightens a person's reactions to factors 1-3. Because each factor has been researched and described in numerous other texts, they are only briefly described here.

Factor 1 - Threat Response

Humans respond to threatening situations with various activating or inhibitory responses. The fear responses are generally considered: preemptive avoidance of threat, freeze (to avoid detection), flight, fight, and fold (appeasement, submission, or helplessness to elicit caregiving). Most *DSM* diagnoses can be viewed as one or more of these various threat responses.

Anxiety, mania, and ADHD are activation of the sympathetic nervous system, resulting in hyper-vigilance and over-reactivity to threats. The inhibitory or dorsal vagal system of the threat response is labeled as depression with behaviors of helplessness, hopelessness, and low motivation. Bipolar disorders are a vacillation between the dorsal vagal (depression) and the sympathetic response (mania or anxiety).

Clinicians must teach clients about the neurobiology of threats, especially how this same system is used to respond to social or emotional threats. Humans are social animals with an innate desire to be accepted by others.

When victimized, rejected, or shamed, connection to others is at risk and the threat response may be activated. As a result, the limbic system, not the more objective and reflective regions of the brain, is used to appraise the situation (Gilbert, 2020).

The resulting social fears decrease empathy, compassion, and caring—toward others or *toward oneself*. In the dorsal vagal state, one may even turn away from caring for oneself with apathy, dissociation, and emotional numbness.

It is important to teach that threat responses are triggered by self-critical thoughts; it is not possible to feel safe with yourself if you loathe yourself. Compassion-based interventions are effective because they decouple shame and fear by providing a warm, non-judgmental response to experiences of inadequacy or failure. Shameful acts can then be experienced more matter-of-factly with healthy shame tolerance, rather than triggering fear with its accompanying emotional dysregulation, cognitive shutdown, and poor coping.

Despite volumes of research on the threat response and its primal influence on human emotions, cognitions, and physiology, the *DSM* largely ignores this concept.

Factor 2 - Fear of Social Exclusion

Evolutionary advantages accrue for groups of animals that cooperate and share. Resource gathering, protection, and caregiving are much easier as a community. The resulting benefits of safety, procreation, and communal resources promote survival. Human ancestors with an ability to get along with others were less likely to be excluded from the tribe, which increased their survival odds. As a result, prosocial "tend-and-befriend" behaviors, such as caregiving, protection, altruism, reciprocity, and conformity are deeply engrained in human behavior.

Humans also have a strong desire to avoid feeling ashamed and cast out. As a result, when we believe we may be ostracized, those with healthy shame tolerance generally have predictable reactions including humility, submission, compliance, and accountability. When anticipating social disconnection, the primal brain believes survival is at stake and responds, for some, in an exaggerated manner. Many people feel unworthy, leading them to anxiously expect, readily perceive, and overreact to social rejection, conceptualized as "rejection sensitivity" by Downey & Feldman (1996).

Neuroscientists now know that the same parts of the brain that evaluate physical pain are used to judge the emotional pain of social rejection (Ochsner et al., 2008). Feeling alone and excluded triggers feelings of fear, hostility, and shame that may result in physical symptoms such as high blood pressure and heart disease (Hawkley & Cacioppo, 2010). Considerable research has been done on the power of social isolation and its links to social anxiety and depression (Downey & Feldman, 1996; Baumeister & Tice, 1990) and increased susceptibility to low self-esteem (Ayduk et al., 2001; Gailliot & Baumeister, 2007).

However, the *DSM* never mentions the influence of rejection sensitivity on human behavior or uses it in diagnostic criteria. Fear of social exclusion is a natural human condition; therefore, loneliness and the need for human relationships should never be considered a mental disorder.

Factor 3 - Shame as an Attempt to Prevent Social Exclusion

Throughout human history, a person's reputation has been an important asset to survival. We came to fear negative evaluation by others: "Humans have evolved to want to create positive feelings about the self in the mind of others" (Gilbert, 2010, p. 83). These social affiliation needs underlie the prosocial behaviors of honesty, cooperation, reciprocity, obedience, and altruism.

Shame, guilt, embarrassment, and humiliation are self-conscious emotions that serve an evolutionary purpose: to encourage moral conduct and prevent or control inappropriate behavior, such as injustice, greed, or violence. By feeling guilty when we do something wrong, we are primed to apologize and choose different behavior in the future, leading to repair of relationships and enhanced social reputation. Those of our ancestors who failed to learn from shame might be disciplined or expelled from the tribe, possibly resulting in death and reduced reproduction opportunities.

Shame is so powerful it triggers a survival-related dread of social exclusion that is encoded in neurobiological reactions. Shame signals the adrenal gland to release cortisol, the primary stress hormone, leading to increased heart rate and flooding of major muscles with glucose (Lewis & Ramsay, 2002).

For those with poor shame tolerance, shame as a primary emotion often triggers secondary fear. The tendency to be hyper-vigilant for rejection and fearful of shaming experiences is especially prevalent in those who have been exposed to interpersonal trauma (factor 4) or who lack secure attachment (factor 5). Shame, trauma, and childhood sexual abuse have even been considered a cause of auditory hallucinations (Woods, 2017). Those diagnosed with schizophrenia often hear voices that are self-evaluative or that focus on the judgments of others.

Poorly tolerated shame creates rejection sensitivity that hinders self-acceptance. Consider that the typical behaviors associated with shame are avoidance, abject slinking away, downcast eyes, and submissive postures. However, when the source of shame is the self, it is impossible to escape. The self is the attacker *and* the attacked — and there is no safe haven. Feeling "never good enough" creates an untenable situation that provokes chronic judgment, inferiority, and anxiety.

In essence, shame is the opposite of love since disconnection is the opposite of the primal need for belonging. It is no surprise that shame is the foundational emotion that fosters so much dysfunctional human behavior — it drives us away from love and acceptance.

Fortunately, compassion allows humans to moderate guilt by offering forgiveness and repair following immoral behaviors. Paul Gilbert, the originator of compassion-focused therapy, has written extensively about the role of evolutionary motivations and strategies. "[R]ather than focusing on a clustering of 'symptoms' or suggested 'attributes,' the evolutionary approach seeks the origins of compassion in the evolution of caring motives and behaviors" (Gilbert, 2020, p. 2).

Why is shame completely ignored in the *DSM* as a cause of emotional distress? Could it be because there are no drugs to sell to treat shame, and it would further bolster the notion that the biomedical model was wrong all along?

Factor 4 – Trauma

Trauma became one of the most widely recognized external causes of psychological suffering following the Adverse Childhood Experiences Study (ACES) (Felitti et al., 1998). This landmark study found that childhood abuse and neglect predicted emotional, behavioral, and physical health consequences throughout life. Notably, most adverse events are relational. One of the original ACES assessment questions even asks about chronic shaming in childhood: "Did a parent or other adult in the household often or very often swear at you, insult you, put you down, or humiliate you?"

Relational trauma is devastating for a child because it interferes with the formation of a secure attachment bond between child and caregiver (factor 5). Victims conclude that caregivers are not willing or able to protect them, and that the world and relationships are frightening.

Acute trauma (factor 4) and attachment trauma (factor 5) combine to heighten the sensitivity of our primal alarm system that signals social exclusion (factor 2). Those who have been harmed, neglected, or rejected by others will be especially attuned to that rejection in the future. They may also develop self-rejecting strategies of excessive guilt and attempt to "fix" the self that was found unworthy by caregivers.

Jeong et al. (2021) reported that childhood maltreatment sensitizes the threat system and causes structural brain changes such as "differences in cortical thickness and volume in key regions associated with attention/executive functioning, emotion regulation, and self-referential processing. Thus, childhood trauma exposure may be a risk factor for structural aberrations in the developing brain…" (p. 11). Children who have experienced trauma show significantly reduced grey matter in the cortex, an area related to decision-making and self-regulatory skills, and in the amygdala, or fear-processing center (Sheridan et al., 2012).

Cook et al. (2005) also conclude that exposure to chronic trauma has the potential to alter children's brains in many areas. Those relevant to this discussion are:

1. attachment problems
2. emotional regulation
3. lack of consistent sense of self, body image issues, low self-esteem, shame and guilt
4. difficulty controlling impulses

Even psychosis is being proven to have connections with trauma. A 2017 study found that childhood emotional abuse, physical neglect, and high perceived stress were significantly associated with "ultra-high-risk" for psychosis in adulthood (Fusar-Poli et al., 2017).

Factor 5 - Attachment Status

Attachment theory explains that humans learn relationship patterns starting at birth based on the emotional attunement, responsiveness, and warmth of primary caregivers. When optimal parenting practices are used, optimal child development occurs resulting in a child's secure attachment relationship or bond with parents. A secure attachment pattern teaches a child a positive model of how another person feels about them, allowing them to accept care from others—and later, from oneself—permitting healthy, loving relationships with others and with oneself.

In contrast, being emotionally or physically cut off from others is the ultimate danger signal to a helpless, dependent child. Adding insult to injury, if the child's stress is not co-regulated by the unavailable parent, she does not develop the skills to self-soothe or turn to others for soothing. With an abusive parent, the child internalizes the confusing experience of seeking care and soothing from a parent who is also a source of threat. These attachment injuries cause an ongoing psychological experience of increased need for reassurance and safety, but also distrust of potentially undependable caregivers. The DSM might label these disorganized attachment patterns as borderline personality disorder or bipolar disorders.

Relational trauma also causes a child to conclude she is unwanted, inadequate, unlovable, and shameful. As DeYoung writes: "[F]amily members will feel shame when what they need to feel human is withheld and there's absolutely nothing they can do about it" (2015, p. 65). Rejection sensitivity stems from early attachment relationships and parental rejection (Butler et al., 2007).

Too many people today rely on social approval too heavily for a sense of their self-worth, leaving them at the mercy of others for validation which could be labeled as insecure anxious attachment (factor 5). Research has linked insecure attachment patterns to lower measures of self-compassion (Jeong et al., 2021; Mackintosh et al., 2018) and fear of compassion from others (Gilbert et al., 2014). Hyper-sensitivity to rejection is directly related to reactivity to criticism and poor shame tolerance.

Insecure attachment patterns in childhood often prompt substitute attachments to depersonalized rewards in adulthood like addictions to drugs, sex, work, or achievement. This is in contrast to the myth of the medical model that addictions are a genetically linked disease.

A non-warm, unavailable, addicted, or abandoning parent trains rejection sensitivity in a child in the form of fears of interpersonal criticism, failure, or disappointment. The result may be one or both of the insecure attachment patterns:

1. avoidant attachment pattern with guarded withdrawal and avoidance of intimacy
2. anxious attachment pattern with over-compliance and a tendency to appease and please others to gain approval and prevent rejection

Those with insecure attachment history often have blocks to developing self-compassion and secure self-attachment, making compassion-based interventions the ideal treatment.

Connecting the Five Causative Factors

The power of a shame-informed model is that it considers the five causative factors as connected and cumulative in creating sensitivity to shame, leading to impaired behavioral and emotional functioning (shame management strategies). Factors 1, 2, and 3 are naturally occurring tendencies. A childhood filled with love, safety, and acceptance predisposes a person to have resilient responses to negative life experiences.

However, trauma (factor 4) and insecure attachment (factor 5) can increase maladaptive behaviors, including hyper-vigilance to criticism and rejection and blame-shifting behaviors. Emotional resilience and an ability to respond with self-soothing may be underdeveloped. For someone with a history of non-attentive or abusive relationships, "tend-and-befriend" urges may even be experienced as a danger leading to difficulty with regulating emotions, seeking reassurance from others, and giving or receiving compassion.

The resulting schema that one's intrinsic self is unlikeable, unworthy, and even a source of threat is fundamentally a self-betrayal, creating fear of failure, fear of social rejection, and anxiety. Poorly tolerated shame can trigger maladaptive emotional and behavioral responses that may be labeled as "mental illness." The *DSM* completely ignores the self-conscious emotions as foundational in evolutionary processes that relied on moral behaviors of cooperation, caregiving, and reciprocity for our species to succeed. In fact, most *DSM* diagnoses could be more accurately considered "shame disorders."

The *DSM* also ignores issues of causation or psychosocial context, such as developmental or attachment trauma. However, most mental health symptoms are actually descriptions of reactions to the prospect of being inter-personally harmed or shamed combined with an inability to self-soothe.

The Impact of Shame on Interpersonal Relationships

The vast majority of people who have been adversely affected by the five factors respond to feelings of shame with maladaptive secondary fear reactions. The conundrum of shame is that it was designed to improve social relationships, yet when poorly tolerated it provokes irrational fear responses that block human connections. "This shame was once a useful response to interpersonal danger, but now a sense of being worthless or unlovable turns up in response even to minor interpersonal trouble" (DeYoung, 2015, p. 58).

Poor shame tolerance causes three predictable behavioral responses in interpersonal relationships that can be easily identified via the behavior of blame shifting. A simple, but powerful assessment is: How does the person handle criticism or being held accountable? Do they:

1. Blame others (externalize, deflect, or deny guilt)
2. Blame self (internalize or feel excessive guilt)
3. Avoid blame and shame (passive denial of blame, social withdrawal, conflict avoidance, or emotional dissociation)

(For a detailed description of each strategy, see:
http://www.harperwest.co/handle-shame/)

While blame-shifting strategies are coping mechanisms intended to protect the individual, they cause difficulties in relationships. In contrast, those with healthy self-acceptance have accurate perceptions of critical messages from others and can tolerate experiences of embarrassment or failure with appropriate levels of guilt. Shame does not trigger significant fear. As a result, they can hold themselves accountable for mistakes, learn and grow, which improves relationships with others and with oneself.

Clinicians must avoid using a pejorative lens when considering the blame-shifting strategies, and they should adopt a compassionate approach. These behaviors are learned, self-protective traits that arose out of exposure to emotional neglect and abuse.

Relationship problems are a major reason for seeking therapy; therefore, an understanding of the shame management strategies can bring significant benefits to the clinical setting. Fortunately, blame-shifting is easy to observe and assess. It is highly indicative of the person's inner world and predictive of difficulties in interpersonal behaviors. However, the *DSM* ignores the impact of blame-shifting strategies on interpersonal relationships and does not even consider relational problems as possible reasons for psychological distress.

Case Assessment and Formulation

Unlike the *DSM*, a shame-informed model directly and logically links etiology, assessment, case formulation, and interventions. Assessment relies on the five causative factors. Therefore, clinicians must make a paradigm shift from viewing a client's behaviors as symptoms of disease to considering behaviors as adaptive and self-protective responses to life experiences.

Written assessment tools should be used sparingly, as clients may infer that these tests are measuring symptoms of a "disease." Clinicians who regularly use written assessments train clients to over-focus on their emotional reactions in judgmental, comparative, and stigmatizing ways in opposition to a compassion-based approach that encourages a curious, accepting, and warm response to thoughts and feelings in the present moment.

Interventions in a Shame-Informed Model

A major downfall of the disease model of mental health is that it blames most maladaptive human behavior on a biological failure of the brain, leaving medications as the most common treatment option. Psychotherapy is conceptualized as a way to provide coping mechanisms and manage "symptoms." In contrast, a shame-informed model offers a logical progression from causation to interventions that provide permanent modification of maladaptive psychological processes, not merely a temporary reduction in symptoms.

Because of the trans-diagnostic nature of shame, compassion-based interventions can be applied to nearly all clinical presentations. Interventions can include those in Paul Gilbert's Compassion-Focused Therapy model and Kristen Neff and Christopher Germer's Mindful Self-Compassion model. Compassion-focused therapy is linked to decreased distress, interpersonal problems, and personality difficulties, and improved secure attachment patterns (Macbeth & Gumley, 2012; Navarro-Gil et al., 2018; Schanche et al., 2011).

Interventions can begin in the first session with clinicians evoking a warm, compassionate, non-judgmental attitude toward the client and their struggles. It can be helpful to use direct, orienting language that acknowledges the experience of embarrassment and gives clients agency to manage their shame: "Most people are very nervous coming to therapy, so I imagine that you are too. Please let me know if anything I ask you makes you especially uncomfortable. We may have to address difficult topics, but I want to do it only in a way that is helpful to you."

Many clients come to therapy previously diagnosed by another clinician or self-diagnosed via internet searches, priming them to feel ashamed and stigmatized. Clients may have been told they need medications to manage a lifelong "brain malfunction." They may over-analyze and judge changes in mood, resulting in feelings of inferiority and anxiety. The very presence of the medical model establishes a shame-based, blame-based way of thinking about psychological experiences that creates a negative spiral of shame and fear.

Clinicians should listen for expressions of shame around a presumed diagnosis or directly ask about a client's beliefs on this topic. Clinicians should be very circumspect about compounding this by sharing diagnostic labels. Education about the failures of the disease model and the lack of scientific rationale for medications often provokes feelings of relief in clients.

Clinicians should assess attachment history as it informs how a client internalized the acceptance or rejection of caregivers and their view of others as a source of compassionate care. Watch for the history of a narcissistic parent or sibling who models shame sensitivity through lack of accountability. Clinicians must inquire about a client's history of involvement in coercive, abusive, or exploitative relationships in childhood or adulthood since these relationships can activate the threat response, exacerbate self-blaming, and weaken propensity toward self-protective boundaries with other-blamer personalities.

Normalizing the human experience of emotional suffering is done by educating on the five causative factors and their impact on the development of unhealthy shame strategies. Clients usually become hopeful and motivated when the emotion of shame is identified as a core cause of their distress and when told that compassion-based therapies are an effective intervention. Compassion-based interventions teach mindfulness meditation practices to regulate the threat system and re-engage an underperforming soothing system.

Clients also learn to use compassionate thinking to decrease social comparative fears and social threat responding. In essence, compassion-based interventions decouple the reactive connection between primary shame and secondary fear/anxiety. As a result, clients learn to experience embarrassment or guilt as freestanding emotions while remaining calm, which enables the neocortex to remain online and permitting more rational responding and activation of self-soothing.

Clinicians should be attuned to shame-based affect or body language. These expressions give opportunities to engage in embodiment or mindfulness exercises, emotional heightening or regulating, or psychoeducation. By identifying shame intolerance patterns, clinicians can choose various styles of psychotherapy.

Notably, those with other-blaming traits are best treated in session with partners or family as they tend to be inaccurate reporters and may use individual therapy to deflect accountability onto others, misrepresent facts, and garner unwarranted approval from an unwitting therapist. For example, an adolescent other-blamer may need a parent in session so that two narratives are heard, and relationship dynamics can be observed. The shame defensiveness of other-blamers makes them sensitive to direct challenges, so clinicians must slowly and patiently develop a therapeutic alliance before exploring deeply hidden issues of self-doubt.

For those who have childhood relational traumas and subsequent adult patterns of insecure attachment, self-compassion builds earned secure attachment by developing an inner sense of self as a secure base and safe haven. Through learned self-soothing, it provides emotional self-safeness and self-connection when distressed.

Conclusion

Mental health professionals are ethically bound to protect and help clients. It could be considered unethical to unthinkingly adhere to the medical model with all its harmful effects and lack of efficacy, and to ignore other solutions that can reduce harm.

A shame-informed model would provide a logical explanation for the underlying cause of secondary emotional responses of externalized anger (other-blaming), internalized anger (self-blaming), and withdrawal/avoidance (blame avoidance). It normalizes our human need for love, connection, and worthiness—and provides tools to build inner resources toward self-acceptance by reducing shame/fear reactivity and enhancing self-soothing.

The good news is that self-compassion is a skill that humans already possess. We are not born to live chronically with shame, anxiety, insecurity, and hostility. By uncovering our inherent self-attachment, one can have loving relationships with others and with the self—the most important relationship of all.

References

American Psychiatric Association. (2022). *Diagnostic and statistical manual of mental disorders (5th ed., text rev.).* Washington, DC

Ayduk, O., Downey, G., & Kim, M. (2001). Rejection sensitivity and depressive symptoms in women. *Personality and Social Psychology Bulletin,* 27(7), July 2001, 868-877.

Baumeister, R.F., & Tice, D.M. (1990). Point-counterpoints: Anxiety and social exclusion. *Journal of Social and Clinical Psychology:* 9 (2), 165-195. doi: 10.1521/jscp.1990.9.2.165

Butler, J. C., Doherty, M. S., & Potter, R. M. (2007). Social antecedents and consequences of interpersonal rejection sensitivity. *Personality and Individual Differences,* 43, 1376–1385. doi:10.1016/j.paid.2007.04.006

Cook, A., Spinazzola, J., Ford, J. D., Lanktree, C., Blaustein, M., Cloître, M., DeRosa, R., Hubbard, R., Kagan, R., Liautaud, J., Mallah, K., Olafson, E., & Van Der Kolk, B. (2005). Complex trauma in children and adolescents. *Psychiatric Annals*, 35(5), 390–398. https://doi.org/10.3928/00485713-20050501-05

Deacon, B. (2013). The biomedical model of mental disorder: A critical analysis of its validity, utility, and effects on psychotherapy research. *Clinical Psychology Review*, 33, 846-861.

DeYoung, P. A. (2015). *Understanding and treating chronic shame: A relational neurobiological approach.* New York, NY: Routledge.

Downey, G., & Feldman, S.I. (1996). Implications of rejection sensitivity for intimate relationships. *Journal of Personality and Social Psychology*, 70 (6), 1327–43. doi:10.1037/0022-3514.70.6.1327

Felitti, V. J., Anda, R. F., Nordenberg, D., Williamson, D. F., Spitz, A. M., Edwards, V. J., Koss, M. P., & Marks, J. S. (1998). Relationship of childhood abuse and household dysfunction to many of the leading causes of death in adults. *American Journal of Preventive Medicine*, 14(4), 245–258. https://doi.org/10.1016/s0749-3797(98)00017-8

Fusar-Poli, P., Tantardini, M., De Simone, S., Ramella-Cravaro, V., Oliver, D., Kingdon, J., Kotlicka-Antczak, M., Valmaggia, L., Lee, J., Millan, M. J., Galderisi, S., Balottin, U., Ricca, V., & McGuire, P. (2017). Deconstructing Vulnerability for Psychosis: Meta-Analysis of environmental risk factors for psychosis in subjects at Ultra High-Risk. *European Psychiatry*, 40, 65–75. https://doi.org/10.1016/j.eurpsy.2016.09.003

Gailliot, M.T. & Baumeister, R. F. (2007). Self-esteem, belongingness, and worldview validation: Does belongingness exert a unique influence upon self-esteem? *Journal of Research in Personality*, 41(2), 327-345. https://doi.org/10.1016/j.jrp.2006.04.004.

Gilbert, P. (Ed.) (2008). *Compassion: Conceptualisations, research and use in psychotherapy.* London, UK: Routledge.

Gilbert, P. (2010). *Compassion focused therapy.* London, UK & New York, NY: Routledge.

Gilbert, P., McEwan, K., Catarino, F., & Baião, R. (2014). Fears of compassion in a depressed population implication for psychotherapy. *Journal of Depression & Anxiety*, S2(01). https://doi.org/10.4172/2167-1044.s2-003

Gilbert, P. (2020). Compassion: From its evolution to a psychotherapy. *Frontiers in Psychotherapy*, Dec. 9, 2020.

Hawkley, L.C., & Cacioppo, J.T. (2010). Loneliness matters: A theoretical and empirical review of consequences and mechanisms. *Annals of Behavioral Medicine*, 40(2), 218–227. doi:10.1007/s12160-010-9210-8

Jeong, H. J., Durham, E. L., Moore, T. M., Dupont, R. M., McDowell, M. G., Cardenas-Iniguez, C., Micciche, E., Berman, M. G., Lahey, B. B., & Kaczkurkin, A. N. (2021). The association between latent trauma and brain structure in children. *Translational Psychiatry*, 11(1). https://doi.org/10.1038/s41398-021-01357-z

Kapur, S., Phillips, A. G., & Insel, T. R. (2012). Why has it taken so long for biological psychiatry to develop clinical tests and what to do about it? *Molecular Psychiatry*, 17(12), 1174–1179. https://doi.org/10.1038/mp.2012.105

Kinderman, P. (2014). *A prescription for psychiatry: Why we need a whole new approach to mental health and wellbeing.* New York, NY: Palgrave Macmillan.

Lewis, M. & Ramsay, D. (2002). Cortisol response to embarrassment and shame. *Child Development*, Jul-Aug, 73(4), 1034-45. doi: 10.1111/1467-8624.00455. PMID: 12146731

MacBeth, A. & Gumley, A. (2012). Exploring compassion: a meta-analysis of the association between self-compassion and psychopathology. *Clinical Psychology Review*, 32, 545–552.

Mackintosh, K., Power, K., Schwannauer, M., & Chan, S. W. Y. (2017). The Relationships Between Self-Compassion, Attachment and Interpersonal Problems in Clinical Patients with Mixed Anxiety and Depression and Emotional Distress. *Mindfulness*, 9(3), 961–971. https://doi.org/10.1007/s12671-017-0835-6

Navarro-Gil, M., López-Del-Hoyo, Y., Modrego-Alarcón, M., Van Gordon, W., Shonin, E., & Campayo, J. G. (2018). Effects of Attachment-Based Compassion Therapy (ABCT) on self-compassion and attachment style in healthy people. *Mindfulness*, 11(1), 51–62. https://doi.org/10.1007/s12671-018-0896-1

Ochsner, K. N., Zaki, J., Hanelin, J., Ludlow, D., Knierim, K., Ramachandran, T., Glover, G. H., & Mackey, S. (2008). Your pain or mine? Common and distinct neural systems supporting the perception of pain in self and other.

Social Cognitive and Affective Neuroscience, 3(2), 144–160.
https://doi.org/10.1093/scan/nsn006

Schanche, E., Stiles, T.C., Mccullough, L., Svartberg, M., & Nielsen, G.H. (2011). The relationship between activating affects, inhibitory affects, and self-compassion in patients with Cluster C personality disorders. *Psychotherapy, 48.*

Sheridan, M. A., Fox, N. A., Zeanah, C. H., McLaughlin, K. A. & Nelson, C.A. (2012). Variation in neural development as a result of exposure to institutionalization early in childhood. *Proceedings of the National Academy of Sciences,* 109(32), 12927-12932. doi: 10.1073/pnas.1200041109

Vanheule, S. (2014). *Diagnosis and the DSM: A critical review.* London and New York: Palgrave Macmillan.

Whitaker, R. (2010). *Anatomy of an epidemic.* New York, NY: Broadway Paperbacks.

Whitaker, R. (2019). *Mad in America: Bad science, bad medicine, and the enduring mistreatment of the mentally ill.* New York, NY: Basic Books.

Whitaker, R., & Cosgrove, L. (2015). *Psychiatry under the influence: Institutional corruption, social injury, and prescriptions for reform.* New York: Palgrave Macmillan.

Woods, A. (2017). On shame and voice-hearing. *Medical Humanities,* 43, 251-256.

How Can We See ADHD From Another Angle, and What Can We Do for Our Kids?

Ann Bracken

Abstract: *Every your, a large number of parents in the United States are told by teachers, friends, or doctors that their child might have attention-deficit/hyperactivity disorder (ADHD). According to Centers for Disease Control (CDC) data from 2016-2019, 6 million children or 9.8% are diagnosed every year using the criteria found in the Diagnostic and Statistical Manual of Mental Disorders (DSM-5). According to some estimates, between 38%-81% of those children are given stimulant drugs and 39% to 62% receive some form of behavior treatment. This chapter will explicate the research behind the diagnosis, the use of stimulant drugs to control ADHD behaviors, and the long-term outcomes of such a treatment plan. Alternatively, this chapter will propose other ways of viewing behaviors classified as ADHD symptoms and will explore two approaches to behavior management that have proven helpful to both families and teachers.*

Acknowledgement: A version of this chapter was first published by Mad in America on June 27, 2023.

In 1987, after my son Connor's first-grade teacher told me that he had attention-deficit/hyperactivity disorder (ADHD) because he stuffed his unfinished schoolwork in his desk, I decided to wait and see how second grade in a new school went. When school started, Connor made new friends, got along with his teachers, and seemed to be completing his work, but things rapidly declined when he stuck his foot out and tripped a classmate. I was called to the school office where I found a scared looking Connor.

"I didn't mean to hurt him, Mom." he told me. "And I apologized right away." As we were leaving the building, Connor's teacher said his classmate was fine, but she was tired of Connor's antics—so I assured her we'd talk to Connor, and he'd do better. But the principal had other ideas.

He approached me as I was leaving and said, "Either you medicate that boy or I will."

At that point, our story followed the same trajectory as many of the parents' stories I read today. Connor's pediatrician gave us a checklist to fill out with a home component and a school component. I didn't have much to report on the home front, but Connor's teacher had some concerns, so the doctor recommended we start him on Ritalin for impulse control. We told Connor he'd be taking some pills to help him pay more attention in school, but when he asked me one night, "Will those pills make me better?" I felt a heavy anchor on my heart and decided to seek another opinion.

Long story short, the psychologist with whom we consulted worked with Connor for a few weeks, and after giving him several assessments, he had this to say: "Connor doesn't have ADHD; he's bored. Just get him involved in some more enrichment activities and he'll be fine. And stop giving him Ritalin."

Connor never saw any urgency about finishing his schoolwork, and it took me much longer than it should have to realize how deep his boredom ran. Thankfully, we encouraged his musical abilities and all of his artistic and mechanical talents—and today, Connor is an accomplished musician and audio engineer, a photographer, and a skilled woodworker and carpenter.

That's Connor's story and mine. (Read my blog post about it at Mad in America.[1]) Readers out there have their own stories and questions regarding ADHD, their own reasons to be skeptical of the advice they're receiving about their kids' behavior. I'm going to do my best to anticipate some of those questions and answer them in a way that, I hope, can inform parents' decisions as they strive to do what's best for their children—and maybe give them some hope in the process.

But haven't things changed since the 1980s?

Even though Connor's "diagnosis" of ADHD occurred in 1987, little has changed in the way we diagnose that cluster of behaviors we refer to as ADHD. Parents, pediatricians, and teachers still use a checklist of behaviors to determine if a child does, indeed, qualify as having ADHD. And in many schools and families across the United States, stimulant drugs[2] such as Ritalin, Adderall, and Concerta are still the first line of treatment for children over six with an additional recommendation for behavior therapy both at home and in school.

If you do a quick search on the internet, you'll find many articles claiming that ADHD is a brain disorder and is due to problems with dopamine transmission,[3] which stimulants correct. But since most children's dopamine levels are never checked, the idea that their brains are deficient in the neurotransmitter is simply conjecture based on the way we know stimulants work: by increasing the amount of dopamine in the brain to give people a boost of motivation to pay attention.

But what about the checklist of symptoms to diagnose ADHD?

I found such a checklist on the ADDitude[4] website run by the magazine of the same name,[5] whose tagline is "Strategies and Support for Attention Deficit and Related Conditions." They offer an ADHD Symptom Checker[6] based on the criteria found in the *Diagnostic and Statistical Manual of Mental Disorders (DSM-5)*[7] of the American Psychiatric Association (APA).

For every symptom, you have a choice of answering "very often," "often," "sometimes," "rarely," or "never." Some of the symptoms listed include forgetting things, interrupting conversations and activities of others, fidgeting, difficulty focusing on homework, losing things, and making careless mistakes. Many would consider the list of symptoms above to be normal childhood behaviors.

"Normal"? Really? Isn't that all pretty official, like a real medical diagnosis?

According to the APA,[8] the *DSM* is "a handbook used by healthcare professionals in the United States and much of the world as an authoritative guide to the diagnosis of mental disorders. The *DSM* contains descriptions, symptoms, and other criteria for diagnosing mental disorders."

Note those two words: "descriptions" and "symptoms." That's it. No hard science about it. No lab tests involved. The book is a handbook of labels, each one listing behavioral characteristics and other signs for practitioners to assess (and, as is often the case, disagree on).

But isn't time of the essence? Shouldn't I take action quickly for when my child is diagnosed?

You can pause and reflect when faced with new information, especially when it involves the use of any kind of pharmaceutical. All you really know after going through the checklist is that your child has a certain set of behaviors that are supposed to indicate a condition called ADHD. But what caused these behaviors?

And if doctors can't tell you the cause, why do they so often tell parents that the child has a chemical imbalance in the brain? And how does a doctor know, based on a checklist of behaviors, that a stimulant drug is the correct measure needed to help the child?

But what about those drugs? Where can I find some detailed information about them? And won't they help my child in the long run?

Mad in America published a guide called "Psychotropic Drugs in Children and Adolescents: Stimulants, ADHD, and Other Behavioral Disorders"[9] that gives an overview of ADHD, provides a diagram of how drugs act on the neurons in the brain, and details both the long and short-term research on using stimulants to help manage ADHD symptoms.

It would be understandable to think of stimulant drugs as a magic bullet for ADHD behaviors if you read and watch ads from the drug companies. But interestingly, after looking at studies from the previous 14 years, the 1994 edition of the APA's Textbook of Psychiatry has this to say about long-term effectiveness[10]: "Stimulants do not produce lasting improvements in aggressivity, conduct disorder, criminality, education achievement, job functioning, marital relationships, or long-term adjustment."

The National Institute of Mental Health (NIMH) then commissioned a study called the **Multisite Multimodal** (MTA)[11] to provide more information on the long-term use of stimulants. People still cite the study today as proof that stimulants are effective for long-term treatment of ADHD, but let's dig a little deeper into the results:

- At fourteen months of treatment, researchers said that treatment with stimulants was superior to behavioral treatment in reducing symptoms and possibly improving reading scores.
- At three years of stimulant use, the results were the opposite: children who had taken stimulants had more symptoms than those who were unmedicated—and were also shorter, weighed less, and experienced more delinquency.
- At six years, those who were using medication showed worse hyperactivity, impulsivity, and oppositional-defiant behavior, and more symptoms of depression and anxiety.

According to MIA's guide, other long-term studies (including results from Australia and Canada) have shown that long-term use of stimulants results in increased "unhappiness, a deterioration in relationships with parents, more anxiety and depression among girls, and a deterioration in educational outcomes." It seems clear that the results (of the MTA study) being touted as showing the stimulants' effectiveness are limited to the results for fourteen months, not the three- and six-year results.

Besides the poor behavior outcomes associated with long-term stimulant use, some of the more serious problems with stimulants can be found on manufacturers' package inserts. For example, the package inserts for Adderall[12] posted on Drugs.com contains this list of common adverse effects:

- Loss of appetite
- Weight loss
- Mood changes
- Feeling nervous
- Fast heart rate
- Headaches
- Dizziness
- Sleep problems
- Dry mouth

The serious adverse effects of Adderall include seizure, muscle tics or twitches, circulation problems, aggression, hostility, paranoia, chest pain, trouble breathing, and feeling like you might pass out.

So, if the drugs don't help much, and ADHD is not due to a chemical imbalance in the brain, how can I understand it? Where else can I look for a cause?

Dr. Thomas Armstrong,[13] psychologist, speaker, and author, thinks we need to consider this idea: "What if ADHD children are not disordered, but we live in a disordered culture?" In this sense, we can look at our American culture with its emphasis on materialism, high achievement, and busyness as being part of the waters we swim in that seep into our skin and our bodies.

Roman Wyden, father, entrepreneur, and host of the podcast *ADHD is Over*,[14] has interviewed many experts in psychology, child development, trauma, and education. I love the tagline he uses at the beginning of each podcast when he says, "The struggle is real. The label doesn't have to be." Wyden's not denying that the behaviors can be problematic—he's just looking at them with a different lens.

He's also put together a wonderful "ADHD Survival Guide"[15] that you can download from his website. Based on his own experiences and what he's learned from his guests, Wyden said this about possible causes of ADHD:

> I don't think there's one main cause, but in general, we can look at the environment's impacts on our lives—things like a stressful birth, heavy metals in our food and water, past and present trauma, and family dynamics can all impact a child's nervous system so that they develop some of the behaviors we associate with ADHD.

Just to be very clear about trauma, I want to place that word in a context that I've found personally helpful. Canadian family practice physician and author Gabor Maté[16] has a special interest in childhood development and the potential lifelong impacts of trauma. Maté explains how he interprets it:

Trauma is a Greek word for wound...Trauma is not the event that inflicted the wound. So, the trauma is not the sexual abuse, the trauma is not the war. Trauma is not the abandonment. The trauma is not the inability of your parents to see you for who you were. Trauma is the wound that you sustained as a result.

Maté goes on to talk about his own life in 1944 Hungary when the Nazis invaded and his mother gave him to a stranger to keep, for a while, so that the Nazis couldn't harm him—because he was Jewish:

So, my wound wasn't that my mother gave me [away temporarily] to a stranger [when I was a child]. My wound was that I made that mean that I wasn't lovable and I wasn't wanted and I was being abandoned, which is a good thing. . . [because] if the trauma wound happens inside you, the wound that you're carrying? That can heal at any time.

I've heard Wyden say in some of his podcast episodes that he and his wife took a hard look at their family dynamics when their older son, Khai, was diagnosed with ADHD. And I don't detect any notes of blame in his approach, like blaming themselves for being bad parents:

Well, there's a difference between blaming yourself and taking responsibility for the way things are. My wife and I were both working a lot, I wasn't very present in the marriage, and the kids had a nanny, so we realized that one thing we could do to help our sons was to remove as many environmental stressors as possible...The more we looked into the idea of trauma, the more we realized our son Khai likely felt traumatized when he was taken from us after his birth and then kept in the hospital for several days so he could be treated for jaundice. The separation from parents, the strange voices of the nurses and doctors, the lights and noises in the nursery—all of that is overloading the infant's nervous system and likely felt as a traumatic event.

The Wydens eventually decided to homeschool both of their sons—Khai and Etienne—and now the boys enjoy a hybrid education—two days at a public school that offers a homeschool program[17] and the rest of the time learning from home. Khai passed the entrance exam for a prestigious high school and will be starting there in the fall. It looks like the road the Wydens took has been successful for their sons in many ways.

I often hear teachers and parents refer to a child who struggles with ADHD behaviors as "an ADDer" as if that label gives you a complete picture of the child. Should I be concerned about people using a label like that?

These days, all of society seems to trade in labels because they serve as a shorthand way of describing individuals, especially in the realm of any kind of emotional distress or differing abilities. We even refer to ourselves this way as if our "diagnosis" is the totality of who we are: "alcoholic," "addict," "borderline," "emotionally disabled," and "ADDer."

Yes, it takes more words to talk about people without labels. But I believe that it also makes them *more fully a person* with much less focus on any kind of difference. Think about the different picture you form of a person who "self-medicates with alcohol" as opposed to the more succinct label of "alcoholic."

Years ago, when I worked as a special educator in a high school, I was assigned to work with the "ED" kids—"emotionally disabled." Now when I think about that label, the term itself doesn't even make sense. And when I close my eyes and see each one of the faces of my former students, I also remember their stories of abuse, abandonment, and family disarray.

I realize that what we were doing was, as researcher Vicky Plows[18] put it, "[locating] the problem within the child, individualizing issues, and shifting the focus away from the larger context. This [kind of labeling] can make it hard to tackle problems holistically." And labels can certainly harm children in other ways, leading to bullying, stigmatization, and marginalization in schools.

Sometimes labels and diagnoses are a necessary component of getting services for a child, such as when they are diagnosed with a learning, hearing, or vision disability. Such information can also be used by teachers to seek out the most effective forms of teaching for a given child. But we all know any child is *more than the label* of their particular problems.

The question I ask myself now is this: Does anyone need to know what a child is diagnosed with? We can probably all remember kids who were labeled when we were in school, and those labels seem to stick forever. Worse than that, a child who is constantly referred to by their symptoms or diagnosis can internalize the negative connotations that people ascribe to certain categories, limit themselves unnecessarily, or develop a very wounded self-image.

If the labels don't help, and the drugs aren't the answer for my child, what can I do to help him succeed in life and in school? Despite our best efforts to be loving and positive, we constantly argue and remind him about homework and chores, and his teachers are frustrated as well.

I remember well how challenging my son was as a child in the sense that we operated on different timetables, and both his teachers and I were perplexed and frustrated with his lack of urgency in following directions or completing school and classwork. I would have welcomed a new approach to working with him that could have eased our mutual frustration.

To give parents an overview of some holistic ways to help children learn self-management skills, I've also looked at two different approaches to helping children learn self-regulation skills—because many ADHD behaviors fall into three main areas[19] that children need assistance with:

1. executive function (planning, breaking down tasks into chunks, blocking out distractions)
2. emotional and social skills (difficulty managing frustration and irritability age-appropriately, starting conversation, waiting your turn to talk, and seeking inappropriate attention)
3. language and cognitive flexibility skills (getting confused with following directions, trouble expressing needs, seeing situations in

black and white, having trouble with transitions and schedule changes, and negative self-labeling based on one experience)

What's an extremely structured, step-by-step approach to helping kids and families deal with such behaviors?

There are two I want to share with you. The first is detailed is Avigail Gimpel's book *HyperHealing: The Empowered Parent's Guide to Raising a Healthy Child with ADHD Symptoms* which is accompanied by an overview of the data behind ADHD in a concise book called *HyperHealing: Show Me the Science*.[20] Her program involves establishing clear family rules and punishments, a collaborative approach to developing better social-emotional skills, and addressing the importance of a healthy diet and adequate exercise for growing children.

Gimpel's book *HyperHealing* is nearly 400 pages long, well-researched, and written in a conversational style that makes you feel as if you're talking with a wise friend who seems to have found a good solution to a difficult challenge. She goes into extensive detail in each chapter, providing supporting research and detailed examples of problem behaviors, possible explanations, and solutions that have worked for her personally and in her professional life.

I'm providing a brief summary of her work, and if you feel that her approach resonates with your parenting style, I'd recommend her books so that you have a complete picture of her program. Gimpel first asks you as a parent to look at the "habit loops" you are in as far as your child's behavior and how you respond. We often find ourselves in patterns of behavior that we don't know how to get out of, and she spends a good deal of ink on helping you figure out your situation. As long as we remain in the loop and respond vigorously to the outburst, we are actually rewarding the tantrum — in the sense of giving energy and attention to the behavior: "The way we communicate either reinforces negative behavior (like giving in to a tantrum or nagging request from a child) or builds positive momentum."[21]

Understanding your family's habit loops and triggers opens the gateway to the rest of the program: compliment positive actions, establish clear ground rules, and punish when rules are broken. Gimpel thoroughly explores the most effective ways to compliment people that will reinforce positive behaviors: "Let's raise our voices with joy when she does something right and be bland when responding to negative behavior."[22] She recommends compliments to be specific (*You made my day when you came in the house with a big smile. . .*); for you to give them right away when the event happens *and* don't add a "but" (. . . *but you forgot to take off your wet shoes*); and reinforce the compliment with touch—a high five, a shoulder squeeze, or a hug—as long as the child is open to that.

From compliments, Gimpel goes on to talk about punishment and family rules. She recommends three rules to explain to children: respect parents, respect siblings, and not putting yourself or others in danger. Each rule has several specifics that you could discuss as a family. What I take away from her presentation is that the compliments show your child how to behave in the world and get along with others, the rules are there as guardrails for everyone, and the punishments are for when the child makes a bad decision and breaks one of the guardrails.

Punishments should be respectful, and one way to accomplish that is to let the child do something to correct the situation. If a child speaks disrespectfully to his sibling, you can tell him calmly and respectfully that he broke a rule—and now he needs to go and water the plants on the porch or fold a few items of laundry. If the child refuses to comply, Gimpel recommends either taking away an item or a privilege—offer half a treat or none at all.

Gimpel spends a considerable amount of time giving real-life examples of how to implement her ideas as far as discipline and compliments go. The rest of the book is devoted to helping the child develop better self-management, social, and cognitive skills. I found her approach highly structured, warm, and caring—and I can see how families might resonate with what she offers.

What's another way to help challenging kids?

If you're looking for another modality, consider Howard Glasser's Nurtured Heart Approach. His books **Notching Up the Nurtured Heart**

Approach and *Transforming the Difficult Child Workbook: An Interactive Guide to the Nurtured Heart Approach*[23] offer more streamlined guidance on working with challenging kids in both the school and at home.

As I read the book for educators, I could immediately see that Glasser's three-step approach to working with kids in schools could also work at home, and I found the workbook for parents to be written in a comprehensive, step-by-step manner that presents all the ideas for parents in small steps with wide-ranging examples. Glasser breaks down his approach into what he calls three "stands":

- *I will purposefully create successes for my child.*
- *I refuse to be drawn into accidentally energizing and rewarding negativity.*
- *I will provide a true consequence when a rule is broken.*

Before leading us through the stands with detailed examples, he presents an interesting concept that he calls "Video Game Therapy." Glasser says kids weather the challenges and setbacks of video games because they have well-defined rules, and the rewards and punishments are clearly laid out ahead of time. A player knows exactly what's expected in order to keep scoring well and play within the rules. Most importantly, video games provide a constant state of now.

Glasser, like Gimpel, discusses the need for family rules to be clear and consistent, and to have the kids know what the rules are. He also suggests framing them in the negative—no lying, no disrespecting parents, siblings, and peers—because doing so removes ambiguity (whereas saying "be respectful" can open you up for debate and creates an unclear situation). Posting the rules is not necessary, and unfailing application—without issuing warnings—is the key to his approach.

Here's how Glasser might approach a sibling argument: Suppose your two children have been teasing each other all morning, and they finally come to you and ask for help resolving the situation. You notice that your daughter has managed not to hit her younger brother even though she's clearly angry. Glasser suggests you say something like: "Thanks for not taking your anger out on anyone. That's really good self-control. I also notice that you decided to solve the problem in a safe way. I'm proud of you for asking for help and managing such intense feelings." This example exemplifies stands one and two: choosing to energize success and refusing to energize negativity.

The third stand — providing a true consequence — is where I got a little hung up because it seems to be the antithesis of the way so many of us parent. Most of us, myself included, would opt for punishment. Instead, in the example above of the two siblings, if the older sister had ripped up her brother's painting or tossed his half-finished puzzle on the floor, Glasser recommends saying to her — so long as she stops her negative behavior: "Sherrie, thanks for putting yourself back in the game." That can be followed with a sincere compliment: "Right now you are helping your brother and being kind."

Glasser talks about the need to "get out of the way" and let the child be successful. He maintains that ALL kids can behave appropriately if you put the bar in the right place. He reminds us that Shamu the whale learned to leap into the air only after he was rewarded for swimming over a rope on the bottom of the pool. In essence, we can make it impossible for our kids to fail using that same approach.

Glasser emphasizes that success is due to giving consequences every time a rule is broken, maintaining a neutral and calm stance when delivering the consequence, doing away with giving warnings, and then rewarding positive behavior as soon as the child completes the consequence.

What else should I know?

In conclusion, I would encourage every parent or teacher who may be reading this chapter to consider the research presented, question any assumptions they may have had about a given child, and explore the resources I've gathered to help you find your own solution.

We all want to help our kids or our students, and sometimes finding the right key to unlock a child's gifts is a matter of time, patience, trial, and error. I encourage you to trust yourself, hold your child in a positive light, and know that you will find the right answer.

References

American Psychiatric Association. (2023). Psychiatry Online, DSM Library. https://dsm.psychiatryonline.org

Bracken, A. (2022). *Parenting Changed My Perspective on "ADHD".* Retrieved from Mad in America website: https://www.madinamerica.com/2022/03/parenting-changed-my-perspective-on-adhd/

Centers for Disease Control and Prevention. (2022). *My Child Has Been Diagnosed with ADHD—Now What?* Retrieved from: https://www.cdc.gov/ncbddd/adhd/treatment.html

Childs, J. H. (2022). *The Relationship Between Dopamine and ADHD.* Retrieved from *Very Well Mind* website: https://www.verywellmind.com/the-relationship-between-dopamine-and-adhd-5267960

Drugs.com (website). Adderall. [2022, Nov. 8]. 2023 May 30, 2023. *https://www.drugs.com/adderall.html#side-effects.*

Gimpel, A. (2021). *HyperHealing: The Empowered Parent's Guide to Raising a Healthy Child with ADHD Symptoms.* Columbus, OH. Gatekeeper Press.

Gimpel, A. (2021). *HyperHealing: Show Me the Science: Making Sense of Your Child's ADHD Diagnosis.* Columbus, OH. Gatekeeper Press.

Glasser, H. & Block, M. (2011). *Notching Up the Nurtured Heart Approach: The New Inner Wealth Initiative for Educators.* Tuscon, AZ. Nurtured Heart Publications.

Heyl, J. C. (2023). *The Relationship Between Dopamine and ADHD.* https://www.verywellmind.com/the-relationship-between-dopamine-and-adhd-5267960

Mad in America. (2019). Psychotropic Drugs in Children and Adolescents: Stimulants, ADHD, and other behavioral disorders. https://www.madinamerica.com/adhd-info/

Plows, V. (2014). *Labelling kids: the good, the bad and the ADHD.* Retrieved from *The Conversation.* https://theconversation.com/labelling-kids-the-good-the-bad-and-the-adhd-31778

Rogers, S, (2022). CBC Radio, The Next Chapter (radio). "Are we mislabeling our trauma? Why Dr. Gabor Mate believes we need to change the way we think about pain." https://www.cbc.ca/radio/thenextchapter/are-we-mislabeling-our-trauma-why-dr-gabor-maté-believes-we-need-to-change-the-way-we-think-about-pain-1.6661540

Saline, S. (2023). *Does My Child Have ADHD? Symptom Test for Kids.* Retrieved from *Additude* website: https://www.additudemag.com/adhd-symptoms-test-children/?src=embed_link

Wyden, R. (2023, May 26). Personal Communication. (personal interview).

Wyden, R. (Host) (2020-2023). *ADHD is Over.* https://www.adhdisover.com/podcast-1

Resources for Parents and Teachers

Armstrong, T. "American Institute for Learning and Human Development."https://www.institute4learning.com/thomas-armstrong/

Chris Rowan Pediatric OT "Reconnect Webinars—Balance Between Teaching and Moving to Learn", Zone-in Workshops. https://www.zoneinworkshops.com/index.html

"17 Ways to Help Students With ADHD Concentrate," by Youki Terada. August 17, 2015; Updated June 28, 2018. Teacher-tested ideas to help students with fidgeting. HTTPS://WWW.EDUTOPIA.ORG/DISCUSSION/17-WAYS-HELP-STUDENTS-ADHD-FIDGET

Jeanine Mouchawar, certified life coach for parents of teenagers. https://www.jeaninemouchawar.com

Endnotes

[1] Bracken, A. (2022). *Parenting Changed My Perspective on "ADHD".* Retrieved from Mad in America website: https://www.madinamerica.com/2022/03/parenting-changed-my-perspective-on-adhd

[2] Centers for Disease Control and Prevention. (2022). *My Child Has Been Diagnosed with ADHD—Now What?* Retrieved from: https://www.cdc.gov/ncbddd/adhd/treatment.html

[3] Childs, J. H. (2022). *The Relationship Between Dopamine and ADHD.* Retrieved from *Very Well Mind* website: https://www.verywellmind.com/the-relationship-between-dopamine-and-adhd-5267960

[4] Saline, S. (2023). *Does My Child Have ADHD? Symptom Test for Kids.* Retrieved from *Additude* website: https://www.additudemag.com/adhd-symptoms-test-children/?src=embed_link

[5] Ibid.

[6] Ibid.

[7] American Psychiatric Association. (2023). Psychiatry Online, DSM Library. https://dsm.psychiatryonline.org

[8] Ibid.

[9] Mad in America. (2019). Psychotropic Drugs in Children and Adolescents: Stimulants, ADHD, and other behavioral disorders. https://www.madinamerica.com/adhd-info/

[10] Ibid.

[11] Ibid.

[12] Drugs.com (website). Adderall. [2022, Nov. 8]. 2023 May 30, 2023. https://www.drugs.com/adderall.html#side-effects.

[13] Armstrong, T. "American Institute for Learning and Human Development." https://www.institute4learning.com/thomas-armstrong/

[14] Wyden, R. (Host) (2020-2023). *ADHD is Over.* https://www.adhdisover.com/podcast-1

[15] Wyden, R. (2023, May 26). Personal Communication. (personal interview).

[16] Rogers, S, (2022). CBC Radio, The Next Chapter (radio). "Are we mislabeling our trauma? Why Dr. Gabor Mate believes we need to change the way we think about pain." https://www.cbc.ca/radio/thenextchapter/are-we-mislabeling-our-trauma-why-dr-gabor-maté-believes-we-need-to-change-the-way-we-think-about-pain-1.6661540

[17] RockTreeSky. https://www.rocktreesky.org

[18] Plows, V. (2014). *Labelling kids: the good, the bad and the ADHD.* Retrieved from *The Conversation.* https://theconversation.com/labelling-kids-the-good-the-bad-and-the-adhd-31778

[19] Gimpel, A. (2021). *HyperHealing: The Empowered Parent's Guide to Raising a Healthy Child with ADHD Symptoms.* Columbus, OH. Gatekeeper Press.

[20] Gimpel, A. (2021). *HyperHealing: Show Me the Science: Making Sense of Your Child's ADHD Diagnosis.* Columbus, OH. Gatekeeper Press.

[21] Gimpel, A. (2021). *HyperHealing: The Empowered Parent's Guide to Raising a Healthy Child with ADHD Symptoms.* Columbus, OH. Gatekeeper Press. p. 76

[22] Ibid. p. 77

[23] Glasser, H. & Block, M. (2011). *Notching Up the Nurtured Heart Approach: The New Inner Wealth Initiative for Educators.* Tuscon, AZ. Nurtured Heart Publications.

Addressing Ethical Loneliness in the Psychiatric Clinic: Creating Healing Spaces Through Acknowledging Personhood and Agency

Michael O'Loughlin

Abstract: *Arguing for the importance of the clinical encounter as a site of bioethical inquiry, I focus particularly on persons experiencing severe psychic distress. Acknowledging the historical wrongs that have been done to persons with severe psychic distress, I suggest that the contemporary colonization of psychiatric care by the medical model and by neoliberal values that prioritize accountability, metrics, and cost over personhood are doing a grave disservice to such patients. I draw on the writings of social theorists including Agamben to argue that the treatment of psychiatric sufferers produces a risk of causing patients to experience bare life and relegation to the status of nonpersons. Drawing on Stauffer's concept of ethical loneliness, I illustrate the kind of harm that is done when the institutions that we design to listen to patients and receive suffering fail in that responsibility. In the second half of the chapter, I offer implications for an ethical, humane, and politically aware sensibility in assisting persons with severe psychiatric distress.*

Acknowledgement: Portions of this chapter were first published in O'Loughlin, M. (2020). Ethical loneliness in the psychiatric clinic: The manufacture of non-belonging. *Ethics, Medicine and Public Health*, 14, July-Sept. and used here with kind permission of the publisher.

Seeking to delineate the scope of bioethical inquiry, Hull points out that the "most obviously ethical moment in medicine is the clinical encounter itself" (2017, p. 2) and that bioethics is, therefore, necessarily about the process of subjectification—about helping us understand and experience who we are becoming. Because healer and patient are drawn together by what Zaner (1988) calls the "moral chance" of illness and the necessarily affiliative nature of the clinical encounter, the clinical meeting is driven by a moral imperative. However, as Hull notes, the moral valence of the clinical encounter is tempered and complicated by the institutional imperatives of modern medical practice such that the relationship is inherently asymmetrical.

This asymmetry has led Foucault (1973) to formulate a theory of how subjectivity is constituted within a nexus of power relations that, in the case of medicine, cause the patient to come to understand her- or himself in a very particular way as subject of and subject to medical practices. Hull notes that in the case of technologically intensive western medicine, and in the context of the increasing commodification of the practice of medicine as a neoliberal capitalist enterprise focused exclusively on individual metrics and parameters at the expense of social context (Dalal, 2018; Fraser, 2016; O'Loughlin, 2018), the ramifications for subjectivity are enormous. Following Crawford (1980), Hull argues that technocratic managerial approaches to medical practice lead to the "medicalization of everyday life" (2017, p. 8) and an individualization of the experience of illness.

Complementing this discussion, Young (2019) suggests that personhood is a core human value, and that for all humans an acknowledgement of personhood ought to be a fundamental human right. In reviewing the status of the person in psychology, Young points to a chasm between the predominant diagnostically driven approach to treatment embedded, for instance, in DSM and ICD classification systems, and holistic, humanistic, and narrative approaches that seek to embrace the totality of human experience. Young suggest that a reductionist medical model, with an emphasis on diagnostic categorization and the reduction of symptomatology to neurobiological and physiological processes "treat(s) the symptoms rather than the whole person" (2019, p. 96), thereby negating personhood.

Critics of the "chemical imbalance" hypothesis of psychic distress, and of the pharmaceuticalization of suffering, echo this critique and argue for a reclamation of the notion of personhood and life narrative as the foundation of ethical psychiatric care.[1] The intrinsic value of personhood is augmented by entrance into validating, respectful, and reciprocal relational processes, as Young notes (2019). The inverse is also true. Environments which, notwithstanding any official rhetoric of "care," negate personhood, deny competence, or reduce a patient to the position of object create conditions of abjection in which agency is denied and the patient's capacity to be fully human—in a relation of reciprocity or mutual recognition—is foreclosed.

An ethics for psychiatry

In his discussion of an ethic of "mental illness"[2] Holm (2019) argues that this is a particularly important yet fraught area of ethical inquiry because of the historical legacy of the field. This legacy includes unorthodox, bogus, morally repugnant, and ethically problematic treatments that have been carried out—often coercively—in the name of psychiatry. Lobotomy, electroconvulsive therapy, forced sterilization, psychosurgery, and the indiscriminate use of drug cocktails to create a "chemical lobotomy" are only the most recent exemplars of a long history of coercive and cruel "treatments" that have deprived psychiatric sufferers of their humanity (Foucault, 1973, Whitaker, 2001).

Holm also points out the thorny ethical issues involved in coercive treatment, and the ethical implications of construing persons with psychiatric distress as "incompetent." Further, he notes that "(b)ioethics emerged, at least in part, as a deliberate reaction to the perceived powerlessness of patients in relation to the paternalistic practices of the medical profession" (2019, p. 2). Part of that power, in a psychiatric context, comes from the health professional's capacity to define psychiatric distress

---

[1] For critique see, for example, Healy, (1993); Mackler (2009); Moncrieff (2013); O'Loughlin, (in press); O'Loughlin, Arac-Orhun & Queler (2019); Whitaker (2001, 2010)

[2] My personal preference is not to use terms such as "mental illness" because it is not at all clear that severe psychic distress is an illness, nor do I know of any definitive evidence that such distress is chemical or biological in origin. I should note that Holm, although employing the term "mental illness," demonstrates a critical awareness of the limitations of the terminology.

as disease, as opposed to as *dis-ease,* a condition brought on by what I call elsewhere "problems in living" (O'Loughlin, Arac-Orhun & Queler, 2019).

Once construed as disease, psychiatric suffering can be reified as a fact, as "mental illness." This "illness" can then be subjected to a medicalized course of treatment. In addition to the diminution of patient subjectivity and the negation of personhood, Holm points out that this kind of delimiting of psychic suffering as an "illness" located in the individual— and often, more specifically, in the brain—removes the patient entirely from the social constellation of family, friends, etcetera within which psychic distress might be understood and ameliorated.

As Holm notes, "analysis that focuses only on the patient is at best incomplete and at worst seriously misleading" (2019, p. 3). The Open Dialogue approach to psychiatric treatment, pioneered in Western Lapland by Seikkula and colleagues (Seikkula & Olson, 2003: Seikkula et al., 2003), as well as observations in cross-cultural psychiatry demonstrate the value of more familially-based, culturally and contextually inclusive approaches to addressing psychic distress.[3] Conventional medicalized approaches essentialize the psychiatric patient as diseased or ill, and this leads to a slippery slope where the patient comes to be viewed as incompetent and lacking in agency and, therefore, requiring coercive treatment.

The chasm between narrative and psychodynamic approaches to psychiatric treatment on the one hand and biologized or medicalized approaches may be unbridgeable, Holm remarks. Bioethics, however, has an obligation to articulate an understanding of psychiatry that is attuned to the phenomenology of human suffering, and that thereby avoids becoming an unwitting enabler of conventional medicalized approaches to psychiatry that serve to negate personhood.

Psychiatric "care": A zone of social abandonment?

Writing almost fifty years ago, noted psychiatrist Harold Searles expressed apprehension about the world turning its back on persons with significant

---

[3] See, for example, Droždek & Wilson (2017); Fassin (2011); Good et al., (2018); Pandolfo, (2018),

psychiatric difficulties and he worried that an excessive reliance on pharmaceutical solutions could lead to even greater isolation for persons already vulnerable to fearing social contact. He suggested that while persons with what he called "schizophrenia"[4] may...

> have written off their fellow human beings as not kin to them...their fellow human beings have come to accept this as functionally true. If the psychoanalytic movement itself must take refuge in what I regard essentially as a phenothiazine-and-genetics flight from this problem, then the long dark night of the soul will have been ushered in... (1975, pp. 227-228)

The hegemony of neoliberal healthcare with its managerial and commodified approach to behavioral health (Dalal, 2018; Vaspe, 2017) raises concern that the dark night of the soul may be upon us. Neoliberal care, driven relentlessly by capitalist concerns for commodification, efficiency and profit, is entirely incompatible, as Fraser (2016) notes, with an ethic of care and justice. Straitened by neoliberal pressures, how do we advocate for the kind of humanistic, receptive, and life-changing care that narrative, psychoanalytic, and humanistic approaches have historically offered and can continue to offer to persons with severe psychic distress brought on by apparently intractable problems in living?

This, I should note, is not an issue delimited to psychiatry alone as Vaspe (2017) and Frank (2013) make abundantly clear in their discussions of physical medicine. Neither is an emphasis on relationality new to psychiatry as pioneering interpersonalist psychoanalytic work by analysts such as Fromm-Reichmann (1960), Karon & Vandenbos (1977), Mosher (2004), Searles (1986) and Sullivan (1968; Wake, 2006) makes clear.

---

[4] Searles used the term "schizophrenia". Although that term still holds wide currency in medical practice, I no longer use it, preferring terms such as "severe psychic distress" that does not carry the individualistic, biological or disease connotations of "schizophrenia". There is sufficient disquiet around the term "schizophrenia" that a petition is currently circulating seeking to persuade the American Psychiatric Association and the World Health Organization to drop the term because of its stigmatizing consequences. See https://www.change.org/p/american-psychiatric-association-apa-who-drop-the-stigmatizing-term-schizophrenia for details.

João Biehl's study of a community of psychiatric sufferers who had sought refuge in a garbage dump in Brazil offers a limit case for the reduction of psychiatric sufferers to "life in a zone of social abandonment" (2005). Speaking of one particular resident, Catarina, Biehl describes her voice as having been "annulled by psychiatric diagnosis" (2005, p. 3), and he describes the excessive use of medication among these sufferers as "the pharmaceuticalization of disarray" (2005, p. 4). He poses a question that is core to my own concerns about how we manage persons with severe psychic distress: "How can we allow such persons to become "unknowables, with no human rights, and no one accountable?" (2005, p. 4).

Biehl raises troubling questions about how societies compose destinies for people like Catarina, and he suggests that pharmaceuticals are moral technologies that redefine a sense of being and help delimit the subjectivities of those we deem mad or abnormal — people, Biehl says, who are patterned into an identity of exclusion and non-belonging. Biehl lays out the *social* bases for what mental health workers all too often conceptualize narrowly as individual intrapsychic or behavioral issues, speaking not only of a *social psychosis* produced by the nexus of life forces that may generate severe psychic distress and hence impact subjectivity, but also of a more catastrophic consequence, namely the production of *social death*.

Social death refers to policies and practices that led, in the particular case of Catarina, for example, to her proclaiming, "Nobody wants me to be somebody in life" 2005, p. 21). Describing Catarina's life in Vita, Biehl illustrated the manufacture of social death:

> *Vita* is a progressive unraveling of the knotted reality that was Catarina's condition — misdiagnosis, excessive medication, complicity among health professionals and family members in creating her status as a psychotic — and the discovery of the cause of her illness, which turned out to be a genetic and not a psychiatric condition. It charts the domestic events and institutional circumstances through which she was rendered mentally defective and hence socially unproductive and through which her extended

family, her neighbors and medical professionals came to see the act of abandonment as unproblematic and acceptable. (2005, p. 4)

Biehl's argument fits into a larger biopolitical argument about what societies do with their unwanted Others—be they refugees, unwanted economic migrants, throwaway children, or psychiatric sufferers. In my larger project on the construction of psychiatric sufferers as abject, I draw on theoretical arguments from Mbembe's (2003) notion of *necropolitics,* Scheper-Hughes' (1997) description of *rubbish people,* and Agamben's (1998) notion of *bare life,* Khanna's (2003) discussion of *human disposability,* and Bauman's (2004) concept of *wasted lives.*

Too often, systems of "care" seem premised on the capacity of societies to identify some categories of people as nonpersons, thereby eliminating the expectation of respect, dignity, and an invitation to narrative and agentic participation to which all humans should be entitled. Persons with chronic and severe psychiatric distress have been and continue to be subject to violent and carceral regimes of treatment, and to pejorative labeling systems embodied in terms such as *schizophrenia, borderline personality disorder, bipolar disorder* etc., as well as to the construction of their subjectivities as *diseased* by the bitter pills of pharmaceutical regimens (Burstow, 2015; Moncrieff, 2013; Whitaker, 2010).

The writings of distinguished professors Lucy Newlyn (2018), Erin Soros (2015), and Ellyn Saks (2008), psychiatric sufferers all, illustrate the systemic misrecognition and social violence too often at the heart of psychiatric "care"—a system that, as Dalal (2018) and Vaspe (2017) document, is increasingly enacting anti-human, managerial, and neo-liberal systems of delivery. There is decidedly less room for narrative, phenomenological, or humanistic therapeutic relationships in this brave new neoliberal world.

For a last word on pharmaceutical annihilation, and how it can negate personhood and render therapy moot, consider this comment by distinguished clinician Christopher Bollas:

A common reason why breakdown results in a broken self is the use of psychotropic intervention. Although such medication may help relieve the person in the immediate situation, the ingestion of such drugs negates meaning. Discovery of the unconscious reasons for the breakdown, and the opportunity for sentient understanding and tolerance of it within a human and therapeutic situation, are denied in the person. The patient may visit the doctor for repeat prescriptions, they may see a psychiatrist briefly every few weeks, but all this does is to seal over the structuralized breakdown and unwittingly ensure its permanence. (2013, p. 18)

Ethical loneliness

Soros (2015) suggests that the institutional blinders of psychology and psychiatry can engender a sense of misrecognition that is catastrophic for the psyche of a person who is in an extreme state and seeking holding, containment, or respite. People seek treatment because of symptoms that mark insufficient interest in their *becoming*.

Unresolved mourning, as Newlyn (2018) illustrates, can leave a person decompensated with no firm foundation on which to stand. Recognizing that dilemma helps the clinician to take a stand for the importance of beginning where one is, rather than where one would like to be. A failure by supposedly therapeutic systems and hospitals to acknowledge this can lead to what Stauffer (2015) calls "ethical loneliness":

Ethical loneliness is the isolation one feels when one, as a violated person or as one member of a persecuted group, has been abandoned by humanity, or by those who have power over one's life possibilities. It is a condition undergone by persons who have been unjustly treated and dehumanized by human beings and political structures, who emerge from that injustice only to find that the surrounding world will not listen or cannot properly hear their testimony—their claims about what they suffered and about what is now owed them—on their own terms. So ethical loneliness is the experience of having been abandoned by humanity compounded by the experience of not being heard. (2015, p. 1)

This argument is reminiscent of Agamben's (1998) notion of *bare life*, and particularly of Fassin and Rechtman's application of *bare life* to psychiatry

(2009). Stauffer remarks on how "unintended ironies surface whenever institutions designed for hearing fail to hear well" and she shows "how the effects of those ironies tend to weigh most heavily on those with the least power to endure bad outcomes" (2015, p. 6). Ethical loneliness, therefore, is a form of abandonment in which whole groups of people are reduced to a non-status so that processes of dehumanization and even annihilation can be enacted without qualms.

Oxford professor and poet Newlyn understood these dynamics well when she remarked that at the time of her breakdown, the attuned listening that she found most soothing came not from her psychiatrist but from her family doctor: "In the day to day management of mental illness I've found GPs to be more helpful than psychiatrists, since they are not committed to any particular methodology: one just talks to them as to another human being" (2018, pp. 4-5).

Reclaiming suffering: Toward a new ethics of psychiatric distress

The core ethical issue in psychiatric care is how we come to understand suffering. As Dalal (2018) noted, Cognitive Behavioral Therapy (CBT) is now a mainstay of the British National Health System, and it is rapidly establishing hegemony as the treatment of choice for psychic distress throughout the Western world and beyond. Contrary to, for example, Buddhist philosophy and Buddhist psychotherapy (Epstein, 1997, 1998), which embrace suffering and loss as central to the human experience, the foundational assumption of CBT is that positivity and happiness is the normal state of affairs, and any experience of loss or pain is caused by a "mental illness" and must be removed by engendering a shift in thought process around the precipitating loss (1997, p. 15). As Dalal (2018) has noted, in this framework psychiatric struggles are symptoms or disorders that one *has* and that can be given up, rather than fundamental existential struggles with being and loss that must, in Freud's (1914) immortal words, be painstakingly *worked through.*

In her foreword to a recent volume of psychiatric narratives written by my research team (O'Loughlin et al., 2019), Soros (2019) suggested that we ought to consider symptoms of madness not as wound or disorder but rather as a way, however artfully disguised, for the sufferer to communicate his or her location. Dorman's (2003) eight-year psychodynamic treatment of Catherine Penney, a young woman who experienced a lengthy period of catatonia, represents an example of the kind of deeply attuned listening that leads to such working through. Cardinal's (2000) autobiography offers comparable insight into the deep existential journey recovery from breakdown necessitates.

Meeting the Other existentially: Story matters

Severe psychiatric distress represents a form of dissolution, an unwinding of the structures that give humans the ability to navigate life, to go on being (Epstein, 2009). The result can be psychic breakdown, intractable depression, debilitating anxiety, or crushing somatic symptoms—all of which are communications about a deep malady of the soul. In some respects, these symptoms might be considered manifestations of a failure to mourn in the face of catastrophic loss.

This loss could be immediate (e.g., bereavement); it could be an ineffable echo of an archaic loss or trauma from as early as infancy or the prenatal period (Piontelli, 1992; Fraiberg et al., 1975); or it could represent an echo of an archaic ancestral wound of the kind that is often described in terms of the sequelae of intergenerational trauma (Abraham & Torok, 1994; Davoine & Gaudillière, 2004). Without the means to render such losses speakable or representable so that working through is possible, there can be no mourning and the inevitable outcome is absence, silence, flight, or dissolution. Speaking of bereavement, Freud (1917) characterized a failure to do the work of mourning as yielding a deep-seated melancholia.

My colleague Marilyn Charles and I (O'Loughlin et al., 2019; Charles & O'Loughlin, 2012) have come to conceptualize a psychic crisis as producing an impasse—a difficulty which the patient cannot resolve. This impasse brings the patient into therapy or into a psychiatric facility, and a positive prognosis appears to be very much related to the capacity of the patient to grapple dynamically with the experience of *being in relation* with an interested Other.

Kristeva (1982) conceptualizes the loss that is at the core of melancholia as a turn inward, a turn toward emptiness or abjection arising from an inaugural loss of significant proportions. André Green (1986; Kohon, 1999) speaks of blank psychosis as a radical solution to catastrophic object loss. Such a loss, rather than leading to repression, results instead in a massive decathexis of emotion and a state of breakdown.

Drawing inspiration from Arthur Frank's (2013) exploration of major physical illnesses as life ruptures, my research team collected 39 hours of interview with persons with long-term psychiatric struggles for a book entitled *Lives interrupted: Psychiatric narratives of struggle and resilience* (O'Loughlin et al., 2019). We opened the book with Lucy Newlyn's description of her induction into emergency psychiatric care in England:

> In her frank and moving autobiography, poet and Oxford professor Lucy Newlyn (2018) charts the course of a significant psychiatric disturbance that she first experienced in her forties, while she kept vigil as her father lay dying. Newlyn offers a harrowing account of the fifteen years since she first experienced psychosis, was sectioned, and was forcibly taken to the emergency room (known in U.K. as Casualty or A & E) in a state of frightened confusion, exacerbated, perhaps, by the precipitous manner in which she was inducted into the psychiatric system:
>
>> Arriving in Casualty I thought I had been put prison. When a psychiatrist interviewed me I didn't know who I was or even what time of day it was. I had turned into a strange thing I couldn't recognize as myself. I sat on a seat which was also a toilet in a large white empty room on my own where a strong bright light shone on me perpetually. I shouted for a long, long time. When I was let out of the observation room I saw the A & E area, where people were lying on stretchers or trolleys. I was sure they were war-victims; there was one whose face was bloated – her whole body was swollen, and it seemed to be in a sack. She looked like my mum. There were other people whose heads I could see over the tops of screens, and I thought two of them were my sisters. I kept hearing their voices and they seemed to be lying

about me – their accounts of me were a tissue of lies, designed to show that I was no carer. They wanted me punished. I kept screaming at the top of my voice: "LISTEN". (Newlyn, 2018, as quoted in O'Loughlin et al., 2019, p. 2)

Newlyn's narrative charts unsparingly the many ups and downs of her condition; her struggles with socially sanctioned stigma and institutional anomie in her workplace; her battle with medications that flattened her symptoms but at the cost of also flattening out the creative spikes that were so vital to her poetry-making; and, of course, the monkey wrench that her psychic struggles threw into the personal and professional relationships she was seeking to stabilize and maintain. Newlyn lifts the veil on the complex and often downright perplexing nature of psychic suffering.

Benefiting from her experiences in counseling and from her struggles to articulate self-understanding in her poetry, Newlyn offers a deeply reflective, nuanced account that serves as a counter-narrative to simplistic, reductionist diagnoses and classifications as well as to the idea that there is any single, simple "magic bullet" or single pill to "cure" severe psychic suffering. It says a lot about Western societies' attitudes to mental distress that a distinguished author such as Newlyn—struck by a form of madness that is just a whisper away from being triggered for any one of us, given straitened circumstances—must frame her work as a coming-out story with all the connotations of overcoming shame and stigma that this implies.

The narrative tone of Newlyn's work is also worthy of note. Modern, industrialized, corporatized medicine with its constant pressure for automation, for cost-cutting—and for the generation of putatively "evidence-based," cost-conscious treatment protocols and the completion of time-consuming records—places enormous billing pressures on medical providers to see as many patients as possible. Too often there is neither time nor interest in listening to the patient—in *getting the story* of human suffering.

The patient narrative that frames the origin and meaning of a medical or psychological/spiritual crisis is at risk of disappearing from general medical practice and, indeed, from psychiatry. Even strictly medical conditions come with attendant spiritual and existential crises that merit attention and anxieties that should be recognized so they might be assuaged. With the notable exception of her general practitioner, Newlyn noted that despite the essential help her carers offered, for the most part there was little interest in the total circumstances of her distress, in the meaning of her experience, or in the effects these aberrant and terrifying intrusions were having on her daily living (O'Loughlin et al., 2019, pp. 2-3).

Implications for practice

Drawing on my clinical experience, particularly in a portion of my practice reserved for persons who have struggled with psychic collapse; my experience supervising clinical psychology externs; my experience teaching and conducting clinical research; and my conversations with hospital personnel, here are some principles that guide my work:

1. I recognize that persons in acute distress need holding, containing and respite care. While pharmacological stabilization may be called for, in the short- or medium-term, medication in and of itself cannot be a solution, or indeed the only solution to psychic suffering. We need to bear in mind Bollas's warning that medication negates meaning making possibilities—or that, as Nikolas Rose (2003) put it, it produces "neurochemical selves."

2. Persons in acute states of distress are suffering, and a first response must be to offer respect, empathy, reassurance, and love. As Erin Soros (2019) noted, in introducing our book, we must honor the voices, the beauty, and the pain of persons in distress. One of the startling findings of our field research (O'Loughlin et al., 2019) is how little talk therapy is offered, even to people with striking levels of suffering over their lifetimes.

3. While diagnosis is foundational to neoliberal care, and metrics-based "treatment" planning is built around econometric assumptions, we must bear in mind that psychologizing human suffering necessarily negates human subjectivity. This is even more true for those who, by virtue of class, race, gender, age, perceived abilities, previous psychiatric breakdowns, unhoused status,

migration status, or carceral histories are already marginalized in our societies and are very vulnerable to mechanisms of social death.

4. Trained as a psychoanalyst, I assume that all human actions and utterances have meaning. Our purpose is to seek the meaning that lies beneath manifest symptoms. This requires, as Lucy Newlyn (2018) noted, listening with an attuned ear. This listening ought to include not only immediate life history and traumatic experience, but genealogical links to ancestral history and what Judy Atkinson (2002) called intergenerational trauma trails and the sweep of history (see also O'Loughlin, in press).

5. Recovery ought to be emphasized instead of an unstated—or sometimes even explicitly stated—expectation of chronicity and medication dependence. Drawing on her own lived experience, psychiatric survivor and psychologist Eleanor Longden (2011) has noted forcefully the problematics of prioritizing medication compliance over recovery. Recovery entails re-storying experience—exploring the triggers that led to fragmentation and breakdown and doing so in the presence of a therapist with a capacity to bear witness patiently (O'Loughlin, 2007a, b). We need to be able to make the road by walking with our patients (cf., Horton & Freire, 1990).

6. We psychotherapists need to build relationships with psychiatrists who understand how medications flatten affect and creativity and foreclose futures. We must seek psychiatrist and physician partners who are committed to working collaboratively with persons suffering psychic distress to taper medications, and create a potential space for agency, meaning-making, and recovery as soon as possible.

7. We must be holders of hope. Therapists must have the stamina and commitment to stay with people in distress for as long as it takes— and must also imagine recovery and a return to a community of care and relational possibility. Bollas's (2013) work is inspirational in this regard.

8. We would be wise to acknowledge that madness can be produced by societal and sociohistorical factors, and that even the hospital

itself may be a driver of madness as Ellyn Saks's (2008) cautionary tale reminds us.

I will conclude with Leanh Nguyen's call to therapists to find the human and to stay human. Nguyen poses the existential problem of our work this way:

> Buried in these fragments of despair is a story about dying and "surviving." When it is established that I am willing to hear their despair and am capable of visiting their living death, these patients would then make the following questions central to our encounter: How is life worth living? What is it that you do with/for me? The ethics and poetics of psychoanalysis have helped me live in these questions with my patients, and also to metabolize them into my own: What makes one human? What and why do I practice psychoanalysis? (2012, p. 309)

At the conclusion of her essay, Nguyen sums up the ethical and political imperatives of work with distressed humans:

> Psychoanalysis has not yet created a cure for cruelty and suffering...But the implicit pledge of our profession is that each life counts. Each story needs to be found and retold, and each telling matters infinitely and effects profound ripples in the world—and in our own individual psychic waters. My proposition is that psychoanalysis requires us to be ethical as well as political. The ethical stance lies in our commitment "to illuminate silence and render it audible" (Grand, 2000, p. 36) and to never give up on the preciousness of the patient's mind. The political act lies in enforcing a vision of life that acknowledges pain and death, and that attempts to work out an ethics of dying and loving. (2012, p. 317)

References

Abraham, N., Torok, M. (1994). *The shell and the kernel*. Rand N. (Ed. & Trans). University of Chicago Press.

Agamben, G. (1998). *Homo sacer: Sovereign power and bare life*. Stanford University Press.

Atkinson, J. (2002). *Trauma trails: Recreating song lines*. Spinifex Press.

Bauman, Z. (2004). *Wasted lives: Modernity and its outcasts*. Polity Press.

Biehl, J. (2005). *Vita: Life in a zone of social abandonment*. University of California Press.

Bollas, C. (2013). *Catch them before they fall*. Routledge.

Burstow, B. (2015). *Psychiatry and the business of madness: An ethical and epistemological accounting*. Palgrave Macmillan.

Cardinal, M. (2000). *The words to say it*. Women's Press Ltd.

Charles, M., & O'Loughlin, M. (2012). The complex subject of psychosis. *Psychoanalysis Culture & Society, 17*(4), 410-421.

Crawford, R. (1980). Healthism and the medicalization of everyday life. *International Journal of Health Services, 365-388*.

Dalal, F. (2018). *CBT: The cognitive beahvioral tsunami*. Routledge.

Davoine, F. & Gaudillière, J-M. (2004). *History beyond trauma: Whereof one cannot speak, thereof one cannot stay silent*, (S. Fairfield, Trans.). Other Press.

Dorman, D. (2003). *"Dante's cure": A journey out of madness*. Other Press.

Droždek, B., Wilson J.P. (Eds.). (2017). *Voices of trauma: Treating survivors across cultures*. Springer.

Epstein, M. (1997). *Thoughts without a thinker: Psychotherapy from a Buddhist perspective*. Basic Books.

Epstein, M. (1998). *Going to pieces without falling apart: A Buddhist perspective on wholeness*. Basic Books.

Epstein, M. (2009). *Going on being: Life at the crossroads of Buddhism and psychotherapy*. Wisdom Publications.

Fassin, D. (2011). Ethnopsychiatry and the postcolonial encounter: A French psychopolitics of otherness. In Anderson W., Jenson, D., & Keller R.C., (Eds.). *Unconscious dominions: Psychoanalysis, global trauma, and global sovereignties* (p. 223-246). Duke University Press.

Fassin, D & Rechtman R., (Eds.). (2009). *The empire of trauma: An inquiry into the condition of victimhood.* Princeton University Press.

Foucault, M. (1973). *The birth of the clinic: an archaeology of medical perception.* University of Notre Dame Press.

Fraiberg, S., Adelson E., Shapiro, V. (1975). 'Ghosts in the nursery, *Journal of the American Academy of Child Psychiatry, 14,* 387-421.

Frank, A. (2013). *The wounded storyteller: Body, illness, ethics.* University of Chicago Press.

Fraser, N. (2016). Contradictions of capital and care. *New Left Review, 100,* July-August.

Freud, S. (1917). *Mourning and melancholia. (Standard Ed.* Vol. 14. pp. 243-258).

Freud, S. (1914). Remembering, Repeating and Working Through: Further Recommendations in the Technique of Psychoanalysis, (*Standard Ed.* Vol. 12. pp. 147-156).

Fromm-Reichmann, F. (1960). *Principles of intensive psychotherapy.* University of Chicago Press.

Good, M., Hyde, S., Pinto, T., Good, B., (Eds.). (2018). *Postcolonial disorders: Ethnographic studies in subjectivity.* University of California Press.

Grand, S. (2000). *The reproduction of evil: A clinical and cultural perspective.* Hillsdale, NJ: The Analytic Press.

Green, A. (1986). 'The dead mother' in *On Private madness* (pp. 142-173). Hogarth Press.

Healy, D. (1993). *Psychiatric drugs explained.* Mosby.

Holm, S. (2019). Bioethics and mental health —An uneasy relationship. *Ethics, Medicine and Public Health, 10,* 1-7.

Horton, M. & Freire, P. (1990). *We make the road by walking: Conversations on education and social change.* Temple University Press.

Hull, G. (2017). The subject and power of bioethics. *Ethics, Medicine and Public Health,* 3(4), 10-419.

Karon, B. & Vandenbos, G. (1977). *Psychotherapy of schizophrenia: The treatment of choice.* Jason Aronson.

Khanna, R. (2003). *Dark Continents: Psychoanalysis and colonialism.* Duke University Press.

Kohon, G. (1999). *The dead mother: The work of André Green.* Routledge.

Kristeva, J. (1982*). Powers of horror: An essay on abjection.* Columbia University Press.

Longden, E. (2011). *Knowing you, knowing you.*[DVD]. Intervoice: The Hearing Voices Movement.

Mackler, D. (2009). *Take these broken wings* [DVD]. http://wildtruth.net/films-english/brokenwings/.

Mbembe, A. (2003). Necropolitics. *Public Culture, 15*(1), 11-40.

Moncrieff, J. (2013). *The bitterest pills: The troubling story of antipsychotic drugs.* Palgrave.

Mosher, LR. (2004). *Soteria: Through madness to deliverance.* Xlibris.

Newlyn, L. (2018). *Diary of a bipolar explorer.* Signal.

Nguyen, L. (2012). Psychoanalytic activism: *Finding and staying human. Psychoanalytic Psychology, 29*(3), 308-317.

O'Loughlin, M. (2007a). Bearing witness to troubled memory. *Psychoanalytic Review, 94*(2), 191-212.

O'Loughlin, M. (2007b). On losses that are not easily mourned. In L. Bohm, R. Curtis, & B. Willock (Eds.). *Psychoanalysts' reflections on deaths and endings: Finality, transformations, new beginnings.* Routledge.

O'Loughlin, M. (2018). Book Review: *Psychoanalysis, the NHS, and mental health work today,* by Alison Vaspe (Ed.). *Psychoanalysis, Culture & Society, 23*(4), 459-462.

O'Loughlin, M. (In press). Cultural ruptures and their consequences across generations. In I. Lambrecht & A. Lavis, (Eds.), *Culture and psychosis.* Routledge.

O'Loughlin M, Arac-Orhun S., Queler M. (Eds.). (2019). *Lives interrupted: Psychiatric narratives of struggle and resilience.* Lexington Books.

Pandolfo, S. (2018). The knot of the soul: Postcolonial conundrums, madness and the imagination. In Good M, Hyde S, Pinto T, Good B., (Eds.),

Postcolonial disorders: Ethnographic studies in subjectivity (p. 329-358). University of California Press.

Piontelli, A. (1992). *From fetus to child: An observational and psychoanalytic study.* Routledge.

Rose, N. (2003). Neurochemical selves. *Society, November/December,* 46-59.

Saks, E. (2008). *The center cannot hold: My journey through madness.* Hachette.

Scheper-Hughes, N. (1997). People who get rubbished. *New Internationalist,* October, 295. *https://newint.org/features/1997/10/05/people/*

Searles, H.F. (1975). Countertransference and theoretical model. In: Gunderson J.G, Mosher LR. (Eds.). *Psychotherapy of schizophrenia.* Jason Aronson.

Searles, H.F. (1986). *Collected papers on schizophrenia and related subjects.* Routledge.

Seikkula, J., & Olson, M. (2003). The open dialogue approach to acute psychosis. *Family Process, 43,* 403–418.

Seikkula J., Alakare, B., Aalotonen, J., Holma, J., Rasinkangas, A., & Lehtinen, V. (2003). Open Dialogue approach: Treatment principles and preliminary results of a two-year follow-up on first episode schizophrenia. *Ethical Human Sciences & Services, 5*(3), 163–182.

Soros, E. Foreword. In O'Loughlin M, Arac-Orhun S., Queler M., (Eds.) (2019). *Lives interrupted: Psychiatric narratives of struggle and resilience.* Lexington Books.

Soros, E. Eyes! Birds! Walnuts! Pennies! (2015). In Tansley L. & Maftei M. (Eds.). *Writing creative non-fiction: Determining the form* (pp. 155-166). Gylphi Press.

Stauffer, J. (2015). *Ethical loneliness: The injustice of not being heard.* Columbia University Press.

Sullivan, H.S. (1968). *The interpersonal theory of psychiatry.* Norton.

Vaspe, A., (Ed.). (2017). *Psychoanalysis, the NHS, and mental health work today.* Karnac.

Wake, N. (2006). "The full story by no means all told": Harry Stack Sullivan at Shepherd-Pratt 1922-1930. *History of Psychology, 9*(4), 325-358.

Whitaker, R. (2001). *Mad in America: Bad science, bad medicine, and the enduring mistreatment of the mentally ill.* Basic Books.

Whitaker, R. (2010). *Anatomy of an epidemic: Magic bullets, psychiatric drugs and the astonishing rise of mental illness in America.* Crown.

Young, G. (2019). Personhood across disciplines: Applications to ethical theory and mental health ethics. *Ethics, Medicine and Public Health, 10,* 93-101.

Zaner, R.M. (1988). *Ethics and the clinical encounter.* CSS Publishing.

The Inviting Lure of Madness

Ronald Bassman

Abstract: *The many forms of suffering may be the price we pay for the enhanced consciousness that is the blessing and the curse of being human. The search for simple solutions to the mysteries of life has often resulted in a brief buzz of excitement for a new promising solution which will later be dumped into the huge overflowing garbage bin of psychiatric history. Psychotherapy is the treatment that has passed the test of time. Psychotherapy does not work for everyone, but it is the best service that can be offered to those who are in emotional pain and turmoil. The challenge to the absolute mistaken belief that those who are experiencing an altered state of consciousness cannot benefit and grow from a genuine interpersonal relationship is central to understanding psychosis. This chapter will explore some of the false myths and erroneous paths of treatment innovations that are both formulaic and minimize the power of compassion and relationship. Recognizing that reality is subjective and can only be defined and understood by the experience of the individual allows for open assessment on the part of the practitioner and promotes genuine connection. Explored further will be how the primary effectiveness of a therapist resides in her or his own self-awareness and openness to seeking understanding of the client's evolving knowledge of their experience moving through the world.*

If you save one person you save the world. (Hebrew Talmud)

Not being the person I wanted to be, and who I believed that I should be, compelled me to try just about anything to numb my unbearable emotions. I purposely dipped my foot into the mysterious ocean of madness expecting a bone-chilling cold, only to discover the surprisingly warm attraction of a new and different way of being. Although the short plunge into madness seems to be simply a taste of the mad journey, it is extremely difficult to withdraw once you discover the thrill of reveling in your newfound power to create a universe where you are the absolute master—a God.

The spiritual mystic often differs from the mad mystic by the dedicated preparation to transforming oneself into an enlightened being. Depending on how one's discipline pursues and defines the journey and destination, the task is Herculean. The pains and emotional turmoil of the desperate unguided seeker will propel her or him into ignoring the inherent risks. Existence in a lonely immaterial prison with its unbearable suffering cannot compete with the seductive promise of unlimited possibilities.

Unfortunately, it is easy to locate the entrance chute that allows one to slide down into the ocean of playful madness, but virtually impossible for most of us to slide back up the chute or to find a door that enables control of the passage back and forth between madness and consensual reality. The question I think a lot about is how many of us have been smothered by the mind-numbing and spirit-breaking of psychiatric drugs that deprive us of our potential—to learn how to swim in an expansive consciousness.

What if we could have experienced therapists or teachers who genuinely understood the power of mad experience and could provide guidance? Spiritual and religious teachers need not be the only qualified guides. I wonder why we cannot do better. Why must institutions rely on health-damaging drugs and incarceration that only succeeds in obliterating the hope for a better life? How much human potential has been sacrificed by an "us and them" culture that is intolerant of those who look, act, feel and think differently?

What is the relationship between madness and altered states of consciousness? John Weir Perry, a psychiatrist who studied with Carl Jung and founded the alternative treatment center Diabasis (Crossing over) suggested that madness may be nature's way of providing one with the means for renewal and the capacity to reorganize the self on a higher level.[1] Must the quest for enlightenment described in the diverse paths of the mystics be sidetracked into the arbitrary mental prison called "schizophrenia"? Zen Buddhist tradition describes the powers that so enthrall us as Makyo and dismisses them as the toys and games of magicians. The Zen master warns the disciple to guard against being seduced by illusions of power and becoming diverted from a more desirable and meaningful path.

When too much emphasis is placed on the paranormal abilities that entice, it interferes with and clouds awareness.[2] The egoism of pride and power, influenced by the need to impress, stagnates the growth process. To Christians, the elevated state of consciousness arises from an encounter with a higher level of Being above the human level. The universal advice of knowledgeable people in such matters is *not* to seek the extraordinary experiences that often occur when any intensive inner work is undertaken. E.F. Schumacher informs us that those who have not had personal experience of a higher level of consciousness cannot understand the language of those who are trying to tell us about it and, therefore, they conclude that the mind is then disordered by madness.[3]

Lucid dreaming is a pleasant harmless experience if it occurs naturally while you are safe at home sleeping in your bed. But being able to experience such a phenomenon while going about your daily waking life requires a major revision in your thinking. When fascinated by new abilities, you are enticed to withdraw from the problems of the external world and spend your time enjoying the exciting imagery of your internal life. The adventure and thrill of the mind's creativity can release a torrent of energy. The high is self-sustaining. As you move deeper and deeper into almost exclusively valuing internal life, the demands and obligations of the external world are ignored.

In his book, *The Seven Story Mountain* (1948), theologian Thomas Merton writes of his admiration for the peaceful freedom of the Trappist monks. Rather than being lauded for accomplishments that make one rise above one's peers, the most successful monk is he who best blends in and is never noticed. Merton writes that the Trappist monk is free from the constraints of being vigilant of what they anticipate being the judgments of others.[4]

Without any training, guidance or requisite cultural initiation rituals, there can be an overwhelming attraction for expanding and then grandly misinterpreting the meaning of powerful new experiences. The freedom, excitement, and adventure can block out one's chronic struggles with life's disappointments. Feeling as if you can do anything furthers the belief that you are beyond submitting to the criticism or judgments of others. The realities of the mind become stronger than any popular view of reality.

Precious are our memories. I wish I could say with conviction as most people easily do that "I'll never forget that." I have worked relentlessly to recapture and secure lost memories from that reality-bending period of my life. I have found some dim flickering lights in the foggy storage space allocated to that pre-hospital summer where I first flirted with and then embraced my madness. I have mourned and let go of the magic, but I will not absolve or excuse responsibility for the psychiatric treatments (40 insulin comas) inflicted on myself and others. The few of us who have been able to survive insulin coma and electroshock treatments and have regained the capacity to speak out must provide testimony to counter the newest, latest, greatest invasive "healing intervention" inflicted upon us "for our own good."

Friedrich A. Kekule, who had searched for many years to find the molecular structure of benzene, awoke from a dream with an insight that revolutionized modern chemistry. His dream of a snake getting hold of its own tail led to his discovery of the construction of the benzene ring. Robert Lewis Stevenson reported that his stories were created in nocturnal dreams by his little dream people and that he merely transcribed them when he was awake. Interesting that his "sleep brownies" gave him a story that hints of the erroneous split-personality portrayal of schizophrenia, *Dr. Jekyll and Mr. Hyde*.

Brief flashes of insight illuminate the dots and dashes of human history. Those discrete visionary moments of clarity or artistic inspiration elevate us. But suppose you misinterpret and/or ignore the context of those pure lucid moments. Or worse, the world doubts your credibility and rejects your new knowledge. During Nostradamus' lifetime, the regard for his visionary ability vacillated several times, alternating between reverential worship and heretical treason depending on shifting political winds. Joan of Arc's prophesies were relied upon to guide her country to victory but later—with the war won—she was sold to her country's enemies. Refusing to renounce her *voices* and absent her former political protection, she became a victim of the Inquisition and was executed for heresy.

The founding of any new religion breaks with the prevailing reality. Moses, Jesus, Gautama Buddha, Muhammad, revered and honored visionaries, were not conventional. Psychiatrist Havelock Ellis spoke to the vagaries of shifting contextual perspectives when he wrote:

> Had there been a lunatic asylum in the suburbs of Jerusalem, Jesus Christ would infallibly have been shut up in it at the outset of his public career. That interview with Satan on a pinnacle of the Temple would alone have damned him, and everything that happened after could but have confirmed his diagnosis.[5]

The argument may be made that all religious beliefs are irrational in their orthodoxy since they make claims that go beyond scientific evidence. In the early days of the Society of Friends, when members felt the inner light of Christ shine on them, they were moved to loud outbursts and violent trembling from which the name Quaker was derived. Would considerations of madness detract from George Fox's legacy as founder of the Quakers? Like many great spiritual leaders who preceded him, he had to confront the inner and outer perils of self-examination in his absolute commitment to discovering truth.

Is it possible to reconcile revelation with reason? Visions and other extraordinary phenomena continue to be reported throughout the world and, despite the scientific skepticism of the past, the faithful remain convinced of their authenticity. And what of the many great artists—those who have been seen in their lifetimes as being touched with "madness" and whose works have later come to be praised by historians as insightful masterpieces capturing the essence of the human condition?

A story in the New York Post newspaper by Adam Miller titled "Psycho Theory on Birth of Jazz" would be subject to a different interpretation by me than that proffered by psychiatrist Dean Spence. He stated that Buddy Bolden, widely recognized as the founding father of jazz, couldn't read music due to being schizophrenic. According to him, Buddy Bolden's need to improvise resulted in the technique we have come to know as jazz. Dr.

Spence goes on to say that modern drug treatments would have helped Bowden, who died in 1931 in a Louisiana insane asylum.[6] Makes me wonder what Buddy would have chosen if he had been fully informed of the cost-benefit ratio involved in taking psychiatric drugs to "cure" his schizophrenia at the expense of his creativity.

How do you react to being trapped? Do you permit the frustration and hopelessness to expand and permeate all parts of your being, to take over your whole life? Feeling or being different, whether you see yourself as blessed with a gift or suffering a curse, sets you moving on an uncharted course. Too easily, stress, life circumstances, temperament and motivations can lead you to misconstrue meaning and misapplied knowledge. With a combination of naiveté and desperation, and lacking supportive and empathic anchors, you might easily aggrandize this gift/curse and twist it into an overgeneralizing, all-powerful escape that is desperately needed to replace an undesired self and an accumulation of unsatisfactory life choices.

Madness and Therapy

Without context, is there agreement as to what is normal? Who among us is not familiar with pain, be it physical or emotional—and, perhaps, we need to include spiritual pain? At some point in our lives, we must confront the knowledge of our mortality and adhere to the belief system that seems to make death palatable. Our early ancestors had an easier time believing in the dominant ideology of their tribes. Small tribes with less diversity had fewer choices.

The availability of more choices can create greater dissatisfaction with the choice one has made—always with the lingering doubt that one could have made a better choice. Conversely, more choice augers more freedom. But is it healthier, less problematic to have less freedom but more certainty? The historical trajectory of the search for healing includes oracles, shamans, witchdoctors, medicine men/women, priests, and sages. They are overlooked and disparaged when evaluated and compared with the research methods of the physical sciences.

Persuasion and Healing, written by Jerome D. Frank, was first published more than 50 years ago and retains its significance today. In this qualitative study of diverse modes of healing, topics ranging from the role of the shaman and the revivalism of communities to psychotherapy are addressed. He along with his daughter, Julia Fank M.D., published the third edition of this book.[7] Its message is still very relevant, perhaps being even more important today. Father and daughter contend that many indigenous healing practices share common elements that improve the morale of distressed people. The various forms of successful healing confront the demoralization people attach to their experiences. The authors argue that many of the non-medical therapies are surprisingly like rhetoric, the art of persuasion.

Today, the medical doctor has become the acknowledged authority designated to battle the grim reaper. Few travel through life on a smooth path without confronting small and large potholes. The assistance one needs takes on many forms dictated by each unique individual's needs and preferences. Psychotherapy is life-affirming when learning and personal growth for therapist and client flows through a dynamic relationship-driven process. The pursuit and attainment of self-knowledge, regardless of path, may be the ideal credential for working with people who are locked in chaotic conflicts generated by their untenable personal constructs of reality.

Too often, what is encountered by most in the throes of madness are therapists who have been taught to prioritize stabilization at the expense of understanding and finding meaning in such an altered state of being. I suggest that the dynamics and etiology of madness are diverse and cannot be understood and treated in a predetermined formulaic manner for those who demonstrate similar symptoms. Madness can be a response to internal and/or externally caused distress. The person may be trapped by events, perhaps a lost or unrequited love, with concomitant internal reactions where denial prevents the integration of the experience.

Stuck with the choice of succumbing to the pain or finding a way to be different (symptoms), one may create a reality that conflicts with the accepted consensually validated reality. I am certain that when I entered my own altered state of being, I had made a conscious choice, a choice to not continue to live my life within the unhappy tiny box that was squeezing out of me any chance to pursue my potential. For a therapist to work with me at that time, I needed someone who could viscerally understand me and have the motivation and courage to be present with me in a quest where the maps had not yet been created. I did not wish to be stabilized only to recover and return to an unhappy "normal."

The Therapist-Client Connection

The principles for my therapy practice are based on my belief that transformative change is always possible. My ideals for best practice:

- **Creating core trust** – avoidance of all forms of force and coercion
- Believing in the **essential goodness** of all who seek help unless clearly demonstrated otherwise
- Being **flexible, adaptive, and creative**
- Knowing your own **limits**
- **Courage**
- **Openness to Learning from Each Other**

The Australian Aboriginal Activist, Lila Watson, offered profound guidance in a statement recognized as a credo for working alongside another rather than assuming the role of expert: "If you have come here to help me, you are wasting your time, but if you have come because your liberation is bound up in mine, let us work together."[8]

Distressed hurt people, who seek a psychotherapist, have come to believe that they will be seeing an expert who has a special skill that will help to overcome their problems. The relationship begins in a hierarchy. Yet the desired outcome for the therapy becomes more accessible as the relationship shifts into becoming the reaching across of two equal searchers. It is not an easy task for both therapist and client to give up the wish for the presence of the *Expert*. Because of our interdependence, relationships are critical to our development. If the needed relationships are not available in family, social network or within the community at large, the help and guidance may be provided in psychotherapy.

It is critical to understand the factors involved in a person's choice for you to be this particular individual's therapist. Was it a choice among genuine options? Was there coercion—subtle or powerful? Past and present conflicts, expectations, reactions, and experiences with mental health professionals can make it easier or more difficult to establish rapport and be open. Nothing is more important than the development of trust. That trust must go in both directions. When working with someone who is or has been dealing with what the professions label "psychosis," it is important to be cognizant of the unique sensitivities arising from her or his present and/or past experiences.

One of the too familiar trust betrayals is when hospitalized patients learn that the nurse or therapist who appears warm and kind will have their medications increased and/or being placed on lockdown after giving into the coaxing for the disclosure of suicidal thoughts—assurances of confidentiality notwithstanding. Several times I have heard inpatients at state psychiatric institutions relay a conversation that is usually limited to other patients in the re-telling of what was unsaid in an interview: "I may be mentally ill but I'm not stupid," when recounting their responses to an interviewer's probing questions.

If one's intense experiences resulted in psychiatric services that resulted in confinement and being forced to take strong psychiatric drugs, resistance might be considered among the healthiest reactions. For those of us who had been involuntary patients and later used those experiences when going on to work in helping professions, some of us had become aware of a counter-intuitive phenomenon. We, who were non-compliant and most resistant to our forced treatment and the denial of our personal agency, were treated the most harshly. Yet if we were not destroyed, we often made the most remarkable long-lasting recoveries and transformations.

Coping with severe psychosocial problems can sharpen the need to develop survival skills. I asked a peer specialist I supervised how she dealt with all the different psychiatrists who she had seen during her many years in the public mental health system. She told me that whenever she had to see her newly assigned psychiatrist, she looked around the office at his pictures and art objects to see if she could identify a particular interest or hobby.

If she saw a picture of a sailboat, she would ask him about boating and strike up a conversation about his hobby. Why? Because she wanted that psychiatrist to recognize and remember her so that she would not be treated like any other widget he would see for ten minutes and offhandedly prescribe drugs without really listening and quickly dismissing her. She knew that the quality of her life was dependent on how well she developed such skills.

A Wu Wei Therapist

The Taoism of 6th century Chinese sage Lao Tzu[9] emphasized the importance of non-action, non-resistance, "going with the flow" as essential to living an elevated and transformative life. He described Wu Wei as non-doing or doing nothing. It is a gentle invitation to relax. This concept is key to the noblest kind of action according to the philosophy and practice of Taoism. It is at the heart of what it means to follow Tao or The Way. More than forty years ago I began studying with a Tai Chi grandmaster who helped me evolve as a therapist and a person.

Psychotherapy can be transformative when both client and therapist join in a quest to learn from each other while each is grounded in a relationship of trust and mutual respect. Each owns, shares and is responsible for communicating their respective areas of knowledge and wisdom along with their deficiencies. Unlike the reliance on forcing a client into the procrustean bed of *diagnosis* at the cost of intuition and insight, the practice of Wu Wei expounds the virtue of *No Force*. One joins with the other's energy and gently moves her/him in a more mutually positive direction.

A similarity to Wu Wei can be seen in how psychologist Mihaly Csikszentmihalyi theorizes about Flow.[10] When you are in flow, you enter a form of high functioning effortless attention. Flow is believed to thrive when goals are clear—feedback is immediate, and a balance exists between opportunity and capability. I believe that psychotherapy thrives when the emptiness of Wu Wei is present.

I am not suggesting that there is no need to acquire knowledge, learn different psychological theories, and the securing of a university education, degrees, and licenses. Rather I am attributing value to the model of Wu Wei. A Taoist or Tai Chi student learns to practice a discipline's fixed forms until they are mastered, and then they learn to trust their non-conscious integration of what they have developed. To a flow theorist, this might be the over-learning that is necessary for the emergence of Flow. When you become truly proficient and have genuinely integrated all past training, you are able to respond to unfolding contingencies without relying on the rote dredging up of practiced techniques.

Conclusion

The analytical critical mind revels in its aptitude for constructing questions. I may never find the answers, but I am glad that I can continue searching. When I examine what I choose to call my transformation rather than my recovery, I find it extremely difficult to separate and prioritize the significant factors. Even attempts to classify into broad categories, like external/internal, seem contrived and artificial.

The importance of a spiritual, mystical, karmic, or divine intervention in the change process is a major component of many of the world's healing traditions. Even devoted practitioners of modern medicine are reluctant to completely shut their minds and hearts to miracles of faith and healing when privately confronting the mysteries of the mind/soul/spirit. Until it's personal, those unknown spontaneous recoveries from all sorts of ailments can be lumped together by scientists into what may be medicine's name for hope—placebo.

Exercising personal agency—the ability and right to make genuine informed choices—fundamental to one's capacity to overcome adversity and grow. Anthropologist Edward Hall in his book, *Beyond Culture*, emphasized that the failure to fulfill one's potential can be one of the most devastating things to occur to a person. Hall writes that "A kind of gnawing emptiness, longing, frustration, and displaced anger takes over when this occurs. Whether the anger is turned inward on the self or outward toward others, dreadful destruction results."[11]

My ascent from madness to my present state of clarity and self-acceptance was and is a journey whose responsibility always resided within me. However, as I try to describe and share with others what wisdom I acquired to aid others in their work, I acknowledge one element that I do not understand or take credit for—something that is named or interpreted according to one's unique beliefs and values as luck, fate, karma, or God's blessing.

I believe that as long as a person is alive, some seed of hope, some possibility is there waiting to be fertilized. Hope fights the fear, nurtures the courage, and inspires the vision and the work required to resist giving up and accepting that your goals are unattainable. Deep in the recesses of our being there are safe sanctuaries, secure hiding places for never fully lost dreams. But sometimes they are hidden so well that we can no longer reach those parts of ourselves. The help we need may come from expected and unexpected sources.[12]

Accepting the difficult, challenging aspiration to help others has its rewards. Among them is letting go of our own fixed dogmatic beliefs in favor of choosing to accumulate and integrate our own experience-based wisdom—working with and embracing the *mystery*.

References

[1] J.W. Perry, *The Far Side of Madness*. (Prentice Hall, 1974).

[2] P. Kapleau, *The Three Pillars of Zen* (Anchor books, 1980).

[3] E. F. Schumacher, *A Guide for the Perplexed* (New York: Harper and Row, 1977).

[4] Merton, *The Seven Story Mountain* (New York: Harcourt Brace, 1948

[5] Havelock Ellis, "Impressions and Comments," *Random House Webster's Quotationary*, ed. Leonard Roy Frank (New York: Random House, 1998) 105.

[6] Adam Miller, "Psycho Theory on Birth of Jazz," *New York Post*, 11 July 2001: 29.

[7] J. Frank & Julia Frank, *Persuasion and Healing: A Comparative Study of Psychotherapy.* (March,1993 Johns Hopkins University Press).

[8] Lila Watson, https://www.azquotes.com/author/26097-Lilla_Watson

[9] Ursula K. Le Guin, *Lao Tzu, Tao Te Ching: A Book About the Way and the Power of the Way* (Shambala, Boulder, 1997).

[10] M. Csikszentmihalyi, *Flow: The Psychology of Optimal Experience* (Harper Perennial Modern Classics, 1990).

[11] E. Hall, *Beyond Culture (Garden City, NY: Anchor Press, 1976*

[12] R. Bassman, *A Fight to Be: A Psychologist's Experience From Both Sides of the Locked Door* (Tantamount Press, 2007).

Time Statues: Alternatives to Harm

Robert F. Morgan

Abstract: *Revisiting cases in California and Hawaii using behavioral prescriptions, contact groups, existential purpose as suicide prevention, David Cheek's hypnosis method, visualizations, and anger reductions. Experiential successes based on insight, education, almost six decades of practice, more than eight decades of lifespan, and considerable luck.*

1) Saying Nothing

Do not go gentle into that good night,
Old age should burn and rave at close of day;
Rage, rage against the dying of the light.
    – Dylan Thomas

Leon was a psychiatrist at San Francisco's Center for Special Problems (CSP). He wasn't viewed as belonging to the group of psychiatrists working there. Instead, he was a member of the group of individuals that belonged to no group (mathematicians' paradox).

Not particularly friendly, this elder man with the trim goatee radiated individuality. That was exemplified by his staunch refusal to ever prescribe damaging psychiatric medications. His prescription pad might otherwise contain a behavioral prescription (*"Buy her flowers and apologize"*) or important notes to himself (*"Fishing with grandson this Saturday: Bring treats"*). Staff usually just left Leon alone.

So naturally, we became friends. I slouched past his office one morning, feeling the weight of my five part time jobs. And the struggles of the patients there at the clinic, plus my own. Leon yelled: "Hey Atlas! Put the earth down and rest for a while." Strange, maybe. But that memory always helped me do just that. Sometimes there *is* a perfect thing to say.

In the 1970s the city was overloaded with special problems, known also as unique individuals. Governor Ronald Reagan had closed major state mental hospitals—hospitals that were unhelpful at best, but failed to pass the financial savings on to us at the community clinics. Many liberated mental patients expanded the homeless ranks in the streets. Some kept from starving by getting arrested. One tried to take a shower in one of our clinic urinals. Many walking along in busy tourist areas were continuing loud conversations with themselves. (If only we had fake cell phones to give them back then, nobody would have noticed.)

Many of these newly lost people on the streets just, actively or passively, took the option of leaving their life. In the mornings, the sidewalk in front of a nearby McDonalds was a favorite spot where their remains would be found. Center for Special Problems staff were often regarded in more traditional mental health centers as special problems in their own right—creative, effective, famous pioneers, and very hard to categorize.

They included pioneers like lesbian couple Phyllis Lyon and Dell Martin, lesbian mother of four (and future Police Commissioner) Pat Norman, bisexuality advocate Maggie Rubenstein, and a vocal raft of gay male psychiatrists. (In a staff meeting, one social worker complained that the gay psychiatrists did most of the talking, to which one replied "And rightly so!")

A social worker named Ron, whose last name I don't recall, was a leader in a successful movement to remove homosexuality as a "disease" diagnosis from the psychiatric DSM manual. I joined in by publishing an article suggesting that if any non-normative sexuality was going to be considered a disease, then celibacy needed to be added and numbered in the DSM diagnostic categories. Ron's next target to remove stigma from the Gay community was the Vatican. Success? Well, not yet.

CSP took on clients the regular centers preferred not to see, even in San Francisco: the newly homeless delusional or suicidal refugees from the defunct mental hospitals, addicts, sexual lifestyle pioneers, and even much sought felons. And while the five other county centers left their empty offices to do community outreach, or traditional medical intervention, our

CSP was the one that still gave face-to-face psychotherapy to the city's citizens.

Leon's reputation rested more than anything else on his evening *contact groups* with self-selected suicidal walk-ins. A contact group was a gathering of people without cost, record, or paper. Even today, the option of walk-in clients—right from the street, including many unable to pay—is a viable form of prevention. Staff sign up voluntarily, usually in the evenings, to lead a group on a specific category of client or problem. This is advertised. Groups are solution-focused.

In fact, CSP was proud to be the last such center in the country to give clients this option to be undigitized. Today, some record keeping is universally required but as a community intervention, that might be minimal.

CSP Director Gene Turrell, formerly with Kinsey's group, specialized in transforming felons wanted by the law to a more peaceful health, including killers, with belief that doing so in absolute confidence, he was saving more victims. Without that, they naturally would not come in. When law officers sat in his office demanding information on any of these, Gene, a chain smoker, would shut his office door and then fill the room with smoke. (Gene looked like Lurch from the Addams family and wore size 18 shoes; law would retreat without what they came for, smoke blown up their visit.)

Leon let me sit in one night with his contact group. One of the 13 people there said: "I have nothing to live for!" Leon: "Yes! That's your reason." Some were confused, other contact group regulars smiled. Leon went on to explain that finding your individual purpose in existing on this earth was the most important thing you can do. "Start looking" he said. Then others reported their progress. Yes, Leon was very existential in his specific approach to a contact group. It worked.

Our staff gathering place was Ernie's, a Chinese restaurant on Polk Street and a block from work. One day I walked in to see something I had never seen before. Leon sat quietly alone at a corner table with tears streaming down his cheeks. A waitress we knew whispered: "His grandson had an accident at school and died yesterday. Very sad." Leon's grandson was the happiest part of his days. Whenever he spoke of him, he would transform into smiles. Clearly, his grandson was Leon's purpose in living. And now...

I sat next to Leon. He acknowledged me with a nod but said nothing. Whatever could I say to this good man that would help him through this trauma? I could think of nothing. So, I just put my hand on his forearm and sat with him in silence. Leon eventually pushed his untouched plate of food away. He quietly said, "Thank you Atlas. I appreciated that."

He left the restaurant and wasn't seen at work for a few weeks. When he returned, his contact groups re-commenced. Leon seemed to have found there another purpose for his existence. And I had learned this: *When you can think of nothing helpful to say, nothing is what to say.*

Note: Leon's actual name was Leonard Miller, M.D. and we miss him.

2) Anger: Three Cases

Years ago, I was a flatlander new to the mountain country of Northern California. As a psychologist in a region with no other psychologists, my work had the range of a country doctor. Time after time I was confronted with new challenges in this practice, some outside my experience and expertise.

Knowing that most of my patients felt that leaving their home territory for a city referral was like falling off the edge of the earth, I acknowledged that whatever I could contribute was likely the best they could get. I learned a lot and was more helpful than I had anticipated. (In fairness, some outlaws did go far enough down-altitude to raid stores in the Chico area.)

Case #1

Let's call him "Range." He was tall, wide, young, and intense—obviously suppressing some rage and sat facing me, scowling. Range said his wife had referred him to me for his uncontrollable violent anger. He was always attacking people for the slightest reason. Just the day before, he had told her that he was going to beat up her hospital surgeon. That's when she insisted he come see me first. And here he was.

It wasn't hard to relax Range. First, I acknowledged that he looked angry. He agreed and stopped looking that way, interested in the conversation now. In a few minutes, he was smiling. He had asked me before we began if I was married and if I loved my wife. After my two yes answers, he unclenched his fists and said that he was ready to begin the session.

I asked him why he wanted to attack his wife's surgeon. Range explained that he loved his wife so overwhelmingly that he just wanted to protect her. She was a little overweight and he felt he had to fight anybody who hurt her feelings about that. The surgeon had given her a diagnostic spinal tap—no problem found—which then caused her continuing pain. The surgeon just told her that she had to live with hurt and not whine about it all the time. Clearly, he had decided that this doctor needed a bloody nose consequence.

As an expert in fighting iatrogenic malpractice (i.e., medical mistakes), I understood his feelings fully. It was important though to help him learn to fight back in a less destructive way to himself and his wife—a goal too often skipped by therapists. We focused on the consequences, following visualizations of that intended fight. Visualizing an attack actually reduced the anger and added control. Nobody ever gets arrested for a private thought (so far).

He liked the technique. We tried it on me as the target. By then the relationship between us had become friendly, and even a mental vision of an attack on me was hard for him to do. He settled for imagining a pie in my face and we both laughed.

Now he came in for a few more once-a-week sessions, glad to share his control. But he still had lots of suppressed rage he carried with him. He asked me why. This was his real goal for therapy: to understand himself. I agreed as it also would give him even more control.

I'm not much of a follower of Freudian doctrine other than saluting him as an essential ancient pioneer for our profession. Most helpful though for me was the emphasis on a problem's origin. "When did this first begin?" and "What was going on then?" are often useful questions. The emotions felt then and now of course.

Range learned to relax in the chair, shut his eyes, and visualize the answer. That took him back to a time in his early years when his mother remarried. The stepfather often beat him as a child. It stopped, as it often does, when Range had grown as big as his stepfather. But the child's rage was still ever with him. Also, the violent model he had learned from his oppressive stepfather.

On reflection, no, he didn't want to be like him. Well, not like the way his violent stepfather had been before. What has changed now?

Oh, he said, they go fishing together at least once a week. They get along okay then.

Has he ever apologized? No.

Did you ever bring the beatings up when you were fishing? Remind him? No.

I suggested he might do that next time they were off fishing together. Range grinned and said he liked the idea. (If I had this to do again, with Range's approval, I would have arranged for the stepfather to come into a session with Range to accomplish this. Hindsight is not always helpful, coming as late as the word sounds, sometimes direct from the hind quarters of our anatomy. Meaning — I was wrong.)

Range entered our next session limping. He had a black eye, cuts, bruises, and a bandage on his forehead. But he was ecstatic. He said he had reminded his stepfather of all that childhood abuse. He said the old boy had put up quite a fight but, in the end, Range won the struggle. The stepfather apologized on his way to the hospital. He recovered a few days later — no more fishing dates though.

On our last session, Range brought his wife. They both agreed that Range was civilized now — said they had never been happier. I didn't ask about the stepfather's opinion.

Case #2

He was a high-ranking law enforcer from another rural county. Let's call him "Shane." Personable and wearing a cowboy hat (no cattle), he sat easily in the guest chair. He said he had come once before to my clinic, but my associate had not impressed him.

That other person doing counseling had no academic credentials beyond a college degree or any psychotherapy training but was a relentlessly nice person. This partner had to do before I got there. After that, it left him more time for his hobby: constructing. Back to Shane.

Shane took off his hat, smiled, and said he had heard about me being helpful to many and, besides, able to keep confidences. Still, psychologists' clients have not the absolute confidentiality enjoyed by lawyers and clergy. I showed him the printed exceptions of state law, including (1) convincing dangerousness to self or others, and (2) convincing confession of serious crime.

(I once counseled an elderly woman who in retirement had pulled off some impressive department store shoplifting as a hobby. Never caught. Yet. And this made *her* happy. Seemed to be seeing me to brag in confidence. We did find an even happier hobby that was without risk of her arrest.)

Shane considered these exceptions carefully, glancing at me several times and rereading the exceptions on the paper. Finally, he carefully phrased the following: "I'm here to see you to help me with my sadness. Losing sleep over it. It's a very cold case. Many years ago a man was killed in a late night fight behind a bar. About then I joined the law but I never caught the killer. I still feel guilty about that. Maybe you can help me shed that guilt."

Shane handed me back the confidentiality exceptions paper—raised an eyebrow to see if I understood. I considered. Seemed like he was the killer he wanted to discuss, but there was no evidence for this to justify any legal intervention. Onward then.

I said I would help him. I had Shane sit back, shut his eyes, and go into a light trance for visualization. The David Cheek hyponosis method was used. (See more on this method at the end of this chapter.) I asked him to imagine he was in the mind of the killer. This he did, signaling he was there.

So I asked him the key question: "Will he ever kill again, then or now?" A vehement no. My relief.

"So exactly what happened the night of the crime. Let him tell us."

Shane described a late night when, leaving the bar at the back, a larger man demanded his money. Rage overcame him, plus maybe he had drunk too much. The rest was unclear. He just remembered standing over the body and then disappearing into the night. He was confused, frightened.

Shane woke up at that point, sitting tall in his chair. He said that was all he could get from this memory. Except that when the body was fouind the next day, this was to be his first case. But no witnesses, never solved. Haunted him still.

Shane came back for his weekly sessions. By the second month he had grown quite adept at describing the thoughts and feelings of his quarry, a man much like himself. Maybe exactly like himself.

He went on to speak in his imagination with the victim. Who in the end forgave the killer. Shane shared his own just and successful law career over the years. Raised a family and became a valued neighbor. He explored the consequences if his killer just confessed the crime. Imagined several different paths.

In the end, he shared that his nightmares had gone away and a blanket of peace slipped over him each night. He said that maybe the killer would confess to law some day but that decision could wait. The probable killer coming out with everything in our sessions had given Shane relief. Time to live in the present.

Our last session.

As to the killer in his mind—he was gone now. His rage had never come back, and he never drank again after that incident. No, Shane said, nor had he himself. He thought the killer might some day want to connect again in his imagination. Maybe at night when he slept.

I asked him how he would react. He said he had already imagined this. The killer would say "Shane! Come back Shane!" But he would just ride off into the horizon, into the decent life where he belonged.

Case #3

This last case takes us to Hawaii in the mid-1960s where I was doing my post-doc internship at the Hawaii State Hospital. My supervisor acknowledged my success so far with adult patients and with my adolescent day program (a therapeutic community for 30 teens) that had never had an unfortunate incident in its yearlong history.

So he said I needed some humility, a failure experience. He assigned me to what he termed a psychotic paranoid patient who would never recover. He was big, Japanese-American and considered dangerous. Scowling as he entered my office, he looked like Toshiro Mifune, the iconic screen samurai. Though we were both only in our 20s. So we'll call him "Tosh."

Tosh had returned to his family after being thrown out of the Marines. Shameful for them already. But then he began to listen for hours to Japanese radio stations. Strange because he knew no Japanese language. He insisted they were talking about him and were truly insulting. Rage built up by the day until he went down to the station and attacked the staff.

At first the police, following a judge's order, just brought him home to await his trial. That didn't last long. A few more rage issues and he was committed to the state mental hospital. Involuntarily in a strait jacket. It took six orderlies. In front of neigjhbors. Overwhelming shame. Loss of face came to any Japanese-American family there and then that included a "crazy" member. So most did all they could to keep their own out of sight and away from the state mental hospital. This meant that fewer ethnic Japanese-American patients inhabited the state hospital, but those that were there were so out-of-control that the families had given up.

Tosh had heard from other patients that my office was a safe place, so he was curious but cautious—suppressing hs obvious anger. The hidden fear below this anger remaining to be discovered. After some small talk, he chose to explain his view. Everybody in the world was out to get him. Or, the few exceptions—maybe me—were just foolishly unaware of that reality. Tosh then took it upon himself to instruct me about this conspiracy that was all around us. I listened carefully and with respect. At the core of every paranoid fantasy was a personal reality. One we needed to find.

Clearly, his view of himself as bravely standing aginst an entire world on his own, well, it functioned as a shield against his sad temporary reality. We shared some light food which also helped Tosh relax. I answered his questions about me and my life to date. This included my honest response that I didn't agree with his conviction that all the world was against him. Instead, I told him that likely he had definitely been wronged at points in his past. This candor built trust as we now agreed to disagree about the nature of his delusion. He said he looked forward to more meetings. And better food next time.

Our second session, with appetizers more to his taste, went better. He now wanted very much to explain to me how he been wronged, what had brought him to this day in the hospital. First, though, he wanted some help in controlling his rage. One doctor had wanted him lobotomized, another favored eletroconvulsive therapy. Clearly, he wanted to avoid these things. If he hurt one more orderly, he would be punished with destructive interventions. He had read about all these "treatments."

I was impressed. There was, in fact, a very good mind hiding in the paranoia. We went through breathing exercises and visualization techniques for more control of his anger. Fight rather than flight had been his remedy. Or maybe both combined. Tosh excelled at these methods, even allowing himself a smile when done. He knew he was a quick study, which I confirmed. Again I was impressed. For him, his success in my office was a minor windfall in the midst of great disaster.

By the remainder of that session and into the next, he shared his life to that point. He labeled this narrative variously as being in "Deep Kimchi" or "Up the Yinyang." Tosh shared an early memory. He was a toddler sitting under a tree when a falling coconut smashed into his young head—a serious potentially lethal hazard, likely a concussion. But when he regained consciousness, his older sisters were there laughing at him. His scalp was full of blood and they thought it was hilarious. It still hurt his head to remember.

Now we were getting to the core of his paranoid universe—the actual world that *was* against him: his family when he was a child. Worse was life growing up with his father. Since his father spoke no English and Tosh didn't understand Japanese, there was literally no communication. Father did do much harsh discipline to his son, though Tosh never knew why. His mother would not help him. Nor his sisters.

Now his actual world was coming into focus. His childhood must have seemed the whole universe to him.—an unjust world demanding he project some meaning into it. He did well in school. He became strong and athletic, and he loved reading. On graduating high school, he joined the Marines, something that he thought might impress his family. Marine basic training is meant to collapse a recruit's personality and rebuild it as a warrior. This occurs by pushing their physical and mental limits to beyond what they can stand.

Tosh, vulnerable to begin with, had an extra problem. His trainers thought he was an American Indian. They called him "blanket-back." Tosh didn't let them know any different for a very good reason. His trainers had served in WW2, in the war against Japan, just two decades before. They remembered Pearl Harbor. Japanese-American trainees would get a whole extra layer of destruction if they were discovered.

Tosh was discovered. He was once more in an unjust world. He fought back. Hard. Dishonorable discharge. Home to his family in Hawaii. There he began listening to those Japanese language radio stations, delusionally thinking he understood what they were saying.

I asked Tosh in our session what he thought they were saying. In this way we could understand the fear underlying his violent anger. They were announcing to the world that he was a "Mahu," which means effeminate or a homosexual. This in 1960s Hawaii, especially to his family and the Japanese-American community, was a blood insult. It was seen as a perversion, either predatory or to be laughed at.

Tosh had used his rage to prove them wrong with violence. That's when he went to one of the radio stations to attack the station manager and DJ—he did the same at the other Japanese language station before the police caught up to him. Charges included several of the hospitalized officers who had trouble arresting him. A psychiatrist had him certified insane so he was transferred to the state mental hospital for an indeterminate time. Possibly for life. Tosh had finished his story. He was calm while in my office and had a request—could he help me with my work?

I was collecting library material on shock treatment's damaging side effects which eventually became a book *Electroshock: The Case Against*. But at that early stage, the task was to gather the science. I did a study comparing patients who had been given ECT with similar ones who had not.

ECT survivors had damaged memories of two kinds. They forgot key parts of their life, sometimes including people they loved. They also forget new information, meaning it was hard to learn. Nor did ECT do any lasting good for their diagnostic condition, even in one case with a violent patient who received 300 shocks (and was still violent). There was a near perfect correlation between when a patient hit a staff memnber and that patient next receiving ECT. A punishment? Clearly so.

Tosh had been threatened with ECT and really wanted to avoid it. So he gladly became my research assistant and haunted the hospital library for material. Now he had a purpose and improved substantially. He had accepted that the reality core for his paranoia was in his own personal world, not in the earth's entire human population. He got very good at understanding his anger and channeling it in an effective but legal manner.

Plus, he really was helpful to my work. So much so that I was able to persuade the staff of my unit to close down any ECT. Our psychiatrist-in-charge had not been there for an extended period of months. On his return he went along, reluctantly, with the ECT ban, though it truly was the only psychiatry he knew how to do. Let's just say that he was far from happy with me.

Tosh eventually had improved so much that I got him discharged to leave the hospital, a "conditional discharge" which allowed him to return once a week so he could continiue our weekly meetings as he worked on assimilating to the community. He enrolled in a university counseling degree program while living in the dormitory there. He managed some decent interactions with his sisters, now also in their own adult lives. Tosh was doing fine.

My supervisor conceded that I had failed to receive sufficient humility. I assured him that I already had more than enough failures in life for humility and expected some valuable learning from much more in the future. I still think he had been rooting for Tosh to get better all along, hence his humility challenge.

One of my own supervisees, intern Jerry Shapiro, made sure I had a humility experience before I left. In my turn to demonstrate psychotherapy with a volunteer patient in front of staff and interns, Jerry chose for me a lobotomized patient. (Volunteer?) Nothing useful came of this demo. Well, maybe some humility.

One week later, Tosh came in for his weekly meeting looking really stressed. He said: "Doc you won't believe this. But on the bus on the way here today some girls were laughing at me. I did NOT imagine this!"

What did he do about it?

"I just waited to tell you about it. I ignored the girls completely."

Feelings at the time?

"I couldn't wait to tell you. I was afraid that I was getting sick again. And I was, well, proud that I didn't get angry. Right?"

"Exactly. You should be proud. Now you can choose what to do with hurt or fear. Still, knowing why they laughed can help. Let's shine a light on it.

Because, you know, I get why they laughed. Look at your tee shirt and shorts."

He did. His shirt and shorts were borrowed from a roommate in the dorm. Both too small, the tee and shorts had Mickey Mouse on them, somewhat incongruous on a powerful samurai-looking man. Tosh looked, considered, and broke out in a loud laugh. He got it. And that laugh meant to me that he was really back to normal.

In another week's meeting, I asked him if there was anything in his recovery that stood out for him. He did have something he wanted to highlight:

> Doc, early on I asked you what I could possbily do when the whole world just gives me a pile of shit! You said "plant flowers." I think you might have been joking but I used that many times as a ladder to climb out into the sunshine, the fresh air smelling of flowers in our Hawaii.

We had our last outpatient meeting as I was on my way to a new job outside Hawaii. I gave Tosh my contact information so he could stay in touch, do follow-ups, and let me know if he needed any other consultation. He returned to his studies.

With me gone, that psychiatrist-in-charge of the unit brought back into the ward his only tool: ECT. He systematically gave shock treatments to as many of my remaining former patients as he could. He had held up Tosh's full discharge long enough to call him back in. There he forced Tosh to undergo a series of three shock treatments. He knew that Tosh would particularly suffer as now he had become an expert on the destructive risks of ECT. Tosh knew it was punitive. As did the shock dotor. Had I still been there, my own anger might well have gone violent. My visualizations worked overtime. I redoubled my anti-ECT work.

Tosh could have reverted to paranoia as this unfair world of punishing involuntary ECT was familiar. But instead he contacted me by phone. I got his discharge to be final through my hospital network, but the damage was done. Tosh had nearly completed his coursework but there were still tests to pass. Now his memory for newly learned material was impaired. So he drew on library resources again. Used memory devices to get him through. Each morning he reviewed his written notes from the day before to restore the memories. He passed his exams.

Tosh moved to another state and took a job as a counselor there. Every Christmas for ten years, Tosh would send me a present with a note of thanks. I knew not to respond with more than a return thank you card. In the culture he grew up in, he was paying what he saw as a necessary debt. On the tenth year I called him long distance at his office. We caught up on life. He finally asked if his gifts were enough. I confirmed that was so. Debt paid.

Tosh continued his work despite the memory challenges and must have helped thousands before he retired back to Hawaii before the 20th century's close. He departed life five years into our 21st century—and a full life it was after all.

3) Trust

Trust is essential for any relationship to survive. Children need trustworthy parents, good marriages require trustworthy partners, employees deserve trustworthy administrators. Effective police departments must earn the trust of their community. Trust is especially important, sometimes life or death, for a doctor's patient. Magnified when the patient is a child.

Dr. David Cheek was just beginning to be recognized as a master hypnotist in 1972. One of my graduate students, Gene Orro, gave me Cheek's phone number and recommended I hire him for a hypnosis workshop. I had already decided that the field of psychology's first free-standing school of professional psychology should offer hypnosis as a first-year core skills class. So, I called.

He had a San Francisco gynecology and obstetrics practice not far from us. He had already made a mark with his respectful client-centered hypnosis approach. Automatic consent or dissent signals from designated fingers for every step. He agreed to do an all-day workshop, so we set a time and date. But he refused to take any pay. He said we were new, just getting started—

and, besides, he was happy to train psychologists in his approach. Medical doctors were uninterested so far, though nurses and dentists were on board.

I told him I would be there at the workshop along with my students. As it was a very large group, I suggested he ask for me before the workshop to sign some papers. Though I was the Dean, I was the same age as my students and, being in San Francisco, dressed the same. I started to describe myself, but he declined since he would know which one I was soon enough.

We assembled for the workshop and waited. Just at the exact time it was supposed to begin, Dr. Cheek, confident in a three-piece suit, walked in. With a friendly smile, he said it was time to begin—said he would catch the Dean at the break. He arranged for us to stand in a large circle, maybe two dozen of us. He had brought enough pencils for each of us to hold one at arm's length. Then he had us, now with finger signing permission, go into a light trance. Eyes shut. We were told that we would know when this autohypnosis was ready by realizing that the pencil had fallen to the floor.

When we were asked to open our eyes, all the pencils were down. Except mine. I was still holding it in my outstretched arm. David walked up to me and said, "Nice to meet you, Robert. So, you're the Dean." (David later told me that I had dropped my pencil at the same time as everybody else, but I had bent down and picked it back up. I had no memory of doing this, so the trance had worked.)

In the workshop afternoon, David divided us into pairs. Each would take turns standing straight and then falling backwards so as to be caught by the partner. This was called a trust exercise. I caught my partner easily. But I could not (with psychologists that meant "would not") fall backwards. With any partner. Therefore, David chose to use me to demonstrate his trauma resolution technique.

He usually did this early trauma memory recovery hypnosis for his female patients, going as far back as needed, even to birth or the trimester before. For me, I only went as far as age three. This was the trauma time statue I revisited that day with David:

I was on my way to the hospital to have my tonsils removed. Fix my sore throat. This was okay because I had been raised and praised for being tough in such situations. And I trusted these giants called doctors. They would make me well, just fine.

Then I was in a hospital bed, ready. In walked these giants (to me) in white coats. The one in front said "Hello Bobby. We are going to take you now to have a nice ice cream cone. For your sore throat. Isn't that nice?"

I hadn't expected this, but sure! They put me on top of something with wheels and rolled me into a dimly lit room. Lifted me onto a table and strapped me down. No ice cream in sight. Put a mask over my face that began hissing. I couldn't speak and they couldn't hear me.

They had LIED to me. I was good at following what a doctor told me. Pain didn't slow me down. Why the ice cream lie? Doctors weren't supposed to lie to children, to me! I got really angry.

I figured out that the hissing mask was supposed to put me to sleep. So I fought it. I still was awake and glaring. They gave me more hissing in the mask. Still awake, eyes open. More hissing.

At some point. I finally passed out. When I woke, my mother was there looking worried. Said I had been asleep for three days. Too much hissing in the mask. Said finally now I could go home. Still no ice cream.

David's intervention was helpful to me, though not 100%. I had, after age three, been damaged eventually in various falls and was still cautious about falling. I, as an adult, knew by then that not every doctor or every other person we meet in life could be trusted. More honor to those who could be.

Bringing this trauma to light though may have explained many things still true in my life. My lifelong work of preventing iatrogenic practice, the doctor's mistakes, may be an outcome—seeking the end of the demonstrably destructive electroconvulsive shock treatment as a prime example. My books along these lines surfaced between 1982 and 2005 with more to come. They should have given me that ice cream cone.

David Cheek's workshop was a big success. The students used self-hypnosis regularly. Overcoming test anxiety, fulfilling skills, speed reading. Research, and many other fresh creative applications. On graduating, they could apply the Cheek method to their practice, for the great benefit of their patients. Today, it's prevalent for hypnotists everywhere.

They also told me that, as the years rolled by, David never raised his $10 an hour fee for them. His methods saved many lives and restored a future to many more. Most central to trust was his Rogerian approach to client permission.

In response to therapist questions, each client did a split second self-induced light trance, allowing separate fingers to signal seemingly independent responses of *yes, no,* or *don't want to say.* These *ideomotor* responses allowed negotiation to a point for a client—ready at a very deep subconscious level—to begin (Cheek, 1993).

Clients were often surprised at their own reflexive but honest finger signals. But, without exception, they appreciated the respect shown to them through this process. Since David's office was close to my work, many secretarial staff were his patients. You could tell by their twitching fingers which let me know agreement or the opposite independent of what was said.

Cheek and I became close friends. It was not the case that he would join me in the 21st century. He remains a heroic time statue in the 20th.

References and Suggested Readings

Cheek, D. B. (1968). *Clinical hypnotherapy.* New York: Grune & Stratton.

Cheek, D.B. (1993). *Hypnosis: the application of ideomotor techniques.* New York: Allyn & Bacon.

Cheek, D. B. & L. LeCron (1968). *Clinical hypnotherapy.* New York: Grune & Stratton.

Morgan, R.F. (1975). Revising the Diagnostic & Statistical Manual (DSM-II, DSM-III) of Mental Disorders by adding iatrogenic categories and recognizing celibacy as sexual deviation. *Journal of Irreproducible Results,* 21(2), 31.

Morgan, R.F. (1982, 2005). *The Iatrogenics Handbook: A Critical Look at Research & Practice in Helping Professions.* Toronto: Morgan Foundation.

Morgan, R.F. (1999). *Electroshock: the Case Against.* (With Peter Breggin, Leonard Frank, John Friedberg, Bertram Karon, Berton Roueche) Albuquerque, NM: Morgan Foundation. (Chapter IV reprinted in Brent Slife's *Taking Sides: Psychological Issues, 13th edition,* Guilford, CT: McGraw-Hill/Dushkin, 2004 and in Richard P. Halgin's *Taking Sides: Abnormal Psychology, 2nd edition,* Guilford, CT: McGraw-Hill/Dushkin, 2002. (First edition: *Electric Shock.* Toronto: IPI Publications, 1985.)

Morgan, R.F. (2012). *Trauma Psychology in Context: International Vignettes and Applications from a Lifespan Clinical-Community Psychology Perspective.* Santa Cruz, CA: Morgan Foundation.

*Morgan, R.F. (2023a). *Time Statues Revisited*: A five book series *"On the Job", "Language & Influence", "Citizenship", "Nonhuman Relatives", "Human Family".* Albuquerque, NM: Morgan Foundation.

*Morgan, R.F. (2023b). *Future Time Statues: Then and Next.* Albuquerque, NM: Morgan Foundation.

Neimeyer, R.A. (Ed.) (2012). *Techniques of Grief Therapy: Creative Practices for Counseling the Bereaved.* London/New York: Taylor & Francis/Routledge. Chapters by R.F. Morgan: "Anticipatory grief through visualization technique: the shaking artist", "Intuitive humor", "Treating traumatic bereavement in conflicted and intergenerational families", "Group treatment of anticipatory grief in senior pseudo-psychosis".

*Selected segments for this chapter have been adapted or adopted with permission.

Can We Move Toward Mindful Medicine?

Natalie Campo

Abstract: *Mad in America's Madison Natarajan interviews Natalie Campo about integrative psychiatry and holistic approaches to drug tapering and withdrawal. In this interview, she discusses her journey through conventional psychiatric training to holistic and integrative approaches and her experiences helping people taper off psychiatric medications.*

Author's Note: A version of this chapter was first published by Mad in America on October 14, 2020. The transcript below has been edited for length and clarity.

Madison Natarajan: To start us off, could you just tell us a bit about your background, such as where you grew up and how you decided to go into medicine?

Natalie Campo: I grew up in a small Midwestern town. My dad traveled internationally for work. He sometimes brought back small gifts, and he always shared stories of his travels. I became interested in cultures outside of the one I was growing up in. Once on my own, I traveled internationally whenever I could afford it.

During my fourth year of medical school, having finished my required rotations, I spent a month traveling in India and another in France. At a young age, I had decided to go into medicine long before I had any of my own travel experiences. But when I think back, many of my international hosts happened to be physicians willing to share their homes and experiences with me.

Natarajan: So, these experiences abroad with different cultures really informed your interest in wanting to go into medicine. What led you to become interested in the subject of psychiatry?

Campo: I had this desire to learn about perspectives outside of my own. It also arose in part out of certain travel experience. In between my first and second years of medical school, I went to the Amazon jungle to study a viral encephalitis (inflammation of the brain) caused by a specific virus.

I was interested in the work, but I was really motivated to apply for the grant because I wanted to see Peru. I joined some students from Johns Hopkins and helped out with their study tracking the infectious spread of another disease. The time in the jungle was transformative for me. I left Peru knowing that I wanted to study the brain and the mind. I don't think I could have articulated it at the time, but I had a felt sense of the interconnectedness of life while I was in the jungle.

Natarajan: It sounds like that really broadened your perspective to see things a bit more holistically, which led you to think more about psychiatry.

Campo: It did. That experience was so much more important than I could have ever known because I was nearing my clinical years—years in which many medical students lose empathy. Medical students going into medical school often are more empathetic than the general population, but, unfortunately, we find that as medical students go through their clinical years and move into their residency training programs, they actually have less empathy than people in the general population.

Teaching medical students and residents about resilience led me to these studies on empathy. Empathy is important for resilience. People are more likely to bounce back from the inevitable traumas of life if they have empathy and the ability to see someone else's perspective. But empathy decreases in clinical training. I believe this is partly due to a large number of patients to be seen and how futile some of our tools are at helping those people.

Natarajan: That's really interesting, and I think it brings up an important part of the medical training experience. You often hear people talk about the need for doctors to have a better bedside manner. It's interesting to learn that something occurs during their training experience. Things start to become so clinical that they're not really making those empathetic connections they did initially when they were starting their training.

Campo: I think that the loss of connectedness is so important. Somehow that experience of being in the jungle, surrounded by the trees and animals and having had that felt experience of the interconnectedness, really impacted me in my clinical rotations. In my third and fourth years of medical school, I found myself more interested in the person with the disease than the disease itself. I saw many examples of chronic illnesses that had resulted from failed attempts at coping with emotional distress.

I remember one patient with end-stage liver disease dying because of alcohol use, dying because of an attempt to cope with life. I remember thinking if he had other ways to cope, he wouldn't be dying this painful death, and he probably wouldn't be alone. I saw psychiatry as an opportunity to intervene sooner and offer tools for coping with life's inevitable stressors. I saw it as a hopeful field.

Natarajan: Can you tell us a bit more about your various professional experiences with holistic treatment?

Campo: I need to back up a bit and say how that interest started. I saw holistic treatment work in medical school. I had the opportunity to spend a month working with a physician in private practice where he used integrative medicine. He used conventional medical treatment models and evaluation procedures, and he also used holistic treatment models including acupuncture. He also used lifestyle changes, like nutrition. He was incredibly fascinated and interested in the power of nutrition, and he taught me the skills and understandings of the topic.

Natarajan: In your medical training, were there any parts of it that led you to become skeptical or critical of psychiatry and its research or treatment modalities?

Campo: There were parts of my training that led me to become skeptical. I will also say that I'm incredibly grateful for the training that I had and really believe that the teaching that I received came from the physicians' best intentions.

The skepticism came before I started my psychiatry training. I was still in medical school. I had just come off an elective with a very interesting physician where I learned about nutrition and acupuncture in my fourth year of medical school. The patients that I was seeing with him were happy and healthy and thriving.

Then I took two months where I did two externships. I was really excited because these are my first opportunities to really work as a psychiatric intern even though I wasn't quite ready to go into residency training. But I was also nervous because these were a bit like month-long interviews. I had selected two externships because they were a part of triple-board programs (combined residencies and pediatric psychiatry/child psychiatry).

The first of these externships was at one of the world's most acclaimed psychiatric hospitals. My rotation would include time on an adolescent unit. It was a beautiful campus of trees, and patients spent time outdoors learning mindfulness as part of their therapy. I was impressed. This truly seemed like a thoughtful approach to allow for healing. But once inside, I saw some of these children holding bags of chips and cookies, munching as they desired all day long. Maybe you think that's great—access to familiar comforts—but I was thinking, "We're mindlessly putting toxins into these kids." Most of them were already obese and on medications known to cause metabolic abnormalities and weight gain. And we were encouraging processed food intake.

Maybe I am coming across as a little bit extreme about processed foods. I had recently read a study where students in schools were given simple nutrients, and those students were found to have less violent, aggressive outbursts towards other students. They were given multivitamins and fish oil. This research suggests that nutrients really do change behavior and drive symptoms.

I couldn't help but bring this question to the director of the hospital. And I asked simply, "Can we replace junk food with real food?" His answer was, "I know, and our activities director smokes." It was a frustrating non-answer to my simple, direct question. But looking back, I can see how authentic it really was. He acknowledged that the junk food was addictive and harmful to the body, including the brain, by comparing it to smoking.

But he felt powerless to make changes for the better for his patients. I was critical of that decision, but I also felt powerless and had no authority.

On the same externship, I was working with the physician for one day. Because I was serving the role of an intern (a first-year position in training) even though I was a fourth-year medical student, I was occasionally asked to write medication orders. On this particular day, the plan was for a taper of a medication. Since I had never tapered a medication before, I asked how to do it. The psychiatrist was annoyed by this question and responded, "Just cut it in half, and cut it in half again. It's not rocket science." I remember thinking, "But it *is* brain chemistry."

I made a mental note to learn about medication tapers and not to ask dumb questions. That was about 15 years ago. As you probably know, there is still no consensus on how to taper antidepressants. It's still a good question.

I went into psychiatry training skeptical and critical of conventional practices. I knew going in that I would practice differently. When I was responsible for treatment plans myself, I knew that they would always be integrative, including conventional knowledge and evidence-based holistic modalities and lifestyle changes, especially with real food.

My training experience in psychiatry was unusual because of that intention. While I still learned about SSRIs, I also spent time studying mindfulness-based stress reduction and sitting with Steven Southwick discussing the science of resilience (a pioneer in this field). Because of his generosity of time with me, I was able to create a mindfulness program to help bolster resilience in resident physicians.

I went into my psychiatry residency training skeptical of conventional medical practices, determined to learn what I could about psychopharmacology, and then to go beyond that and to think about ways to thrive and heal.

Natarajan: How often would you say clients are coming to you after being on antidepressants for extended amounts of time and are interested in getting off them?

Campo: This does happen. People call requesting consultations for assistance coming off of medications. It probably happens a few times a month. I think I've noticed it more as public awareness has grown about how difficult it can be, thanks to people doing work like you're doing to help bring that to public awareness. Public awareness has grown around how coming off of these medications can be very difficult as conventional consensus on how to taper these medications has stalled.

Natarajan: Since there is no standard consensus on the best way to do this, I'm wondering what your personal guidelines are for when and how to prescribe psychiatric drugs to clients. Do you typically engage in conversations about side effects and long-term use?

Campo: My guidelines for prescribing pharmaceuticals are really my guidelines for the way that I work in general. The integrative approach is always collaborative. I'm only bringing knowledge of certain modalities, including medication, but it's really the patient who's bringing the questions, the intentions for the treatment, the distress, the life experiences. It is only through that partnership that we can create an effective treatment plan at all.

To answer your question, when I'm thinking about prescribing pharmaceuticals, I'm always discussing alternatives. I'm always thinking about risks and benefits because medications can have so many implications and many unknown risks. I will often discuss medication with a person as a last resort, but not always. I do find them to be helpful tools.

I will often include a partner or a family member in the discussion of a medication trial. We might even look at a list of common side effects of medication together, but then since the lists are often so long for potential side effects, I will encourage a patient to think about it and read about the medication on their own in between sessions, and then to come back and sit and again and discuss potential alternatives to reassess where they are at in their life at the time, even if it's only a few days or weeks later.

Natarajan: I think there are so many people who have the experience of coming in to meet with a psychiatrist, having a 15-minute conversation, and walking out with a prescription. You do a thorough job of getting a full evaluation of the psychosocial factors impacting this person and empowering the patient to have agency over their own decision around what types of medication they might be on.

New research shows that tapering over the span of months or possibly even years is more successful at preventing withdrawal symptoms than the quick discontinuation of two to four weeks. I'm curious about what your experience has been helping clients taper off their medications.

Campo: My experience with helping clients taper has been as individual as the interactions with the patients themselves. That's really because there's so much more to what we're doing than just tapering a medication or even just starting a medication. I really think of it as such a small part of our plan. Sometimes an incredibly helpful and effective part of our plan, but really such a small part.

It's hard to say with certainty what effects the taper itself has on the patient. But I will say that my experiences with helping people come off medications have taught me to go as slowly as we can. It's not always that we go slowly, but I agree with you that it's weeks and even months or years for some people, many people.

Oftentimes these medications have been used for a very, very long time. If we want a very effective, smooth taper, it's often most helpful to go as gradually as possible to create as few waves or shifts as possible in the biochemistry or even the person's habits.

Natarajan: Anecdotally, what results do you see when clients come off their medication? What changes do you witness or do your patients report to you?

Campo: These results are also really variable, but I do want to share one example that I remember vividly. This was from years ago, and it's a simple example in some ways because it was just one medication. Maybe this helps to illustrate a point about medication.

This particular patient had been referred to me by an acupuncturist. She was hoping to be able to conceive, and she was taking a benzodiazepine and didn't want to be on the benzodiazepine when she was pregnant. She'd been taking it for 10 years for insomnia. So the acupuncturist called and asked if this was something that I would be interested in helping this patient do.

She wanted to come off before she conceived, and we did a slow taper. She had the time, and she was already doing so many things to support her emotional wellbeing. That is always foundational. If we can do other things to support wellbeing, as we're doing a taper, it's really essential. In fact, I usually don't encourage people to even consider a taper unless life is going really smoothly.

This patient tapered off slowly. It took us a while, but we tapered her off and I can remember the day that she was off completely. She came in, and she stood up. She threw her arms back behind her, and she said, "I'm free!" And I said, "What?" I didn't know what she was talking about.

She said, "I'm free of the medicine. I didn't realize that I wasn't [free]. I didn't realize that it was just helping me to fall to sleep at night; rather, my body actually had become dependent on it. I had needed it. I required it. And I no longer need it!"

It's usually not that dramatic, but that's a fun example of how she felt. She was able to use other ways to care for herself and to allow for sleep at night.

Natarajan: Why do you think psychiatry as a field might be reluctant to confront more of these issues?

Campo: I think that it's actually a bigger issue than just psychiatry confronting it. We really live in a culture where we are interested in quick fixes, and medication can sometimes provide a change—and sometimes a quick change. Sometimes that's very helpful, and I would go so far as to say that sometimes it's essential and even life-preserving—but not always. I think, culturally, we would much prefer a quick fix.

Natarajan: We want to believe that these medications can provide that quick fix. Maybe in an ideal world they could, but it's just not what seems to be happening.

Campo: It doesn't seem to be happening, and it's not sustainable. Even if there is a quick fix because of a state change from a medication, the underlying causes are not being addressed.

If we don't ever address the root causes of depression or anxiety, the healing doesn't happen and it's not sustainable. If we don't ever search, for example, for a vitamin or nutrient deficiency, if we don't see the psychological stressors that a person is dealing with, there's no way. And how can we see that in 10 minutes? We can't.

We can't even get a full picture of the person's life, let alone look for causative agents, and discuss alternatives and risks. We are not allowing physicians time. The systems in place do not allow physicians time to interact with their patients in meaningful ways.

Natarajan: There would really have to be an entire restructuring of the medical field, as opposed to even just pinpointing what psychiatry needs to change. The whole system needs to be reconsidered.

Campo: I do think so. I think, for the most part, when we're thinking about chronic conditions, the answer tends to be more medication because that is a quick answer.

You only have 10 minutes. You really only have time for quick answers. But we have a lot of problems in our society and our culture and now in our world with obesity and insulin resistance, which has led to depression for many people.

Natarajan: You use the word "healing." That the concept of healing is very different than just thinking about symptom reduction. Going back to the question of "What are the root causes?"—and even if we have something that can reduce symptoms—the root causes affecting other areas of people's lives are not being looked at, not being healed. How can you do that in 10 minutes?

Campo: I couldn't agree more. I think that's so well said. I think that there are times when medication might help provide a reprieve or a moment to be able to reflect. But I think that, as a field, we are placing way more hope in medication than it can deliver.

Natarajan: I think it makes sense to look at it from the perspective that perhaps it's less about what's being said, and more about what's not being said. For you to have the time to add these other conversations into your meetings with patients is what could make all the difference and give them a lot more information and agency over their own decision making.

Campo: Absolutely. Mostly the patients that are contacting me are already thinking in that way, and that's why they're contacting me. So that has been a really rewarding experience.

A patient called last week wanting a second opinion. He said that he really liked his psychiatrist that he had been meeting with for years, but he only saw him every six months. He only met with him for ten minutes at a time, and when they met the instructions or the directions were always to either increase his medication or add another one.

The patient said that he was tired of that kind of approach and asked the physician to help him taper. The physician was doing so, but reluctantly. He was hoping for a second opinion, but he had also said that he had been studying on his own and had been starting to eat a real whole food diet and was already feeling so much better. That was really encouraging. It'll be interesting to see how that turns out for him.

Natarajan: Calling yourself an integrative psychiatrist, and the name of your practice, "Mindful Medicine," already kind of brings in a certain type of client. Is it at all professionally difficult or threatening to your career to help people taper from their medication?

Campo: I don't think it's professionally difficult or threatening to help a patient taper from a medication that is causing them harm. It is certainly a different way of practicing, sitting with people for extended lengths of time and thinking through treatment modalities that are outside of conventional treatment plans. For years, it did sort of feel like I was practicing in a very different way, but many people came before me who did this work and whose professional careers were absolutely threatened by the work they were doing.

A very famous example of this is Herbert Benson who studied the relaxation response at Harvard many years ago. He would sneak subjects into his lab in the middle of the night and record their breathing and monitor their blood pressure and show that their blood pressure would go down with this relaxation response. But this was controversial. I mean, we all have to breathe—and it's safe and effective for bringing blood pressure down and for helping with anxiety—but he had to sneak these people in to be able to do this research!

I don't think it's nearly as threatening for me to practice in the way that I practice, because I do practice with so much caution, always thinking about safety and always thinking about the patient's best interest. To me, that is the best type of medical practice that we can have, but it is different and, in many ways, unconventional.

Natarajan: Can you speak more about the different types of treatment modalities that you've seen work best when it comes to treating clients with anxiety and depression?

Campo: It's really hard to talk about this type of treatment without a patient. That's because when I'm sitting with someone, I'm only bringing my knowledge of the modalities, and the person is bringing their experiences and their distress and their intentions. I'm listening very carefully to understand what the person is experiencing and what it is that they're seeking—what type of guidance they might be requesting or thinking about.

In some ways, it is very hard to think about what the treatments are. This type of work is necessarily collaborative. But there are some very specific things that we can do. There are many easily identifiable vitamin deficiencies. People may be struggling with thyroid disease. These issues can present as depression. This *is* conventional psychiatry. This is absolutely taught in psychiatry residencies. However, I don't know how often it's practiced.

I hear lots of clients who will come in and say they haven't had blood work done in a very long time. So I want to be looking for those biological root causes because if they're there, I want to be able to treat it. That's important to keep in mind—that integrative psychiatry *is* conventional psychiatry. It is also holistic psychiatry and it also includes lifestyle changes. The Venn diagram of those three and where they converge is integrative psychiatry.

When I'm thinking about holistic modalities and anxiety, breathing techniques can be very effective. That goes back to what we were talking about with Herbert Benson. There are many different types of relaxation breathing techniques, but they all come down to one key component—and that is extending the exhale.

The reason for this is that every time we inhale, we activate the sympathetic autonomic nervous system. And every time we exhale, we activate the parasympathetic autonomic nervous system. In theory, we're in balance all day long—inhaling and exhaling, inhaling and exhaling. When we inhale, that is the sympathetic part that is getting ready, fight or flight. It is being on guard. As we exhale, the parasympathetic activates to rest and digest. It's ease, being at peace, feeling safe.

All day long, if we oscillate between the two, we are in balance. But what do most of us do? If we're feeling anxious, we inhale, and we hold our breath. Then we're in a state of sympathetic overdrive, and we balance it out by exhaling. If you can really extend your exhale, you can move into that parasympathetic state. You can do that in one or two breaths. You can do it for yourself. You can notice that sensation in your body—you will become calmer.

For depression, it certainly is helpful to be able to use breathing techniques, especially if there is a lot of anxiety with depression—but there are other things that can be helpful as well. Mindfulness or nonjudgmental awareness of the present moment, a curiosity, can be a helpful practice in daily life.

When I'm thinking about depression, I'm often thinking with people about movement. It doesn't have to be a certain type of physical exercise, but some exercise—some physical movement—is absolutely helpful for depression. It increases BDNF in the brain, which is a brain-derived neurotrophic factor. And so with exercise, we will see the mood improve. It might just be momentary, but once we have a habit of exercise, BDNF is building in the brain, becoming more regular.

That brings me to another piece. Habits and rhythm sleep are incredibly important. It's foundational. If that's the only thing I can help someone with, they will feel better. We have to have sleep so that our bodies can heal. We have to have sleep so that we can think and focus and concentrate. If we're falling asleep at about the same time every night, and we're waking at about the same time each day, that helps our circadian clocks. We have circadian clocks in every cell of our body, and that helps reset them. So sleep is important.

Food is incredibly important. We've talked about that already. Breathing is incredibly important. Moving. None of these things are new, right? I'm not telling you anything that you haven't heard before, but it's about actually putting them into practice on a daily basis. Mindfulness or meditation is new for some people to think about, and they are incredibly powerful and effective.

If we can have a rhythm in our life; if we can wake in about the same time every day, check-in with ourselves with a short meditation or a breathing exercise; if we can eat at about the same time every day, and we eat real whole foods as close to their natural way as possible; if we have movement every day, and we allow for sleep again at night; if we have restorative relationships, nurturing relationships.

We talk a lot about consuming toxic things in our lives, but sometimes our relationships can be very painful—and maybe we need help setting up boundaries to protect us from difficult people in our lives. Therapy is incredibly important. Unfortunately, we don't see a lot of that in conventional psychiatric practices. The vast majority of the patients that I work with have therapists, and all of them receive some type of therapeutic intervention when they're meeting with me.

I imagine I'm leaving many things out. I think about yoga with people. I think about biofeedback at times. I've studied lots of different herbs and supplements that have been incredibly helpful, but, again, these are all taken in context. They're all individualized for the person that I'm meeting with. We're thinking about how one thing will interact with another.

Natarajan: This links to what you said earlier about the need for more structural change in medicine. It goes back to the fact that if you don't have the time to be collaborative with your patient and learn all of these things and figure out what's conducive to the lifestyle, you miss so much. There seems to be a culture shift that needs to happen to see more psychiatrists practicing in this way.

Campo: There is kind of a gap between what I was trained for in conventional psychiatry and what I see in common practice. However, my training with integrative work really came even before I started studying psychiatry. I was working with that integrative physician in medical school, learning about nutrition and acupuncture even before I started my psychiatry training. I knew that would be the way that I would practice when I moved into it.

I didn't know a lot of integrative psychiatrists when I finished my residency and started my own journey, but I did know some. Now I am really happy to say that I know many, and there are more every day. Every year when I go to these conferences, more and more people are interested in this way of working because it works.

I'm really encouraged and excited that we are at the beginning of something that is going to be very different. It may take a very long time. I know that there are a lot of people who are really struggling and who don't have a relationship with a provider, but that could change.

Natarajan: It is encouraging to hear that you are encountering more people interested in this perspective in your professional circles. It sounds like you do envision a future where more people are practicing in this way, but the shift may occur at a slower pace because there's a lot of structural change that needs to happen as well to make practicing conducive to this type of work. Thank you for joining us today.

Zen and the Art of Moodcycle Maintenance

David Healy

Abstract: *Depression was slow to come to Japan. Selective Serotonin Reuptake Inhibitors were licensed there a decade later than in the West. Once licensed, the use of antidepressants escalated rapidly. There is now talk of a mental health crisis in children and adolescents in both West and East, in which a younger generation seems to have lost its bearing and psychotropic drug use in this age group in particular is now rampant despite minimal evidence for effectiveness. A Zen approach to life was slow to come to the West. Meditation in the form of Mindfulness arrived in America just before the SSRIs arrived in Japan. Mindfulness, as practiced in the West, shows features of commodification that are antithetical to the 'spirit' of Zen. The marketing of both SSRIs and Mindfulness point to a commodification of techniques that are at odds with the spirit of science. They also point to an encephalization in the way we view ourselves and our problems that may be getting in the way of us seeing how both drugs and meditation are actually acting.*

Acknowledgement: This chapter previously appeared in *Ethical Human Psychology and Psychiatry.*

Introduction

I was invited—through the auspices of Pfizer who were attempting to get Zoloft onto the Japanese market—to lecture at a Japanese neuropsycho-pharmacology meeting in Tokyo in 1997. Prior to going, I read the history of Japanese psychiatry in the limited number of available books in English. Two features stood out. One was a recognition of conditions like *taijin kyofusho* that is common there, non-existent in the West, but was about to become common in the form of social anxiety disorder (Healy 2001, 2004).

Second, while Germany had been historically the primary Western influence on Japanese psychiatric thinking, it was Americans arriving in the 1960s to study the Japanese and Chinese who wrote the story. They brought an assumption that other cultures had to catch up, especially when it came to psychoanalysis. Westerners had minds that could get mentally ill, Easterners were slowly developing minds like this, but they somatized and had concepts like neurasthenia.

Looking for signs of earlier stages of development, Westerners seized on Morita Therapy. This wasn't psychoanalysis. It resembled behavior therapy but it offered hope that these other cultures would learn to value "talk therapy."

The companies making selective serotonin reuptake inhibitors (SSRIs) certainly hoped the Japanese would become more like Westerners. There were no SSRIs licensed in Japan in 1997. The Japanese viewed their nervous problems as anxiety for which benzodiazepines were effective treatments. Their education to have colds of the spirit—*kokoro no kaze*—lay in the future.

Their anxiety was converted to depression during the 2000s and beyond (Kitanaka 2011), leading to a 7-fold increase in antidepressants prescribed between 1998 and 2012.[1] Does this demonstrate the power of pharmaceutical marketing? Or the imprecision of our diagnostic criteria? Many clinical cases can meet operational criteria for depression or anxiety. A decade earlier the West had been the testbed for converting cases of Valium into cases of Prozac (Healy 2004). In addition, the looseness of these criteria makes it possible to diagnose unhappiness or sadness as depression.

With the creation of the third edition of the *Diagnostic and Statistical Manual of Mental Disorders* (*DSM-III*), American psychiatry proclaimed that it was leaving behind the fuzziness of the psychoanalytic era where everyone was viewed as ill or latently ill. This didn't happen. *DSM-III* lists operational criteria for diagnoses and states that meeting them requires an exercise of judgement. But simply listing sets of operational criteria sets up a clash between "opinions" with the easiest default being to let the patient have whatever illness they want. Americans have enthusiastically embraced all drugs. They have bought into the idea of being treated for risk factors, spun

---

[1] Figures from Fuji Keizai medicinal drugs data book

initially as preventative health, and more recently as wellbeing (Healy 2021).

By 1997, psychoanalysis was eclipsed in the United States as a mainstream activity. But some magisterial, even revered figures (like Arthur Kleinman) remained imbued with analytic ways of thinking, and the influence of these figures meant that American mental health culture remained wedded to the idea of talk therapy. Kleinman viewed the Chinese who complained of neurasthenia rather than depression as mistaken and may have unwittingly done a lot to sell SSRIs in China (Kleinman 1988a & 1988b; Healy 1997).

Something similar could be said about another magisterial Harvard figure, Leon Eisenberg, who in the 1960s put Attention-Deficit/Hyperactivity-Disorder (ADHD) (then called Minimal Brain Dysfunction) and its treatment by stimulants, on the map. While viewed by Europeans as almost one of them when he warned against both mindlessness and brainlessness in psychiatry (Eisenberg 1986), like most Americans Eisenberg had no sense of the physical roots of European concepts of introversion and extraversion, which means some of us engage in risk management while others are risk takers without either predisposition being a disease (Eisenberg 2000; Healy 2002).

This sketch of my 1997 impressions of Japanese psychopharmacology seen through the lens of a few American texts is neither exhaustive nor nuanced. I undertook interviews while there and these showed that Japan, like Europe, had had a 1968 moment, in which the Tokyo Department of Psychiatry was occupied by students protesting the dehumanization represented by biological psychiatry (Clark 2000; Toru 2000; Healy 2002). America had nothing like this.

In terms of psychopharmacology, Teruo Okuma and colleagues had already done important research, unrecognized in America, that later underpinned the unfortunate marketing concept of a mood-stabilizer (Okuma 2000; Healy 2008). And the Japanese pharmaceutical industry was also at this time beginning to make its presence felt on the global stage and draw on global marketing strategies (Kobayashi 2000).

Around 2002, Nikolas Rose—contrasting the West and the Rest (especially Japan)—framed the issues in terms of Westerners becoming neurochemical selves, something quite different to physical selves (Rose 2004). In 2004, Kal Applbaum used Western pharmaceutical company efforts to penetrate the Japanese market to chart how business practices were subverting professionalism. In 2011, Junko Kitanaka definitively outlined a post-2000 transformation of Japanese sensibilities from viewing mental disorders (like depression) as rare and shameful, to embracing them and pointing to the ambiguities in recognizing social issues more readily at a potential cost of locating them within the self (Kitanaka 2011).

A Crisis in the Making

This brief account sketches the ground for an emerging crisis. A quarter of a century later, Western countries face a teenage mental health crisis (Richtel 2022; HCFEA 2023). There is alarm at the ten or more psychotropic drugs teenagers are being prescribed. Some psychiatrists claim even more teens are diseased than realized, needing access to psychiatrists and medication. Non-psychiatrists claim the need is for more talk therapy as teens are being put on medication in the absence of talk therapists.

As in the West, Japanese and Korean teenagers are having difficulties. New disorders have emerged like *hikikomori* syndrome, first described in 1998 but perhaps comparable with school refusal syndromes described in the US and Japan in the 1950s. Those affected become recluses, sometimes living indoors for years (Saito 1998). Hikikomori has since spread to the West.

In the West, a contrast between drug and talk therapies is a cliché. Few are aware that for much of the world the idea of fixing a nervous problem by talk therapy doesn't compute. For the Japanese, until recently it made sense for a confused or unhappy teenager to talk to an adult, though an adult who was a teacher or mentor rather than a therapist. This had also been the sensible option in the West three decades prior. When the SSRIs were launched, the belief was children did not get depression (melancholia) and it was difficult to find depressed children for clinical trials of SSRIs (Healy et al. 2020). What is going on?

Zen Buddhism

Buddhism began to migrate to the West in the early 20th century. This was a spiritual movement, not a service for people with mental health problems. The word spiritual is ambiguous here in that Buddhism recognizes no god. "Spirituality" in this context best connotes an attainment of awareness or openness, often termed enlightenment, either through the practice of meditation or by adherence to norms of "right" behaviour. Its reception in America and Europe was very different (Giraldi 2019).[2]

In the 1990s, as some Westerners were figuring the Japanese would soon join the modern world and understand inner life the way "we" did, a form of Zen Buddhism especially adapted for Western mental health purposes—deliberately called "mindfulness"—exploded onto the American scene and diffused rapidly to Europe (Harrington 2009). In 1990, Jon Kabat-Zinn's *Full Catastrophe Living* introduced mindfulness, understood as meditation, as a new way to cope with stress (Kabat-Zinn 1990). Around 2000, no academic articles featured mindfulness; by 2018, there were 1000 per year and tens of thousands per year in the lay press (Giraldi 2019).

Kabat-Zinn discarded the spiritual dimension of Buddhism. Mindfulness became a technique, to be tested for effectiveness in treating conditions defined by the latest *DSM*. In the U.K., it was incorporated into Cognitive Behaviour Therapy (CBT), and Mindfulness-Based CBT (MBCBT) is now formally designated as a psychotherapy. MBCT has flourished as a form of Evidence-Based Medicine (EBM) rather than a form of complementary or alternative medicine. As part of EBM, it is reductionist, mechanistic and far from open (Giraldi 2019).

Mindfulness aims at strengthening a poorly functioning self, whereas Buddhism views the self as an illusion, the source of many of our problems, and not something to be strengthened. For mindfulness, meditation is homework assignment rather than a potential way of life. Mindfulness functions in a world where labels like "bipolar," "depressed," or "autistic"

---

[2] Robert Pirsig's, pre-*DSM-III*, Zen and the Art of Motorcycle Maintenance (1974) offers an early link between Zen and American mental health. This book could never have been written in Europe.

define people and are incorporated into their identity, whereas Buddhism views these labels as aberrations.[3] The contrast can perhaps be brought out by a new movement that has emerged in Japan: Tojisha-Kenkyu. Tojisha refers to a party in a dispute, as in lawsuits or those contesting discrimination. Kenkyu means research.

Tojisha-Kenkyu began in the 1970s when people suffering from a physical disability began to contest their marginalization. It spread to groups suffering from discrimination, and since 2000 has been increasingly picked up by people liable to attract mental health labels (Ayaya and Kitanaka 2023). It encourages people to reflect on their own experience and become, as in the current Western phrase, experts-by-experience.

In Tojisha-Kenkyu, expertise is not simply born from having a condition; it requires research which, in part, means reflection and a contesting of hypotheses by reporting self-observations to others aimed at finding a consensus. There is an assumption that, whatever the label, the person is an individual, and their experience may differ significantly from that of others who might attract a similar label. Individuals, however, are also embedded in a community.

Inner and Outer

Tojisha-Kenkyu raises questions about what we are doing in the mental health domain. First come questions about the wisdom of stripping out the "spiritual" element from meditative practice. Perhaps we should reconceive meditation as a scientific rather than a religious exercise? Like science, Buddhist meditation attempts to grasp the world as it is rather than as we might wish it to be. Tojisha-Kenkyu makes this more explicit by calling on the parties to a dispute in order to test things out and come to a consensus judgement as to the best way to explain a situation. This is the very essence of science in general and central to clinical science.

---

[3] Mindfulness was not the only interface between Western psychotherapy and Japan. Acceptance and Commitment Therapy (ACT) took elements from Morita and Naikan without going down the mindfulness route.

The history of science stresses that science deals in questions that can be "settled by data" rather than questions about the meaning of life. The emphasis in official accounts is on the word "data"—as though the data speak, are guarantors of objectivity, and considering anything else other than data is to introduce values. The word "value" is typically left undefined and, for many, hints at religion from which they step back on principle. Scientific data never speak in this way—not even when processed through endless statistical tests.

The key word in this history of science is "settled." Objectivity comes from the experiment of testing hypotheses in public hoping to achieve a consensus view as a legal trial does in front of a jury or a scientific experiment does when it is carried out in public. Objectivity does not fall out of statistical tests or algorithms. It stems from two or more people attempting to establish the meaning of events, which is what should happen in clinical settings but has almost vanished when the adverse effects of drugs are concerned.

In addition, science from genetics to astronomy is about recognizing individuality rather than generalities. Establishing generalities can help in the scientific process but this is a step on the way—rather than the goal— of science (Healy 2023). Clinical trials can tell us about the average effects of a drug on one parameter, but treating the person in front of me on the basis of average effects is perilous for them, especially if the system denies them the option to dispute what is happening. It is also unscientific in principle and morally hazardous. Moral hazard is used here in a behavioral science rather than a value-laden frame; it implies an alignment of incentives that demonstrably puts patients at risk. In this case, Western clinical professionals get penalized if they acknowledge that pharmaceuticals have adverse effects (Healy 2021).

Tojisha-Kenkyu has overlaps with Open Dialogue, Soteria House, and Peer Respite.[4] All recognize the importance of individuals in crises that do not necessarily stem from their illness or disability but arise in part because our

---

[4] The testing of hypotheses offers an area of overlap with CBT but Tojisha-Kenkyu, at the moment, is less office- and more communally-focused than CBT, and engages with power structures. Patients, whether Japanese or Western, have this need in common.

systems have rendered the person invisible. This crisis affects a growing number of healthy people who health systems have redefined as mentally ill and put on psychotropic and non-psychotropic treatments that produce the features of an apparent mental illness—suicidality, agitation, sexual dysfunction, etc. This is a growing problem as pharmaceutical companies make their money from treating the healthy. Since 2000, the word polypharmacy has entered our lexicon and with it has come falling life expectancies, even among children (Woolf et al 2023), and a huge increase in mental illness (Healy 2021).

Another aspect these developments point to is an encephalization of mindfulness in Western settings—reflected in the use of the word mindful (Van Dam et al 2018). While for many Westerners the word "meditation" is likely synonymous with a mental activity, traditional meditative practices more often refer to a developing awareness of outer and inner. In the 1880s, William James and Carl Lange cited the body as a key site in knowing what is going on within and without. The brain has a secondary role in knowledge, which is to posit possible explanations for arousal or other changes in internal or external milieu. But in the century that followed, Westerners increasingly viewed their brains as a direct interface with the world, looking out from, or down at, a relatively inert body. Lectures on mindfulness present brain scans and electroencephalographic imagery as evidence that it is working, and the brain is the site of its action.

Our skin, by far the biggest organ in the body, is the boundary between outer and inner.[5] Along with our eyes and ears, most processing of what is happening within us and without is done by our sensory systems with skin containing multiple sensory organs. In the last century, enormous progress has been made to look within brains at their functioning. While we still do not understand consciousness, we have a better grasp on how brains

---

[5] The mucosa of our guts and bladders with all their contents lie outside our bodies rather than inside. Our gut and skin have an extraordinarily rich microbiome which many popular texts all but see as capable of cognitive functions in their own right. What is unquestionably the case, our brains' attention is more attuned to our skin, gut, and bladder than to the wider environment. The brain has a role in processing competing interpretations of what might be happening in these domains, but it is our gut, skin, eyes, ears, and other senses that do the initial and critical processing of what is happening.

function than we have about skin, which is extraordinary given how available to explore this boundary is.

When talking about themselves, and the most intimate details of their selves, a wider public—particularly in the United States—talks glibly about their serotonin and dopamine levels. This bio-babble has replaced a prior Freudian psychobabble; none of the terms used from serotonin now (to libido, formerly) are being used in a scientifically meaningful sense (Healy 1997 & 1999). There is a parallel here between drug treatments and mindfulness. For over a century, the treatment of nervous problems was brain-focused aimed at strengthening nerves with tonics or stimulants or damping them down with sedatives (Atigari and Healy 2014). It is assumed that all psychotropic drugs act similarly.

Boundary Drugs

There is, however, relatively little serotonin in our brains. Serotonin is located primarily in skin, gut, blood, and bones. The most common and immediate effect of a serotonin reuptake inhibitor is to produce genital numbing, which it does close to universally, and almost as quickly as rubbing a local anesthetic into genitals (Healy 2020). The immediacy and similarity to a local anesthetic effect suggests an action at sensory receptors in genital skin. This genital numbing is accompanied by a muting of orgasm and, over time, a loss of libido. One consequence of SSRI treatment is that these effects can intensify and remain permanent after treatment stops—post-SSRI sexual dysfunction (PSSD)—leading to suicides (Healy et al 2018; Healy et al 2022). There are no treatments for PSSD. It confounds pharmacological receptor theory.

In many cases, the genital numbing is accompanied by an emotional numbing and, while not linked by those affected to a more general numbing of touch receptors, a numbing of touch receptors certainly happens. Those with PSSD also complain of brain fog. With mental features like emotional numbing, brain fog and loss of libido stemming from drugs marketed as "antidepressants," the almost universal assumption is that something has gone wrong in the brains of those affected. A better explanation may lie in a James-Lange view that reconceives the effects of

SSRIs as acting on sensory systems. They affect touch and affective touch, vision, and proprioception. Within the brain, these effects show up as reduced input. The difficulties in understanding and solving PSSD may lie in the poverty of our knowledge of peripheral sensory systems.

As this quote about emotional numbing brings out, the effects of SSRIs are close to the opposite of the "mind-revealing" effects of the psychedelic drugs which also work on sensory systems:

> The mental symptoms are literally an altered state of consciousness that one absolutely cannot comprehend if he didn't experience it. No words can explain such a thing. Every day I am shocked that such a state is even possible. It has nothing to with a mood disorder although it would make anyone depressed. The best way to describe it is mental anesthesia. Everything in the mind is tuned down so low, even thoughts. The mind is blank, emotions are so muted that they are barely relevant. In a way, it's the opposite of what psychedelics do to the mind. They enhance and amplify what is going on whereas SSRIs completely mute it - so much that one has the impression that everything has been wiped out, and there is no mind anymore (Villeneuve, personal communication, 2023).[6]

This striking testimony suggests relabeling the SSRIs as "psychekleismics" (mind closing), an almost directly opposite action to the mind manifesting effect of the psychedelics.

Psychedelics

The SSRIs have created a public health crisis with roughly 15% of most Western populations taking them, primarily because they are unable to stop. Reproduction rates have now fallen below replacement rates, one factor which may well be the lack of love-making these drugs cause along

---

[6] Similar quotes can be found in an extraordinary podcast from Post-SSRI Sexual Dysfunction (PSSD) sufferers (https://www.youtube.com/@pssdnetwork). This captures the key points being made in this chapter.

with increased rates of miscarriage and birth defects (Healy 2020). This crisis points us toward a previous and, perhaps, future psychotropic crisis.

In 1971, both the use of and research on LSD, psilocybin, and mescaline—drugs that act primarily on serotonin systems—were banned because of threats they posed to the social order. Criminalizing a branch of science runs counter to the view that Western societies lead the world in making progress on the basis of science. The psychedelics, meditation (not mindfulness), and a number of physical techniques that bridge the gap between them (such as holotropic breathing) share points in common. All lead to an awareness of outer and inner, caught in Aldous Huxley's reference to the effects of psychedelic drugs on the Gates of Perception. All lead toward a dissolution of the ego, in some cases to the benefit of what has previously been labelled as a mental disorder. This benefit from experiences has led to a sense that both the psychedelics and meditation might be useful "therapies." But what is a therapy?

Efforts to decriminalize the psychedelic drugs have focused on getting them licensed as therapies. This means adapting them to a world of regulatory standards, algorithmic demonstrations that the standard has been met for *DSM* defined conditions, and above all embodying them in therapy packages (Healy 2023). In practice, embodying the drugs in therapy packages means having a dose that is too low to make a meaningful difference so that treatment has to be given at regular intervals with costly safeguards in place. Treatment like this becomes a predictable profit point for companies and therapists.

As noted above, something very similar happened when mindfulness was commodified. This template changes the psychedelics and meditation to fit society rather than changes society. The template reduces a three-dimensional experience aimed at opening people up, to a two dimensional, closed algorithmic system. The algorithmic approach is billed as objective and scientific but an emphasis on procedure is the template on which business and bureaucracy—rather than science—operates. This business approach is inimical to clinical science. It pretends to be an engineering precision, but increasingly is a source of alienation for those it professes to be in the business of helping—whether with psychotherapy or drug therapy.

In making disputes socially acceptable again and focusing on the resolution of disputes by critical tests involving the individuals affected, as Soteria House once did, Tojisha-Kenkyu restores the judgement calls and openness that are absent in bureaucratic and business procedures. Can healthcare that hinges on making judgements survive and make a difference in a world of health services, or will Tojisha-Kenkyu face an uphill struggle as Open Dialogue and Soteria House have?

Zen and the Art of Clinical Science

It is increasingly possible to make money from delivering "health" services to people who are vulnerable or in distress. Just as a successful clothes business in our day standardizes its procedures and produces clothes for the average person—not for individuals—so, too, with "life science" companies, which are now the biggest business sector on the planet.

There may be no limit to the size of this market. We are not just becoming neurochemical selves, as Rose put it. Health rather than holiness ("spirituality," openness) has become our central concern. While there have been notable scandals around money in the holiness domain, the spiritual and health domains formerly offered an alternative to a business model— a professional model.

Clinicians were once professionals whose job was to deploy their medical knowledge and available resources to help us live the lives we wanted to live. They bore some resemblance to a Zen Master. The relationship between clinician/master and pupil/patient was important. It needed to be good, continuous, and open. Algorithmic health services claim their closed models (that treat clinical components as interchangeable) are more efficient, but studies that test this claim show greater mortality when compared to continuity of care (Gray et al 2003; Gray et al 2018).

This somewhat idealized picture of medicine, and perhaps Zen, faces a problem in our day in that not only has religion been discredited in favor of business, but so has professionalism. The word conjures up images in

Western settings of a white, male, knowledge elite with a bias against openness and capable of abuse, especially in "religious" settings. Many will shrink from embracing a model which seems to advocate a throwback to a discredited past, even at the cost of instead accepting the verdicts of impersonal algorithmic processes.

Delegating our narcissism to a god or father figure is no longer an option but neither is delegating it to an algorithm. We need a relationship-based healthcare in which neither party disputes the validity of the other and treatment is individually-tailored. We need a new breed of "professionals" who are aware of the risks that an alignment with power structures might pose to those seeking their help. Anything less is incompatible with clinical science. Interfering with either the rights or the ability of people and their clinicians to exercise judgement about what is needed in individual circumstances, such as claiming that a drug is causing an adverse effect, is profoundly alienating.

We need to support each other—wherever we live in the world—to resist the Tunics of Nessus that health services offer as solutions when we need Health Care. And we also need to be able to resist these health service offers that are being seen as solutions to other more political problems.

References

Applbaum K. The Marketing Era. From Professional Practice to Global Provisioning. Routledge, London, 2004.

Atigari O, Healy D. Proconvulsant effects. A neglected dimension of psychotropic activity. Aust & N.Z. J Psychiatry 2013, 47, 998-1001.

Ayayais S, Kitanaka J. Tojisha-kenkyu. Japan's Radical Alternative to Psychiatric Diagnosis. Aeon 2023.

Clark D. Community Care. On SamizdatHealth.org. Shipwreck of the Singular, References. Interview in 2000, published on Samizdat in 2021.

Eisenberg L. Mindlessness and brainlessness in psychiatry. Br J Psychiatry 1986, 148, 497-508.

Eisenberg L 2000. Stimulants and Children. On SamizdatHealth.org Shipwreck of the Singular, References. Interview in 2000, published on Samizdat in 2021.

Giraldi T. Psychotherapy, Mindfulness and Buddhist Meditation. Palgrave MacMillan London 2019.

Gray D, Evans P, Sweeney K, Lings P, et al Towards a theory of continuity of care. J R Soc Med. 2003; 96: 160–166.

Gray D, Siddaway-Lee K, White E et al. Continuity of Care: A Matter of Life and Death. BMJ Open 2018 e021161.

Harrington A. The Cure Within. A History of Mind-Body Medicine. WW Norton, New York, 2009.

Haut Conseil de la famille, de l'enfance et de l'âge (HCFEA). QUAND LES ENFANTS VONT MAL : COMMENT LES AIDER? March 13, 2023.

Healy D. The Antidepressant Era, Harvard University Press, Cambridge Ma, 1997.

Healy D. Trouble in the Freudian Gulf. British Medical Journal 1999, 318, 949.

Healy D. The Creation of Psychopharmacology. Harvard University Press, Cambridge Ma. 2002.

Healy D. Mania. Johns Hopkins University Press, Baltimore Md. 2008.

Healy D. Let Them Eat Prozac. New York University Press, New York. 2004.

Healy D. Have drug companies hyped social anxiety disorders to increase sales? Yes. Marketing hinders the discovery of long-term solutions. Western Journal Medicine 2001, 175, 364-365.

Healy D. Shaping the Intimate. Influences on the Experience of Everyday Nerves. Social Studies of Science 2004, 34, 219-245.

Healy D. Antidepressants and sexual dysfunction, a history. J Roy Soc Medicine 2020, 113, 133-135.

Healy D. Shipwreck of the Singular. Healthcare's Castaways. Samizdat Healthwriters' Co-operative. Toronto 2021.

Healy D. If God Does not Play Dice, Should Doctors? Consilium Scientific 2023.

Healy D. Randomized controlled assays and randomized controlled trials. A category error with consequences. Ethical Human Psychology and Psychiatry 2023.

Healy D, Le Noury J, Mangin D. Enduring sexual dysfunction after treatment with antidepressants, 5α-reductase inhibitors and isotretinoin: 300 cases. Int J Risk and Safety in Medicine 2018, 29, 125-134.

Healy D, Le Noury J, Wood J. Children of the Cure. Samizdat Healthwriters' Co-operative, Toronto 2020.

Healy D, Bahrick A, Bak M et al, Diagnostic criteria for enduring sexual dysfunction after treatment with antidepressants, finasteride and isotretinoin. Int J Risk and Safety in Medicine 2022, 1-7.

Kabat-Zinn J. Full Catastrophe Living. Random House, New York, 1990.

Kitanaka J. Depression in Japan. Princeton University Press, Princeton, N.J. 2011

Kleinman A. Rethinking Psychiatry. From Cultural Category to Personal Experience, Free Press, New York, 1988.

Kleinman A. The Illness Narratives. Suffering, Healing and The Human Condition. Basic Books, New York, 1988.

Kobayakawa T. Psychopharmaceuticals in Japan. Interview in 1997, published in The Psychopharmacologists vol 3 in 2000 and on Samizdat in 2021.

Okuma T. The Psychotropic Effects of Carbamazepine. Interview in 1997, published in The Psychopharmacologists vol 3 in 2000 and on Samizdat in 2021.

Richtel M. This teen was prescribed 10 psychotropic drugs. New York Times August 27, 2022.

Rose N. Becoming Neurochemical Selves. Research Gate 2004.

Saito T. *Shakaiteki hikikomori: owaranai shishunki (Social withdrawal: a neverending adolescence)* Tokyo: PHP Shinsho; 1998.

Toru M. Neurotransmitter Research in Japan. Interview in 1997, published in The Psychopharmacologists vol 3 in 2000 and on Samizdat in 2021.

Van Dam N, van Vugt M, Vago D. et al. Mind the Hype: A Critical Evaluation and Prescriptive Agenda for Research on Mindfulness and Meditation. *Perspectives on Psychological Science: A Journal of the Association for*

Psychological Science 2018, 13, 36–61.
https://doi.org/10.1177/1745691617709589.

Villeneuve M. Email to Healy July 2023. See also PSSDNetwork Podcast
Episode 2, 2023.

Woolf S, Wolf F, Rivara E. The new crisis of increasing all-cause mortality in
US children and adolescents. JAMA, 2023; 329, 975-976.

Life Formulation and the Human Experience Specialist

Eric Maisel

Abstract: *In this chapter, the author argues that, despite the large number of categories of helper that already exist (among them psychiatrists, psychologists, psychotherapists, life coaches, clinical social workers, marriage and family therapists, and mental health counselors), there remains a need for a new helper, one the author dubs a "human experience specialist" who is trained to bring a wide-angle lens to the work of healing and helping. At the same time, the author advocates for a particular alternative to the flawed DSM checklist method of "diagnosing mental disorders"—the method of life formulation, amplifying on this well-known model.*

Another way to think about what we are after when it comes to "alternatives" is the following: that we are trying to figure out how to think about what's going on when a human being presents himself or herself for help; that, as a secondary matter, we want to be able to describe what is going on, so as to communicate with our client; for record-keeping purposes, so as to be able to share information with other concerned parties; that we want to know what we intend to do about what's going on—what in the diagnostic model would be called our "treatment plan"; and, fourth, that we want to have a clear picture of what we see as our role, what we see as our mandates and our limits, what we see as the best way to use ourselves, and so on.

This is a mouthful. In this chapter, I want to focus on two ideas. The first idea is that a new helper is needed, someone I'm calling a "human experience specialist"—someone who has a "large" view of life and who can, at the drop of a hat, take the social view with her client, and then switch to a focus on changed circumstances, and then deepen the conversation by diving into the existential, and so on. Second, one tool that this new helper might employ is the idea of "formulation," which we can define as a provisional explanation or hypothesis as why our client is suffering in the way that he's suffering. Let's start with formulation first.

The idea of "formulation" as an alternative to *DSM* diagnosing has been around almost exactly as long as the *DSM* has. George Kelly, father of personal construct theory, argued in the 1950s for the idea of formulation as an antidote to diagnosis. He explained in *The Psychology of Personal Constructs* (1955):

> Much of the reform proposed by the psychology of personal constructs is directed towards the tendency for psychologists to impose preemptive constructions upon human behaviour. Diagnosis is all too frequently an attempt to cram a whole live struggling client into a nosological category. (p. 775)

Formulation as a way of thinking about your client is particularly popular in the United Kingdom, where it has been championed by Lucy Johnstone, Rudi Dallos, and many others. Here is my version of formulation, one that I'm calling a "life formulation model." It nicely disputes the current *DSM* paradigm and also frees us from the tyranny of acting as if we are talking only about "psychology" when we talk about mental health when, in fact, we are talking about all of life.

In this life formulation model, a practitioner would describe her relationship with the person she is seeing in the following six ways:

1. the person's expressed concerns
2. the person's circumstances of note
3. the person's behavioral and emotional considerations
4. the person's challenges as inferred by the provider
5. the provider's concerns
6. the provider's recommendations

There would be no *DSM* or pseudo-medical language used in this model, no new diagnostic language introduced, and everything would be described in "plain English" (or plain French or plain German).

How might this work? Let's consider a 15-year-old girl named Jane who is "brought in" to a service provider by her parents. They believe that Jane is "depressed." They are also worried about her drinking, her insomnia, her school difficulties, her thinness, and the fact that she is cutting herself.

First, the service provider would check-in with Jane about her own expressed concerns. These might turn out to be that Mary likes Elizabeth better than she likes Jane; that the clique that includes Mary and Elizabeth will not let Jane in; that Billy prefers Elizabeth to Jane; that Mrs. Williams in English may well be giving Jane a C, ruining Jane's chances of getting into the college she is dreaming of attending; and that her parents are driving her crazy by always scrutinizing her and criticizing her.

There is absolutely no reason why these concerns can't also come with some sort of number, if that were deemed useful: it would not be hard to create a huge list of concerns and attach a number to each one, if that was wanted. So, let's say that in addition to the words describing Jane's concerns, there were also numbers: let's say 1104, 1931, 2242, 4482 and 5561. It would be child's play to list those five numbers in a "summary report," if a service provider needed to do such a thing. This would look like: Expressed Concerns (1104, 1931, 2242, 4482, 5561). (But I think there is a better way to do this summarizing; see later.)

Next would come an acknowledgment and understanding of Jane's circumstances, gleaned from Jane and maybe from the reports of others. This might sound like:

Circumstances of Note:

> + In Jane's family, a college education and a professional career are required
> + In Jane's family, it is not permitted to date someone from a different cultural or religious background
> + Jane is not permitted to lock her door or any door, including the bathroom door
> + Jane surprised herself by doing much more poorly in freshman year that she had expected to do
> + Jane's older sisters were the stars of her high school

Are these all of the circumstances that one might include? Of course, they aren't. Are these the most pertinent circumstances to include? Who knows? But each is suggestive, and each helps a service provider understand Jane's reality. They may not be exactly the correct circumstances to note or a sufficient number of circumstances to note, but they are important, and they matter.

Next would come behavioral and emotional considerations. In Jane's case this might look like the following:

+ Jane is cutting herself (confirmed by Jane)
+ Jane is drinking excessively (disputed by Jane)
+ Jane is quite sad (confirmed by Jane)
+ Jane is starving herself (disputed by Jane)
+ Jane is sleeping very little (confirmed by Jane)

Next would come inferred challenges; that is, the provider's ideas or hypotheses about what is going on. This might sound like the following:

+ Predictable challenges of adolescent girls in Jane's cultural and socioeconomic situation
+ Special challenges of living in a strict, punitive family
+ Emotional challenges of intense sadness and constant worry
+ Cognitive challenges of self-denigrating and punitive self-talk
+ Behavioral challenges of cutting, drinking, starvation, and sleeplessness

These inferred challenges would be described in the service provider's preferred language: the language of psychological formulation, the language of narrative psychology, the language of CBT, the language of Jung, the language of Freud or contemporary psychoanalysis, the language of existential psychotherapy, in "ordinary" or "everyday" language, and so on.

A service provider could use whatever language she wanted to use, indicating where her language came from: that is, in addition to a long list of everyday inferences (like "the predictable challenges of adolescence") there might be also long lists of Jungian inferences, existential inferences, etc. If a code was needed, coded items might appear as J462 for "Jungian mid-life crisis" or F993 for "Freudian arrested development in the anal stage" and so on. Naturally (and hopefully) these taxonomical niceties would not be needed or wanted. But if they were, they could be accommodated.

Next would come the provider's concerns. These would be expressed in ordinary language in the following sort of way:

+ Concerned that Jane has no one to talk to, given that she's on the outs with her successful siblings and that she has no confidante in either of her parents

+ Wondering if Jane was born a little sad and, if so, if sadness will constitute a lifelong challenge for her

+ Some suspicions of childhood sexual abuse given Jane's particular presentation

+ Want to really focus on the sleeplessness and its causes, as sleeplessness can drive "mania" and "psychosis"

+ Must tackle the cutting, the drinking, and the self-starvation

Next would come the provider's recommendations. This might sound like:

+ Cognitive work around self-esteem

+ Depth work around possible trauma

+ Behavioral work around eating, cutting, and drinking

+ Behavioral work around sleeping

+ Family work around expectations

Personally, I would want a seventh category that communicates the sufferer's life purposes, dreams, goals, aspirations, and other existential and motivational factors. These could be reported in ordinary language and might sound like the following:

+ Jane remembers her camp counseling experiences as particularly meaningful

+ Jane considers that one of her life purposes is to marry and raise a family although she believes that she would be a "bad parent"

+ Jane would like to leave her small town and live in London or Paris

+ Jane sees herself as both "secular" and "spiritual" and would like to find a "spiritual outlet"

+ Jane does not believe that she has a real chance at success

This represents the life formulation model in a nutshell. Let's take a closer look at some of its pluses.

Life Formulation Model Pluses

Some virtues of this life formulation model (and its accompanying Life Formulation Guide, which might eventually replace the DSM) include the following:

+ It not only avoids the word "diagnosis" and the very idea of "diagnosis" (and essentially ends diagnosing), but it also avoids the word "psychological"—and announces that a service provider is helping people in distress with their problems with living, not exclusively with their "psyche." Thus, for example, both "getting a job" and the "psychological consequences of not having a job" become legitimate areas of exploration. A helper could also legitimately work on "job skills" or "social skills" as work on any traditional "psychological" or "psychotherapeutic" issue.

+ It doesn't conflate or confuse the person's concerns with the provider's concerns. Jane may not be concerned about her lack of sleep, her drinking, her cutting or her eating habits, but her service provider may well be. This model allows both sorts of concerns to find a place in the conversation and a way to get both sorts of concerns communicated to third parties.

+ It allows for conversations about, and reporting on, both "causes" (like suspected sexual abuse) and "treatment recommendations" (like, for example, cognitive work on self-esteem or behavioral work on stopping the cutting). No two providers might look at "causes" or "treatment recommendations" in the same way but the life formulation model at least has built-in places for both to appear. "Causes" can appear in both "inferred challenges" and "provider's concerns" and "treatment" has a dedicated home in "provider's recommendations" (with the pseudo-medical word "treatment" studiously avoided).

+ Some items could so-to-speak "auto-fill." If, for example, it is generally accepted that everyone should have a complete medical work-up to see if the concerns presented are organic or biological in nature—to see, that is, if any "real" disease or medical condition is present—then one "standard recommendation" that could "auto-fill" would be "It is suggested that Jane have a complete medical work-up."

Likewise, if it is generally accepted that it is good to have someone to talk to about things, then the recommendation that "Jane should have the chance to talk in an ongoing way with a service provider" might auto-fill. This latter point might seem obvious and to go without saying, yet in the pseudo-medical model that we are disputing it is not at all clear that "talking to someone" is seen as valuable, not when chemicals can be dispensed in a minute and save psychiatrists so much time and idle chit-chat. If we believe that "talking to someone" matters, it should be regularly included in our recommendations.

+ It allows for an interesting "tag" system of reporting. This is an important point. When you search for something on the Internet, you introduce certain words or "tags" that help you find what you are looking for: say "solar system," "planet," and "rings" if you are looking for a planet with rings. This gets you to "Saturn."

Tags are not labels but instead are our attempts to partially describe an entity. You can partially describe a thing in a "list sort of way" by identifying its parts: legs, head, tail, and so on (this is "defining by denotation"). You can also partially describe a thing in an "idea sort of way" through the use of concepts: a horse is a carbon-based living creature descended from some now extinct other carbon-based living creatures (this is "defining by connotation").

Such describing and defining is always incomplete, imperfect, and more arbitrary than we would like to admit. We know from philosophers of language like Wittgenstein that every abstract word (say "war" or "love") has no real definition but rather a huge range of meanings and colorations. Maybe World War II is the exemplary or paradigmatic instance of "war," but it is not meaningless or inappropriate to talk about "the war between the sexes" or "corporate warfare." The same is true of words like ego, dysfunction, abuse, or any other abstract word that can be used to describe human beings, human behaviors, and human situations.

Tags "merely" help describe; they do not amount to a "diagnosis," and they do not pretend to present an exhaustive, complete, or even adequate picture of a life. That is a good thing because we should be tired by now of all that pretension. In Jane's case, you could report on Jane by providing some number of items in the six categories—say five items per category—and produce a one-page report that is thirty lines in length. That is one kind of "description of Jane's situation." But you could also choose from among those various items and select some number of tags—let's say seven—that together provide a kind of snapshot of Jane's current reality.

For example, one provider might choose as her seven tags for Jane and her situation "strict and punitive family dynamics," "low self-esteem coupled with high expectations," "adolescence," "self-starvation," "sadness," "excessive drinking," and "cutting." Naturally each of these tags could come as a number rather than as words, if that was wanted. This snapshot would in no way provide a complete picture of Jane's current reality, but it would do a more sensible and humane job than labeling Jane with a pseudo-medical "clinical depression" diagnosis and some additional "adjustment disorder" or "personality disorder" diagnosis.

What might this tag system sound like in practice? For one person, and according to one service provider, the seven tags might be, "sad; unemployed; mid-life crisis; recently divorced; health issues; 'addicted' to porn; no goals or aspirations." For another person, and according to another service provider, the seven tags might be, "traumatic childhood; issues with food; dramatic relationships; spiritual seeker; creatively unfulfilled; uninspiring day job; lives in 'chaos and confusion.'" These snapshots could be created around any agreed-upon number of tags: three tags, five tags, seven tags, ten tags, etc. The more tags, the more cumbersome the system—but also the more complete the snapshot.

If you decide to set the bar as, "We need one word like 'depression' to capture everything that we need to know about a person's distress and his or her current situation," a tag system does not reach that absurd height. But if you decide to set the bar differently as, "We need a way of communicating a snapshot of a person's reality that includes some important features of a person's life and aims a helper in the direction of helping," a tag system would meet that threshold beautifully.

+ This model would "force" a service provider to inquire about Jane's actual concerns, learn about Jane's actual circumstances, acquire a picture of Jane's behaviors, thoughts, and feelings, come to some conclusions about Jane's situation, and offer up some recommendations as to what might help. This would naturally improve the service. Service providers would become smarter about human nature and about human challenges by virtue of having to think about how "cause and effect" operates in the lives of real people and having to consider what actually works to reduce distress. This model stretches and tests the practitioner in a useful way.

To be clear, as we are not always so clear about this, this life formulation model is not an alternative system *of* diagnosis but an alternative system *to* diagnosis. It allows for providers to chat with one another, either through summary reports or the tag system, and if it were widely accepted it would force those entities that believe they need diagnoses (like, for example, the courts) to begin to change their mind. The courts and other institutions would be forced to accept that "hearing voices," for example, is a reportable thing but does not lead to some made-up "diagnostic label" like "schizophrenia." It would serve our vital communications needs and, at the same time, would act as an agent of change.

No doubt other alternative systems to diagnosis can be dreamed up, and one or another of them might provide even more pluses than this life formulation model. But this is a good start, I think. It could be enacted right now, and were it enacted it would revolutionize how helpers think about and care for the people who come to them in difficulty and distress.

This life formulation model would go a long way toward providing a practitioner who is looking to free herself from the *DSM* model or some other model both with a conceptual framework that honors the richness of life and the naturalness of distress, and an organizational scheme that allows her to report in an honest way on a sufferer's experience. In one sense, no such model is needed: the essence of our task is to lean forward and collaborate, not to report on our efforts. But a model that by its very nature disputes the *DSM*, that helps a practitioner ask the right questions, and that distinguishes her concerns from her client's concerns might well prove extremely valuable.

Now, who *is* this practitioner?

Say that you wanted to be a humane helper who uses formulation and all the other tools at your disposal to help people when they're experiencing emotional distress and problems with life. How might you proceed? Well, your choices are severely limited: limited by the mental disorder paradigm and its reliance on chemicals and by the medical mythology underpinning psychotherapy and mental health counseling.

If you wanted to work with someone in a wide-ranging way, taking everything into account that ought to be taken into account—from her current circumstances to her original personality, from her socioeconomic realities to her lack of life purpose—you would find that there is no job, job description, or job title for that. You would quickly learn that you are mandated and constrained to focus on "treating mental disorders" or "treating psychological issues."

You might have imagined that because we already have psychologists, psychiatrists, psychotherapists, mental health counselors, marriage counselors, clinical social workers, family therapists, life coaches, consultants, and so on, that we do not need a new helper to supplement— or replace—these many practitioners. But we do. I am calling this new, vitally needed helper a "human experience specialist."

A human experience specialist is a helper of a new and special sort. She is someone who casts aside the very idea of "mental disorders" and leans forward into the reality of the person sitting across from her. She brings a wide-angle perspective to her work, knowing for certain that there is bound to be a lot to consider. Rather than limit herself to symptom checklists and to the hunt for a "precise" mental disorder label, she knows to consider her client's circumstances, social and economic realities, original and formed personalities, and much more.

If you are her client, she refuses to reduce your experience to some mental disorder matter or limited psychological issue. That your husband or wife is having an affair, that he or she doesn't like you, that he or she doesn't respect you, or that he or she is snide with you and critical of you, is not a "psychological issue." It is a terrible human experience, one with powerful consequences that might include "symptoms" like anxiety, sleeplessness, despair, and so on—but a terrible human experience that is not reducible to a "symptom picture," a "diagnosis," or a "psychological issue."

Your bad marriage is neither a medical condition nor a psychological issue—it is a bad marriage. Your friends know it, you know it, and yet your psychiatrist isn't interested in your deteriorating marriage and even your psychotherapist may skirt that reality. As obvious as this is, that your bad marriage has human consequences, we have somehow lost this understanding. We have rather lost the way of saying, "Your husband is cheating on you and that is making you sad and angry. That's playing right into your sense of defeat and your belief that life is a cheat. What can we do about all that?"

You would need someone who has a handle on this and a grasp of the whole picture: what life is like, what your life is like, what you are like "inside," and what might actually help you, given your personality and your circumstances. Our new helper, this human experience specialist, would be that person. No one has the superpower to snap her fingers, upgrade our species, and produce emotionally healthier and happier people "just like that." But our new human experience specialist would come as close as we can to possessing that superpower.

Our human experience specialist will almost certainly find no place inside any medical model system. Since she will refuse to "diagnose and treat," she will find herself excluded from the world of managed care, HMOs, insurance payments, insurance panels, professional trusts, "mental health parity" schemes, and the rest of the mental health establishment apparatus. To be excluded is not her desire but simply a fault of the system. Since she will be excluded, she will need to hang out her shingle as an independent practitioner and operate as, for instance, life coaches do—as a needed, unregulated outside practitioner.

Can she actually do this, given that she is forthrightly dealing with "mental health issues"? Will society allow her to advertise her point of view and argue, for example, that "mental disorders" are made-up labels? Would she be wise, from a legal standpoint, to take such risks? Because she positions herself in opposition to what society currently holds as its standard of care—pseudo-medical treatment as provided by psychiatrists, psychologists, psychotherapists, and other licensed mental health professionals—she could easily find herself in too vulnerable a position, exposed to litigation and pressured to refer the person she is helping to someone with the power to prescribe a chemical fix.

These are big and, perhaps, unsolvable issues. But let's imagine for the sake of argument that these issues could be resolved—which, given how odd and diverse the world of helping already is, might not be an impossibility. Today a distressed person might visit a psychic or an astrologer. She might go to an acupuncturist or a homeopath. She might see her priest or her rabbi. She might chat with the woman behind the counter at the health food store. She might follow the advice of a blogger writing for some website. She might consult a self-help book or embark on a shamanic retreat. She might chat with her sister or her best friend. She might do dream work, scream work, past life cleansing, gestalt work … given this weird and eclectic array, is there no room for a human experience specialist? Perhaps there is.

Not only is there this eclectic mix out there already—many psycho-therapists function as de facto human experience specialists; they fib as they fill out the necessary insurance forms when they assert that the person across from them has this or that "mental disorder" and that in six or eight sessions "treatment" will be delivered—but, having done their fibbing so as to get paid, they then go about their business of simply trying to be of help. They ask ordinary questions, make ordinary suggestions, share their observations, ask what hurts, react sympathetically, provide some human warmth, and recognize that life causes distress. They already function as human experience specialists—and maybe some of them will come out of the "mental disorder" closet and affirm that they are already doing this work.

What if the person across from our human experience specialist says, "I am old, I am ugly, no one wants me, I have no reason to live"? Our human experience specialist must have her responses at the ready. This is what she is trained for or what she has trained herself for. It isn't that she needs theories, pat answers, or homilies—and, of course, she would never dream of turning this lament into some sort of diagnosis. But she does need a way of responding, a way of using her heart, her experiences, her savvy, her intuitions, and her training. She can't sit mute and she must go well beyond the too-easy response of the client-centered therapist, "And how does that make you feel?" She must respond—and she can respond effectively by keeping her eye on her posture. She must keep leaning forward. She may have no answers, but she has the radical power of engagement at her disposal.

Given a significant caveat that the person across from her must be at least somewhat available—not too mute, not too disturbed, not too aggressive, not too withdrawn—how will our human experience specialist operate? She will act as a guide of sorts; a teacher of sorts; a problem-solver of sorts; a sounding board of sorts; a coach of sorts; a confidante of sorts; a teammate of sorts.

She will travel with the person suffering through difficult territory where neither knows for sure what they will find or even what exactly they are looking for. She will own a personal menu of tactics that allow her to offer support, frame issues, hold the person across from her accountable, and do the sorts of things that good helpers know to do. In this way, a willing person and a savvy helper enter a certain sort of collaboration, use everyday language like "sadness," "anxiety," and "boredom," and work together to choose and even create language that serves the sufferer. To put it simply, our human experience specialist would do no particular thing except try to be of help.

Of course, a human experience specialist would need to know all the current labels, including the latest fad *DSM* and *ICD* diagnoses, since the world uses them and since it would be silly not to be able to find useful information because you didn't know the lingo. But that is a different matter from believing in the labels or countenancing them. The human experience specialist would know the lingo, would know about the special challenges with which "an anorexic" or "an alcoholic" is likely to be grappling, would know what seems to help best with those special challenges, and so on—she would not be opting for ignorance. But she wouldn't call the girl sitting across from her "an anorexic." She would call her by her name.

Training the human experience specialist

Of course, no training program currently exists to train human experience specialists. Therefore, let's dream one up. Here is one reasonable human experience specialist two-year master's level program, three classes a quarter and eighteen classes in all, with summers for interning. The interning would naturally be vital—imagine a human experience specialist program without experiences!

The main difference between a class presented in a psychology or counseling program and a class presented in a human experience specialist program would be that the class in the human experience specialist program would provide *meta*-analysis or critical analysis of the subject matter presented. If the *DSM* were presented, it would be to analyze it and not to swallow it whole. For anything that might be presented— psychological tests, personality theory, etc.—the twin questions asked would be "What do we really know about this?" and "What have we really learned from this?" Each class would be a lesson in skepticism and not piety.

Here are the eighteen classes I have in mind:

1. Being Human – Who Are We?
2. Sources of Human Distress
3. Personality – What is it?
4. Listening and Speaking: The Art of Dialogue

5. Person as Individual and Person as Social Animal

6. What Helps? – Tactics and Strategies for Helpers

7. Meaning and Life Purpose – What Are They?

8. Qualities of a Helper – How to Be in Session

9. Psychological Formulation – What Do We Know About the Mind?

10. Context: Human Beings and Their Circumstances

11. Psychology Today – What Help is Being Offered?

12. Session Work – What Goes on In a Session?

13. Labels: Dealing with the Language of "Mental Disorders"

14. The Big Five: Sadness, Anxiety, Obsessions, Compulsions and Addictions

15. Relationships: Intimate Relationships and Family Dynamics

16. Lifespan: Being Human Over Time

17. Practice-Building for Human Experience Specialists

18. A Day in the Life: What a Human Experience Specialist Actually Does

Might a good program look different from the above? Of course, it might. One program might take a special interest in life purpose and meaning and have a more existential flavor to it. Another program might take a special interest in social issues and matters of social justice. A third program might include classes about work with children and adolescents and have that as its special focus. One program might include a class on how to ask strategic questions, another class on the differences between short-term work and long-term work, a third a class on ethical and legal responsibilities. None of these differences or variances would prove any sort of problem as long as a careful eye was kept on the central idea—that a person intending to do a new sort of work was being trained.

There might also be some sort of abbreviated training program for therapists and other mental health professionals who want to be released from the grip of the medical model and the constraints of doing "psychology," and who see value in adding a human experience specialty to their current way of working. Many in the profession are doing this work in a de facto way already: they might love a little additional training and a new set of initials to put behind their name. Let us offer them that possibility and see if they are moved to come aboard!

Our human experience specialist is needed for all sorts of reasons. First among them is that virtually all current mental health practitioners—psychiatrists, clinical psychologists, family therapists, mental health counselors, etc.—are by virtue of their training and their very name obliged to focus on the "disordered mind" of their clients and not on their clients' lives. A person is not a brain or mind in a bottle. He has a life, a personality, and a world. He doesn't "catch" depression: he experiences sadness and suffering. Right now, he may ask for a pill because he thinks he is going to some sort of doctor. In the future, if he is provided with a new option, he may choose to visit a human experience specialist and bravely announce, "I need help with living."

Questioning Clinical Technologies: Psychotherapy After Heidegger

Donald R. Marks

Abstract: *Martin Heidegger's essay "The Question Concerning Technology" offers a starting point for examining the implications of mechanistic and functional approaches to clinical psychological science. The upshot of Heidegger's critique of technology for psychological treatment is twofold. On the one hand, it allows for an examination of the consequences of objectification and quantification, including the ways that these analytical methods render a human person as a representative of a clinical population—a kind of "raw material" available for deployment to alternative ends. On the other hand, it suggests the limitations of excluding mystery from discussions of human life. Construing emotional experience as symptoms of illness and the human person as susceptible to analysis as a mere confluence of material forces neglects the most profound dimensions of human experience as a clearing in which being is revealed. This chapter contrasts mechanistic and functional approaches commonly adopted in clinical psychological science with a poetic view of the human person that eschews the reductionism and context-stripping characteristic of scientific analyses, privileges the poetic dimensions of human thought, and prioritizes openness to mystery.*

Questioning Clinical Technologies: Psychotherapy After Heidegger

In his essay "The Question Concerning Technology," Martin Heidegger describes modern technology as a "mode of revealing" that poses a specific challenge for human beings: it orders the real "as standing reserve."[1] In

---

[1] Martin Heidegger, "The Question Concerning Technology," in *Readings in the Philosophy of Technology*, 2nd ed., ed. David M. Kaplan (Lanham, MD: Rowman and Littlefield, 2009), 13-14. Any scholar who draws upon Heidegger's thought must confront the staggering contradiction between his work, which as Harris Bor has noted evokes key Jewish themes of "mysticism, revelation, the embrace of being in the world (*Dasein*), the here and now, the primordial, pre-intellectual, worldly, poetic, and

other words, modern technology treats the world as a kind of inventory of products or storehouse of energy: "Everywhere everything is ordered to stand by, to be immediately at hand, indeed to stand there just so that it may be on call for a further ordering."[2]

Heidegger considers this mode of revealing, which he calls "Enframing," a challenging-forth which "sets upon" human beings and the real, ordering them as standing reserve.[3] Human beings themselves may be challenged in this way, set-upon as nature is for stockpiling—transformation into the accumulation of resources. As Heidegger observes, the organizational language that characterizes people as "human resources" offers one example of Enframing at work. Another, he suggests, is considering "the supply" of patients available to a clinic.[4]

Thinking and acting in this manner, Heidegger argues, subordinates human beings to the orderability of the world, to the technological "challenging-forth" of supply for various industries and activities.[5] Although human beings cannot, Heidegger contends, be fully transformed into "mere standing-reserve," they are ensnared continually into Enframing—a mode of revealing nature as a kind of storehouse.[6] Heidegger notes that Enframing, in its essence, is not technological in itself, though technology poses the challenges that gather human beings into this way of ordering things. The essence of modern technology, he says, "lies in Enframing," and Enframing is a mode of revealing or, more precisely, it is a "destining" —that is, a "sending-that-gathers" —of revealing.[7]

This destining of revealing—the way things are called into ordering—is the most fundamental challenge that human beings face. When destining

---

mythical," and his personal history of antisemitism. For a thoughtful consideration of Heidegger's continued relevance to critiques of technology despite his hateful personal views and political allegiances, see Harris Bor, *Staying Human: A Jewish Theology for the Age of Artificial Intelligence* (Eugene, OR: Cascade Books, 2021), 5-8.

[2] Heidegger, "Question Concerning Technology," 14.

[3] Heidegger, "Question Concerning Technology," 15.

[4] Heidegger, "Question Concerning Technology," 15.

[5] Heidegger, "Question Concerning Technology," 14.

[6] Heidegger, "Question Concerning Technology," 15.

[7] Heidegger, "Question Concerning Technology," 18.

"reigns in the mode of Enframing"—the revealing of nature as standing-reserve—human beings face "the supreme danger."[8] In the mode of Enframing, the "unconcealed," what is revealed or called forth in the world, is no longer a proper object like a work of art or a craftsman's handiwork (Heidegger offers the example of a silversmith's making of a chalice); it becomes, instead, merely a stockpile or inventory of things.[9] Through their reduction to this mere ordering of nature, human beings become subject to viewing even themselves as standing reserve.

Mechanistic approaches to psychology participate in technological processes such as those Heidegger describes in several important ways. Enframing, one could argue, characterizes approaches to human suffering that emphasize the production of scientific knowledge through the amassing and manipulation of human quantities. Proponents of the evidence-based treatment movement, for example, often emphasize the volume of participants involved in clinical trials. Demographic characteristics, such as gender or ethnicity, and even epidemiological variables, such as diagnosis, drop away in the stockpiling process. The specific experiences and unique personal histories and contexts of the patients and clinicians who engaged with one another in therapeutic dialogue are, in this view, nowhere to be found.

Moreover, the hallmark of any evidence-based psychotherapy is its demonstrated utility—the proof that it works and a formulaic explanation for how it works. All human activity in the technological society, including psychotherapy, must be evaluated according to its usefulness and repeatability. The randomized controlled trial (RCT), a "gold standard" of psychotherapy evaluation, relies upon the comparison of group means on measures of symptom distress or psychological constructs. These metrics, which clinical psychological science insists upon, obscure the obstinate, intractable details of human beings' lived experience, defining participants quantitatively on a vector of interest. The unquantifiable yet persistent aspects of human experience (e.g., the temporality of humans as beings-in-time), whenever possible, become the targets of statistical control. They are

---

[8] Heidegger, "Question Concerning Technology," 19.
[9] Heidegger, "Question Concerning Technology," 11.

parceled out from the findings as "confounds," or they are simply ignored. The effectiveness of an intervention lies in its capacity for efficient transformation of quantities deemed clinically relevant.

One might contrast this perspective regarding the cumulative value of clinical trial participants with the narrative method Sigmund Freud adopted in his early psychoanalytic case studies, each of which featured a distinctive individual with a memorable history that unfolded, albeit through the ministrations and interpretations of the analyst, to reveal a dimension of the human psyche. The classic Freudian case, one might say, was an artisanal gathering and bringing-forth—in much the same way that, for Heidegger, a silversmith gathers the material, formal, and final causes of the silver chalice to bring it forth into appearance.[10]

I make this comparison not to dispute the logic of the evidence-based treatment movement or minimize the significance of large-scale participation in clinical trials. Proponents of evidence-based practice in psychology will note that widely tested interventions are, by definition, more reliable than those without such a track record. If nothing else, treatments that can be applied to large numbers of cases must consist of replicable procedures.

Also, proponents of clinical psychological science will contend that tracking a volume of participants helps establish the acceptability of a psychotherapy. If a treatment procedure has the potential to yield negative consequences or adverse effects, these problems are likely to be revealed over the course of treating thousands of cases. Even disseminating an intervention to enough clinicians to treat tens of thousands of people in hundreds of clinical trials, it must be noted, is a significant scientific accomplishment.

The matter at hand here, however, is the effect of the discourse—the way the technological perspective of clinical psychological science "brings forth" human beings. When thinking in this aggregative, quantitative manner, the particularity of the person vanishes. Only the patterns and flows of quantitative data can reveal the relevant truth regarding the

---

[10] Heidegger, "Question Concerning Technology," 11.

therapy: Does it work? Psychotherapy, in this way, becomes a means alone, a technology for which the human object may serve as raw material.

It is not surprising, therefore, that psychologists routinely refer to their particular therapeutic models as forms of technology. The cognitive-behavioral therapists Michael Addis and Neil Jacobson, for example, describe their approach in this manner:

> As CBT technology becomes widely disseminated into practice, studies of therapeutic competence in specific skills such as increasing homework compliance should become an increasing priority.[11]

Julieann Pankey and Steven Hayes refer to ACT in similar terms as a technology for overcoming the patterns of avoidance associated with many forms of psychological distress:

> Rather than attempt to change the content of undesirable perceptions, thoughts, or feelings, RFT [relational frame theory] suggests that the main way to weaken the negative behavioral impact of these events is to alter the context supporting cognitive fusion and experiential avoidance. ACT is a technology designed to accomplish that end.[12]

To be fair, Hayes and colleagues have also described ACT as "not just a technology," noting that it is, rather, a "functionally defined" method for producing "psychological flexibility" and that any method or set of techniques derived from the theory of psychological flexibility on which the therapy relies could be labeled "ACT." In other words, the psychotherapy known as "ACT" is not merely a specific technology or set of techniques but also a matrix of *possible* technologies pragmatically

---

[11] Michael E. Addis and Neil S. Jacobson, "A Closer Look at the Treatment Rationale and Homework Compliance in Cognitive-Behavioral Therapy for Depression," *Cognitive Therapy and Research* 24 (2000): 324.

[12] Julieann Pankey and Steven C. Hayes, "Acceptance and Commitment Therapy for Psychosis," *International Journal of Psychology and Psychological Therapy* 3, no. 2 (2003): 316.

derived from a functional theory.[13] Whatever techniques work in accordance with the theory of psychological flexibility would belong to the larger set of ACT technologies.

There can be no doubt here, however, that psychotherapies are conceptualized as technological means to clinical ends and that they should be evaluated according to specific functional criteria. Ironically, the developers of ACT have identified their proposed technological solution as a means of overcoming "the repertoire-narrowing effects of an excessive reliance on a problem-solving mode of mind."[14] In this sense, what ACT's therapeutic technologies provide are applications of problem-solving methods specifically designed to address the problems that arise in response to the constraining effects of reducing human beings to means and the objects of means.

At the level of the individual, scientific psychotherapies informed by the evidence-based treatment movement have always rested on the quantification of operationally defined psychological processes. A few examples of these—and it should be noted that there are dozens, if not hundreds, in active research—include "emotion regulation," "experiential avoidance," "psychological flexibility," "uncertainty tolerance," and "thought-action fusion."

These processes are defined in terms that are intended for universal application. In other words, there is no one—from the day-laborer in Papua, New Guinea to the high-tech billionaire in Palo Alto, California— for whom these processes would not have relevance. The mission of the clinical researcher is to identify processes, many of which are considered to have served evolutionary functions for human beings, that can facilitate the clinician's ability to—to use one formulation popular among psychological scientists—"predict and influence behavior with precision, scope, and depth."[15]

---

[13] Steven C. Hayes, Kirk D. Strosahl, and Kelly G. Wilson, *Acceptance and Commitment Therapy: The Process and Practice of Mindful Change*, 2nd ed., (New York: Guilford), 97.

[14] Hayes et al., *Acceptance and Commitment Therapy*, 97.

[15] Sean Hughes, "The Philosophy of Science as It Applies to Clinical Psychology," in *Process-Based CBT: The Science and Core Clinical Competencies of Cognitive Behavioral*

Each of these psychological processes is inscribed in a system of quantification using self-report instruments (i.e., questionnaires) on which individuals rate the degree of their engagement in behaviors believed to be indicative of the underlying process. A person who is having difficulty with emotion regulation may be asked, for example, to rate on a scale of 1 (*almost never*) to 5 (*almost always*) a series of statements concerning emotional responding, such as the following from a scale concerning emotional responding:

1. "I experience my emotions as overwhelming and out of control."
2. "When I am upset, I become out of control."
3. "When I am upset, I feel out of control."
4. "When I'm upset, I feel like I can remain in control of my behaviors."
5. "When I am upset, I have difficulty controlling my behaviors."
6. "When I'm upset, I lose control over my behavior."[16]

These six items make up the Impulse Control Difficulties subscale of the Difficulties in Emotion Regulation Scale (DERS). Individuals who reply toward the "almost always" end of the scale on these items would be considered likely to have problems with impulse control, and therapeutic interventions to facilitate either modulation of strong emotions or a heightened sense of self-possession would likely be tried. The measure would also serve as a means of monitoring progress toward alleviating the problem.

Available norms for the DERS indicate that those without clinically significant distress ($n = 808$) have a mean score of 12.22 on those six items, an average score of just above 2 per item on the 1 to 5 scale.[17] That score is

---

Therapy, ed. Steven C. Hayes and Stefan G. Hofmann, (Oakland, CA: New Harbinger, 2018), 35.

[16] Kim L. Gratz and Lizabeth Roemer, "Multidimensional Assessment of Emotion Regulation and Dysregulation: Development, Factor Structure, and Initial Validation of the Difficulties in Emotion Regulation Scale," *Journal of Psychopathology and Behavioral Assessment* 26, no. 1 (2004): 48.

[17] Luciano Giromini, Francesca Ales, Gaia de Campora, Alessandro Zennaro, and Claudia Pignolo, "Developing Age and Gender Adjusted Normative Reference Values

"age- and gender-adjusted," meaning that it is the expected score when gender and age values are controlled or held constant. By contrast, a large ($n = 341$) clinical sample of individuals with diagnoses of bipolar disorder obtains a mean score of 15.37 or just over 2.5 per item, while a similar-sized group ($n = 381$) of individuals with diagnoses of borderline personality disorder, a psychiatric condition associated with severe emotional distress, obtain a mean of 19.35 or about 3.2 per item.[18]

My point in sharing these findings here is twofold. On the one hand, they offer a clear example of the potential utility of quantitative measures in distinguishing between those who are experiencing what one might consider ordinary emotion regulation difficulties and those whose impulse control problems may warrant clinical intervention. On the other, they also illustrate a way of thinking about human beings, and particular aspects of a human being's behavior, that is devoid of any contextual detail. This stripping away of the context in which experiences and behaviors are embedded completes the "bringing-forth" of human beings as standing reserve. In this case, individuals become populations, and populations become storehouses for predictable, standardized quantities of dysfunction.

These quantitative methods, regardless of their clinical utility in alleviating psychological distress, exemplify what Andrew Feenberg has called the "functional rationality" dimension of technology, which "isolates objects from their original context in order to incorporate them into theoretical or functional systems."[19] As Feenberg observes in discussing the "double aspect" of technology, functional rationality is "inextricably intertwined"

for the Difficulties in Emotion Regulation Scale (DERS)," *Journal of Psychopathology and Behavioral Assessment* 39, no. 4 (2017): 710.

[18] Christopher J. Fowler et al., "Differentiating Bipolar Disorder from Borderline Personality Disorder: Diagnostic Accuracy of the Difficulty in Emotion Regulation Scale and Personality Inventory For DSM-5," *Journal of Affective Disorders* 245 (2019): 858.

[19] Andrew Feenberg, "Democratic Rationalization: Technology, Power, and Freedom" in *Readings in the Philosophy of Technology*, 2nd ed., ed. David M. Kaplan (Lanham, MD: Rowman and Littlefield, 2009), 147.

with social meaning, though the functional aspect may be viewed in a decontextualized way so that it is not understood as a social activity.[20]

What is missing from this context-independent view, one might say, is the recognition that a particular mode of revealing (i.e., Enframing) is at work. Even those who adopt contextualist perspectives within clinical psychological science find themselves fetishizing the functional dimension of their efforts. "Utility," the pragmatic means, is all. Techniques and technologies may be drawn from anywhere—they may even prioritize contemplative perspectives or reflective modes of awareness—as long as they contribute to the therapy's "workability." Some social determinants of this functional dimension (i.e., what renders a technique "useful" with a specific population) might be examined on occasion, but the underlying imperative to demonstrate utility is never in question.

The production of scientific clinical knowledge, in the case of the DERS, is contingent upon the construal of responses to verbal prompts—the six "impulse control" items, for example—as the means for calling forth an "object," a latent construct that characterizes a dimension of human experience and behavior. Moreover, this "object" of empirical inquiry replaces the unique occurrences that arise in the hundreds of specific contexts of those individuals whose aggregated data provides the mean scores. One person has been up for three consecutive nights nursing a colicky infant; the other faces daily conversations with a parent with worsening dementia who begs to leave the nursing home; and still another, experienced his first disappointment in love, the break-up of an exhilarating college romance. Their answers on the measure of emotion regulation and impulse control, however, may be similarly elevated.

Likewise, in the clinical setting, the psychotherapist adopting an evidence-based approach to treatment compares the decontextualized score of the individual in treatment to the aggregated norms as a way of ascertaining the progress of treatment or the severity of the problem to be addressed. The unique historical and relational situation in which the individual is

---

[20] Feenberg, "Democratic Rationalization," 147.

embedded falls away as the scientific dimensions of the "emotion regulation problem" are revealed.

The danger here, like the peril that Heidegger identifies in Enframing and modern technology, is that this decontextualized quantification of experience, though contingent on human behavior, is an "already unconcealed" phenomenon into which human beings themselves are called forth. That is, the method of quantification and decontextualization, coupled with the unquestioned valorization of the pragmatic, reveals human experience to have specifiable dimensions; it gathers human beings into the technological mode of ordering, as Heidegger would say, and destines them to constitute themselves as standing-reserve.

Many critics of the evidence-based treatment movement have highlighted the weaknesses of the scientific methods on which the movement's proponents have relied. In *The End of Average*, Todd Rose draws on the work of quantitative psychologist Peter Molenaar to expose the faulty assumptions behind the aggregation of data and comparison of group means as modes of evaluating human behavior.[21]

For example, Rose points out, the statistical analyses that inform the comparison of group means and standardized distributions of data are predicated on the assumptions of the ergodic theorem, which stipulate that: (a) all members of the group to be aggregated are identical, and (b) all members of the group will remain the same in the future. Neither of these assumptions, as Molenaar and Rose have noted, has ever been true for human beings.

Similarly, critics have highlighted the problems associated with evaluating treatments for psychiatric diagnoses that themselves lack an adequate empirical foundation.[22] Still others have pointed to the, at least implicit,

---

[21] Todd Rose, *The End of Average: How We Succeed in a World That Values Sameness* (New York: Harper Collins, 2015), 63-65; Peter C. M. Molenaar, "Consequences of the Ergodic Theorems for Classical Test Theory, Factor Analysis, and the Analysis of Developmental Processes," in *Handbook of Cognitive Aging*, ed. Scott M. Hofer and Duane F. Alvin (Thousand Oaks, CA: 2008), 91-93.

[22] John Cromby, David Harper, and Paula Reavey, *Psychology, Mental Health, and Distress* (New York: Palgrave MacMillan, 2013), 106-107; Allen Frances, "DSM,

medicalization of thoughts, behaviors, and emotions that characterizes the evidence-based treatment model.[23]

When confronted with the inadequacy of group means and standard deviations as methods for predicting behavior, proponents of quantification and the technological articulation of human psychological experience merely shift their focus to momentary ecological assessment, tracking and modeling individuals' idiographic trajectories for later aggregation.[24] The processes of "challenging forth" human beings according to particular predefined, precisely quantified constructs continue unabated, albeit with newer, more robust, and ecologically valid methods.

A psychology that makes use of Heidegger's questioning of technology, however, need not depend on unraveling flawed scientific arguments or rectifying insufficiently rigorous empirical methods. In fact, Heidegger makes clear that his critique of Enframing is not predicated on finding fault with scientific reasoning.

From a methodological standpoint, any miscalculation or violation of assumptions can be addressed through a modification of analytical methods. Science is self-correcting in this regard. As Heidegger concedes, the mode of revealing by which "nature presents itself as a calculable complex of the effects of forces" does allow for "correct determinations."[25] Inaccuracy or scientific error is not what is at issue. The danger that Heidegger identifies is that it is precisely amid "all that is correct" in the

---

Psychotherapy, Counseling and the Medicalization of Mental Illness: A Commentary from Allen Frances," *The Professional Counselor* 4, no. 3 (2014): 282-284; Gary Greenberg, *The Book of Woe: The DSM and the Unmaking of Psychiatry* (New York: Penguin, 2013), 52-53.

[23] Dalal, *CBT*, 59; Cromby et al., *Psychology*, 102-103.

[24] Steven C. Hayes, Joseph Ciarrochi, Stefan G. Hoffman, Fredrick Chin, and Baljinder Sahdra, "Evolving an Idionomic Approach to Processes of Change: Towards a Unified Personalized Science of Human Improvement," *Behaviour Research and Therapy* (2022): 104155. As Hayes and colleagues observe, the overthrow of conventional statistics requiring ergodicity need not defeat efforts to model human behavior and responses to psychological intervention for purposes of scientific prediction and control.

[25] Heidegger, "Question Concerning Technology," 19.

mode of technological revealing that the truth regarding human beings "will withdraw."[26]

That is, human beings find it increasingly difficult to extricate themselves from attending to Enframing and its mode of revealing nature—"the frenziedness of ordering."[27] Other vital human endeavors, including other ways of bringing-forth, are thoroughly subordinated to the technological mode of revealing. The means by which human beings are classified and understood have displaced any possibility of discussing the ends of human life.

Vague considerations such as "psychological flexibility," "emotion regulation," and "psychological well-being" serve as therapy's stated aims, yet it is easy to recognize that these are merely means that have been re-stated as ends. Their meaning, as such, is not open to public debate or poetic evocation in the manner of the human values of prior eras (e.g., "love," "dignity," "freedom," or even "health"), but merely to measurement through ostensibly reliable means.

From "Anti-vitalism" to the "Universality of Illness"

This subordination of the personal to the technological is, I would argue, the danger that confronts clinical psychological science. One problem that has vexed psychology as a discipline since its emergence from philosophy in the nineteenth century is its standing as a science. Countless academic debates and papers have taken as their starting point the question of whether psychology is or can be a science—or whether it is merely a profession with scientific pretensions.[28]

---

[26] Heidegger, "Question Concerning Technology," 19.

[27] Heidegger, "Question Concerning Technology," 22.

[28] Martin E. Morf, "Agency, Chance, and the Scientific Status of Psychology," *Integrative Psychological and Behavioral Science* 52, no. 4 (2018): 494; Christopher J. Ferguson, "'Everybody Knows Psychology Is Not a Real Science': Public Perceptions of Psychology and How We Can Improve Our Relationship with Policymakers, the Scientific Community, and the General Public," *American Psychologist* 70, no. 6 (2015): 538-539; Scott O. Lilienfeld, "Public Skepticism of Psychology: Why Many People Perceive the Study of Human Behavior as Unscientific," *American Psychologist* 67, no. 2 (2012): 111, 115-116.

The consensus among psychologists has been that the more rigorously empirical (and statistical) one's methods are, the more scientific they are. As a result, positivist and post-positivist approaches, both relying on the hypothetico-deductive method, became the field's de facto modes of inquiry.[29] Some, including Valery Chirkov and Jade Anderson, have referred to these disciplinary touchstones as the "myths" of psychological science.[30]

In adopting these methods, scientific psychology also largely adopted a "correspondence theory of truth" (i.e., a view that the scientific knowledge that the field produces accurately reflects the actual nature of phenomena in the world).[31] The contribution of the method and the contextual standpoint of the psychologist to the object of study is considered only as a source of error, something one attempts to account for and control, either statistically or methodologically.[32] More recently, functional contextualist approaches have eschewed concerns with correspondence in favor of a pragmatic scientific problem-solving that does not make ontological claims. Regardless, quantification and the hypthetico-deductive method remain the necessary tools of the trade when construing psychological phenomena.

Indeed, in their efforts to enhance psychology's standing as a science, psychologists have historically insisted upon the terms of Emil Dubois-Reymond and Hermann von Helmholtz's famous "anti-vitalist oath."[33] In 1842, Dubois-Reymond and Ernst Brücke, together with two other leading

[29] Hughes, "Philosophy of Science," 27-28. Mark H. Bickhard, "The Tragedy of Operationalism," *Theory & Psychology* 11, no. 1 (2001): 36-37.

[30] Valery Chirkov and Jade Anderson, "Statistical Positivism Versus Critical Scientific Realism. A Comparison of Two Paradigms for Motivation Research: Part 1. A Philosophical and Empirical Analysis of Statistical Positivism," *Theory & Psychology* 28, no. 6 (2018): 714. See also Leonard G. Rorer, "Some Myths of Science in Psychology," in *Thinking Clearly About Psychology*, ed. Dante Cicchetti and William M. Grove (Minneapolis, MN: University of Minnesota Press, 1991), 71, 75-77.

[31] Hughes, "Philosophy of Science," 27-28; Brian D. Haig and Denny Borsboom, "Truth, Science, and Psychology," *Theory & Psychology* 22, no. 3 (2012): 279-280.

[32] Hughes, "Philosophy of Science," 34-35; Molenaar, "Consequences of Ergodic Theorems," 92-93. Rose, *End of Average*, 124-125.

[33] B. R. Hergenhahn, *An Introduction to the History of Psychology*, 6th ed. (Belmont, CA: Wadsworth, 2009), 237.

European scientists of the time, Hermann von Helmholtz and Carl Ludwig, agreed to constrain scientific explanations to a description of physical or chemical processes. These scientists, all of whom were students of Johannes Müller, a towering figure in nineteenth-century science (who subscribed to vitalist ideas), headed some of the most influential laboratories in Europe; collectively, they came to be identified as the "Helmholtz school."[34]

Sigmund Freud studied physiology with Brücke and chemistry with Ludwig. Wilhelm Wundt, the founding figure of experimental psychology and teacher of William James and G. Stanley Hall, studied with both DuBois-Reymond and Helmholtz.[35] When applied in the context of human psychology, this assumption extends the Cartesian view of animals as machines to human beings. Others had, of course, made this leap already including, famously, Julian Offray de La Mettrie in his *Man, a Machine* of 1747 and Claude Adrien Helvétius in *On the Spirit* in 1758.[36] The anti-vitalist movement, however, systematically installed this methodological assumption in European science.

While figures like Wundt, James, and Freud explored aspects of human experience and behavior that resisted reductionistic explanation and a simplistic correspondence theory of truth, the commitment to identifying, at some point, a "physical-chemical" explanation for psychological phenomena characterized all their work. For Wundt and Freud, though not for James, even the divine and that uniquely human mode of revealing truth, the poetic, could be explained, ultimately, as biological (i.e., physical-chemical) phenomena.[37]

---

[34] Robert R. Holt, "Two Influences on Freud's Scientific Thought: A Fragment of Intellectual Biography," in *The Study of Lives: Essays on Personality in Honor of Henry A. Murray,* ed. Robert W. White and Katherine F. Bruner (Upper Saddle River, NJ: Prentice-Hall, 1963), 372.

[35] Hergenhahn, *History of Psychology,* 264-265, 337, 354.

[36] See John C. O'Neal, *The Authority of the Senses: Sensationist Theory in the French Enlightenment* (University Park, PA: Penn State University Press, 1996), 84-85, 197-198.

[37] George Herbert Mead, "The Imagination in Wundt's Treatment of Myth and Religion," *Psychological Bulletin* 3, no. 12 (1906): 394-395; Sigmund Freud, *The Future of an Illusion,* ed. and trans. James Strachey (New York: W. W. Norton, 1961), 53.

James, who espoused theistic views of an empirical sort, believed that human experience, which could be explained in terms of "reflex action," contributed to conceptualizations of God. Yet he also envisioned a God "behind the universe" outside the scope of science: a "confession of an ultimate opacity in things, of a dimension of being which escapes our theoretic control."[38]

At the same time, over the course of the nineteenth century, the movement toward understanding psychological distress not as mere "madness" but as "mental illness" — reflective of a latent physical disease process — began to take shape. Diagnostic taxonomies for categorizing and specifying psychiatric conditions emerged in the work of Jean-Martin Charcot and Emile Kraepelin, followed by that of Richard von Krafft-Ebing, Eugen Bleuler, and Adolf Meyer.[39]

These figures focused on identifying neurological lesions or other markers of underlying disease as explanations for psychological symptoms. In some cases, these were found, as when Krafft-Ebing and his research laboratory identified syphilis as a potential contributor to various forms of psychiatric illness.[40] Efforts to understand the physiological bases of psychological suffering expanded considerably throughout the twentieth century, and to be sure, biological psychiatry, though beset with ethical and scientific crises, remains a powerful, if not hegemonic, discourse in the mental health field.[41]

Indeed, members of the general public increasingly espouse biological explanations for psychological distress, despite the absence of any recognized biomarkers and lack of supporting empirical research.[42] Yet

---

[38] William James, *The Will to Believe and Other Essays in Popular Philosophy* (New York: Dover, 1956), 88, 93.

[39] Anne Harrington, *The Mind Fixers: Psychiatry's Troubled Search for the Biology of Mental Illness* (New York: W. W. Norton, 2019), 14-18, 30, 38-43.

[40] Harrington, *Mind Fixers*, 30.

[41] Harrington, *Mind Fixers*, 272-274.

[42] Joel Paris, *Overdiagnosis in Psychiatry: How Modern Psychiatry Lost Its Way While Creating a Diagnosis for Almost All of Life's Misfortunes*, 2nd ed. (New York: Oxford University Press, 2020), 9-10; Matthew S. Lebowitz and Paul S. Appelbaum, "Biomedical Explanations of Psychopathology and Their Implications for Attitudes and Beliefs About Mental Disorders," *Annual Review of Clinical Psychology* 15 (2019): 560-561.

these pathologizing and medicalizing discourses have also constituted and construed human beings in a particular way. As Michel Foucault noted, such discourses were "dangerous" — that is, they had unavoidable political dimensions, and they determined what it was to be sick or to be well, normal or pathological. In so doing, they relegated previously uncontrolled dimensions of human experience to the territory of illness and the jurisdiction of the clinical specialist.[43]

Madness, thus, becomes marginalized or, in Foucault's terms, reason "indefinitely repels madness to its outer limits."[44] Nevertheless, its persistent presence, as in the work of great artists and thinkers such as Van Gogh, Nietzsche, and Artaud, demands from rational discourse "an explanation for this unreason."[45] Foucault argues that the patient-clinician relationship ultimately becomes a "monologue by reason about madness" and that the clinically "serene world of mental illness" admits of no dialogue — and no articulation of the irruption in reason that psychological suffering represents.[46]

The "abstract universality of illness," Foucault contends, then serves as the means by which madness or suffering can be tamed and channeled. It also provides the means through which specified human beings are constituted, in Heideggerian terms, as "the supply of patients for a clinic" so that they may then be designated for quantitative assessment and treatment by clinical professionals employing scientific methods and following empirically supported algorithms.[47]

Releasement, Meditation, and Mystery

The combination of the anti-vitalist movement in science and the systematic medicalization of psychological suffering have yielded the technological mode of ordering that contemporary clinical psychological science has become. Even as psychiatry has fallen into crisis with the

[43] Michel Foucault, *History of Madness*, ed. Jean Khalfa, trans. John Murphey and Jean Khalfa (New York: Routledge, 2006), 510.
[44] Foucault, *History of Madness*, 537.
[45] Foucault, *History of Madness*, 537.
[46] Foucault, *History of Madness*, xxviii.
[47] Foucault, *History of Madness*, xxviii; Heidegger, "Question Concerning Technology," 15.

exposure of its systematic collusion with pharmaceutical interests, psychological science has continued to constitute "patients" in the manner of the clinic—through the rubric of illness, diagnosis, and pathological processes.[48]

These processes, I would contend, are examples of Enframing, technology's mode of revealing, at work on human beings. Clinical psychology becomes a rhetoric of well-being, the purpose of which, at least in part, is to ensure assent to the technological order that construes human beings in terms of measurable, operationalized constructs. The technologies of the self that clinical psychological science offers are presented as pathways to improved functioning without questioning their subordination of ends to means.

Moreover, it becomes increasingly impossible to differentiate between the person and the technologies of selfing, well-being, emotion regulation, and the like, through which clinical psychology understands human behavior. As the human person is increasingly technologized, the self comes to be understood as a mere assemblage of techniques, evaluated according to functional parameters (i.e., can I do what I am expected to do?).

Although Heidegger offers no specific alternative to technology's ascendency, he suggests the possibility of identifying such an answer within the essence of technology itself. Quoting Hölderlin, Heidegger intimates, "But where danger is, grows / The saving power also."[49] This "saving power," Heidegger suggests, may appear as Enframing if examined more carefully:

> If the essence of technology, Enframing, is the extreme danger, and if there is truth in Hölderlin's words, the rule of Enframing cannot

---

[48] See Steven C. Hayes, Stefan G. Hofmann, and Joseph Ciarrochi, "Building a Process-Based Diagnostic System: An Extended Evolutionary Approach," in *Beyond the DSM: Toward a Process-Based Alternative for Diagnosis and Mental Health Treatment*, ed. Steven C. Hayes and Stefan G. Hofmann (Oakland, CA: New Harbinger, 2020), 263-266. For a detailed account of the relationship between psychiatry and the pharmaceutical industry see, Robert Whitaker and Lisa Cosgrove, *Psychiatry Under the Influence: Institutional Corruption, Social Injury, and Prescriptions for Reform* (New York: Palgrave MacMillan, 2015), 6-10, 173-174.

[49] Heidegger, "Question Concerning Technology," 20.

exhaust itself solely in blocking all lighting-up of every revealing, all appearing of truth. Rather, precisely the essence of technology must harbor in itself the growth of the saving power. But in that case, might not an adequate look into what Enframing is as a destining of revealing bring into appearance the saving power in its arising?[50]

The tentative language here conveys the exploratory dimension of Heidegger's argument. Ultimately, his explorations of Enframing take him back to *technē*, the Greek word for "not only the activities and skills of the craftsman, but also for the arts of the mind and the fine arts."[51] In this designation, he finds a suggestion of a possible response, one which may have valuable implications for psychology:

> There was a time when it was not technology alone the bore the name *technē*. Once that revealing that brings forth truth into the splendor of radiant appearing also was called *technē*. Once there was a time when the bringing-forth of the true into the beautiful was called *technē*. And the *poiēsis* of the fine arts also was called *technē*.[52]

Heidegger concludes his essay with the cautious suggestion of a tension between the "poetic revealing" of the arts and "the frenziedness of technology."[53] In that tension, I would argue, lies what a psychology that is not entirely beholden to Enframing might have to offer.

In his Memorial Address, delivered in 1955 at a community celebration of the composer Conradin Kreutzer, Heidegger describes the adoption of a stance toward technology, "releasement toward things" (*Gelassenheit*), and advocates a mode of meditative thought, both of which could have significant implications for psychological dialogue. By "releasement," he refers to a simultaneous participation in technology *and* awareness of the implications of its mode of revealing.[54]

---

[50] Heidegger, "Question Concerning Technology," 20.
[51] Heidegger, "Question Concerning Technology," 13. 23.
[52] Heidegger, "Question Concerning Technology," 23.
[53] Heidegger, "Question Concerning Technology," 24.
[54] Martin Heidegger, *Discourse on Thinking: A Translation of* Gelassenheit, trans. John M. Anderson and E. Hans Freund (New York: Harper Perennial, 1966), 54.

The objective, as he describes it, is to "let technical devices enter our life, and at the same time leave them outside, that is leave them alone."[55] The possibility of approaching the technological revealing implicit in clinical psychological science in this way offers the prospect of a dialogue with the person who experiences suffering—a dialogue which does not, or at least does not exclusively, constitute the sufferer as a patient and the suffering as dysfunction. If one could adopt such a perspective, the grip of pathologizing discourses could be loosened, at least to some degree. More importantly, perhaps, the additional suffering that stems from conceptualizing oneself as "ill" or "abnormal"—and hence as a kind of raw material for a clinical industry—might be alleviated.

Amid such a "releasement" from psychological technology, the empirically supported techniques that clinical science has to offer (such as exposure therapy for anxiety, behavioral activation for depression, or even present-moment focus for emotion regulation) could be used in ways that remain practical but, at the same time, entail greater attention to the unique meaning and context of the individual's experience. These techniques need not entail the pathologization of experience and mechanization of the human person that have been the hallmarks of clinical psychological science. They could become one thing among many others rather than a categorical imperative.

In this newly emergent setting, there would be no need to pathologize anxiety, sadness, or intensity of feeling—and therapeutic responses to these experiences might cease to be mere "techniques" applied according to treatment algorithms. Neither the experience of psychological distress nor the therapeutic dialogue through which it is alleviated need be reduced to mechanisms or functional processes. They could become, also, artistic or poetic strategies, like the painting technique of *cangiantismo* or the poetic form of *terza rima*.

In short, techniques could enter therapy and, at the same time, vanish immediately with their application, just as the chisel departs with the appearance of a sculpture or the pen quits one's awareness when the verse

---

[55] Martin Heidegger, *Discourse on Thinking*, 54.

is composed. In this deprivileged sense, psychological techniques and their associated science would tell us little or nothing convincing or definitive about what a human being is, though they might be helpful tools when we are inquiring who a given person is.

In his 1959 essay "The Way to Language," Heidegger suggests that Enframing has a characteristic mode of thinking that distorts the workings of language—specifically, the "propriation," which gives rise to the "clearing" in which things come forth to presence—and the relationship between human speaking and listening.[56] The result is the dominance of calculative thinking, the problem-solving mode of thought:

> The Enframing because it sets upon human beings – that is, challenges them – to order everything that comes to presence into a technical inventory, unfolds essentially after the manner of propriation; at the same time, it distorts propriation, in as much as all ordering sees itself committed to calculative thinking and so speaks the language of Enframing. Speech is challenged to correspond to the ubiquitous orderability of what is present.[57]

In this way, he notes, speech becomes mere "information" as "Enframing, the essence of modern technology that holds sway everywhere, ordains for itself a formalized language—the kind of informing by virtue of which man is molded and adjusted into the technical-calculative creature."[58] Heidegger does, however, suggest another way of proceeding for "mortals, those who are needed and used for the speaking of language," an alternative to the ceaseless ordering and reductionism of Enframing.[59]

Specifically, in the Memorial Address, he offers "meditative thinking" as an antidote to the calculative thought that plans and computes "ever more promising and at the same time more economical possibilities."[60] Meditative thinking, by contrast, "contemplates the meaning which reigns

---

[56] Martin Heidegger, "The Way to Language," in *Basic Writings*, ed. David Farrell Krell (New York: Harper Perennial, 1993), 418.
[57] Heidegger, "The Way to Language," 420.
[58] Heidegger, "The Way to Language," 420-421.
[59] Heidegger, "The Way to Language," 423.
[60] Heidegger, *Discourse on Thinking*, 46.

in everything that is."[61] In this way of thinking, human beings "dwell on what lies close and meditate on what is closest; upon that which concerns us, each one of us, here and now; here, on this patch of home ground; now, in the present hour of history."[62]

Although allusions to "meditative thinking" may evoke psychological processes such as "mindfulness," Heidegger's discussions of "releasement" is, I believe, offering something more than the "nonjudgmental observation" in a "state of non-doing" that one finds in mindfulness-based psychotherapies.[63] Heidegger's description of meditative thinking, for example, suggests a kind of doing that involves "questioning," a questioning that explores the most hidden meanings of experience:

> That which shows itself and at the same time withdraws is the essential trait of what we call the mystery. I call the comportment which enables us to keep open the meaning hidden in technology, *openness to the mystery*.[64]

He goes on to state that "releasement toward things and openness to the mystery belong together."[65] In conjunction, releasement and meditative thinking (i.e., openness to the mystery) "grant us the possibility of dwelling in the world in a totally different way," one that is not "imperiled" by technology.[66] There is, in short, an irreducible mystery about the poetic word, one which reflects the mystery at the heart of the human person. Although poetic language has been marginalized amid the discourses of science and technology, which strive to reduce even language to its functional operations, it offers both continual renewal through the proliferation of possible meanings and intractable opacity that prevents its replacement with mere algorithms or calculations.

---

[61] Heidegger, *Discourse on Thinking*, 46.
[62] Heidegger, *Discourse on Thinking*, 47.
[63] Zindel Segal, Mark Williams, and John Teasdale. *Mindfulness-Based Cognitive Therapy for Depression* (New York: Guilford, 2018), 90-91.
[64] Heidegger, *Discourse on Thinking*, 55.
[65] Heidegger, *Discourse on Thinking*, 55.
[66] Heidegger, *Discourse on Thinking*, 55.

How can we differentiate our meditative or poetic thinking from the persistent machinations of calculative thought? At the close of the Memorial Address, Heidegger indicates that meditative thinking can become a ground for creativity, suggesting the potentially salvific activity of *poiēsis*. Where calculative thinking races from one problem to the next, counting on "definite results" to such an extent that it becomes automatic (or even thought-less), mediative thinking takes both time and "genuine craft."[67] It is a form of doing that is not technological but poetic, not a flight-from-thinking into automation but a "persevering meditation" in pursuit of meaning.[68]

In "The Way to Language," Heidegger observes that "every thinking that is on the trail of something is a poetizing, and all poetry a thinking."[69] Thinking of this kind demands a personal experience with the persistence of mystery, which gives rise to song (another word for the thinking that is a poetizing).

A psychology that practices both releasement toward things and openness to mystery could, in this way, become not merely a technology but also a verbal art, a poetic practice dedicated to the possibilities of mortal life. As a linguistic and, therefore, simultaneously personal and relational endeavor, it would foster not scientific certainty about behavior but the artistic freedom of the "psyche"—the sublime experience of the human person's encounter with mystery.

References

Addis, Michael E., and Neil S. Jacobson. "A Closer Look at the Treatment Rationale and Homework Compliance in Cognitive-Behavioral Therapy for Depression." *Cognitive Therapy and Research* 24 (2000): 313-326.

Bickhard, Mark H. "The Tragedy of Operationalism." *Theory & Psychology* 11, no. 1 (2001): 35-44.

---

[67] Heidegger, *Discourse on Thinking*, 45-47.
[68] Heidegger, *Discourse on Thinking*, 46.
[69] Heidegger, "The Way to Language," 425.

Bor, Harris. *Staying Human: A Jewish Theology for the Age of Artificial Intelligence*. Eugene, OR: Cascade Books, 2021.

Chirkov, Valery, and Jade Anderson. "Statistical Positivism Versus Critical Scientific Realism. A Comparison of Two Paradigms for Motivation Research: Part 1. A Philosophical and Empirical Analysis of Statistical Positivism." *Theory & Psychology* 28, no. 6 (2018): 712-736.

Cromby, John, David Harper, and Paula Reavey. *Psychology, Mental Health, and Distress*. New York: Palgrave MacMillan, 2013.

Dalal, Farhad. *CBT: The Cognitive Behavioral Tsunami: Managerialism, Politics, and the Corruptions of Science*. New York: Routledge, 2018.

Feenberg, Andrew. "Democratic Rationalization: Technology, Power, and Freedom." In *Readings in the Philosophy of Technology*, 2nd ed. Edited by David M. Kaplan, 139-155. Lanham, MD: Rowman and Littlefield, 2009.

Foucault, Michel. *History of Madness*. Edited by Jean Khalfa. Translated by John Murphey and Jean Khalfa. New York: Routledge, 2006.

Fowler, Christopher J., Alok Madan, Jon G. Allen, John M. Oldham, and B. Christopher Frueh. "Differentiating Bipolar Disorder from Borderline Personality Disorder: Diagnostic Accuracy of the Difficulty in Emotion Regulation Scale and Personality Inventory for DSM-5." *Journal of Affective Disorders* 245 (2019): 856-860.

Frances, Allen. "DSM, Psychotherapy, Counseling and the Medicalization of Mental Illness: A Commentary from Allen Frances," *The Professional Counselor* 4, no. 3 (2014): 282-284.

Freud, Sigmund. *The Future of an Illusion*. Edited and translated by James Strachey. New York: W. W. Norton, 1961.

Giromini, Luciano, Francesca Ales, Gaia de Campora, Alessandro Zennaro, and Claudia Pignolo. "Developing Age and Gender Adjusted Normative Reference Values for the Difficulties in Emotion Regulation Scale (DERS)." *Journal of Psychopathology and Behavioral Assessment* 39, no. 4 (2017): 705-714.

Gratz, Kim L., and Lizabeth Roemer. "Multidimensional Assessment of Emotion Regulation and Dysregulation: Development, Factor Structure, and Initial Validation of the Difficulties in Emotion Regulation

Scale." *Journal of Psychopathology and Behavioral Assessment* 26, no. 1 (2004): 41-54.

Greenberg, Gary. *The Book of Woe: The DSM and the Unmaking of Psychiatry.* New York: Penguin, 2013.

Haig, Brian D., and Denny Borsboom. "Truth, Science, and Psychology." *Theory & Psychology* 22, no. 3 (2012): 272-289.

Harrington, Anne. *The Mind Fixers: Psychiatry's Troubled Search for the Biology of Mental Illness.* New York: W. W. Norton, 2019.

Hayes, Steven C., Stefan G. Hofmann, and Joseph Ciarrochi. "Building a Process-Based Diagnostic System: An Extended Evolutionary Approach." In *Beyond the DSM: Toward a Process-Based Alternative for Diagnosis and Mental Health Treatment.* Edited by Steven C. Hayes and Stefan G. Hofmann, 251-279. Oakland, CA: New Harbinger, 2020.

Hayes, Steven C., Kirk D. Strosahl, and Kelly G. Wilson. *Acceptance and Commitment Therapy: The Process and Practice of Mindful Change.* 2nd ed. New York: The Guilford Press, 2012.

Heidegger, Martin. *Discourse on Thinking: A Translation of* Gelassenheit. Translated by John M. Anderson and E. Hans Freund. New York: Harper Perennial, 1966.

———. "The Question Concerning Technology." In *Readings in the Philosophy of Technology,* 2nd ed. Edited by David M. Kaplan, 9-24. Lanham, MD: Rowman and Littlefield, 2009.

———. "The Way to Language." In *Basic Writings.* Edited by David Farrell Krell, 397-426. New York: Harper Perennial, 1993.

Hergenhahn, B. R. *An Introduction to the History of Psychology.* 6th ed. Belmont, CA: Wadsworth, 2009.

Holt, Robert R. "Two Influences on Freud's Scientific Thought: A Fragment of Intellectual Biography." In *The Study of Lives: Essays on Personality in Honor of Henry A. Murray.* Edited by Robert W. White and Katherine F. Bruner, 365-387. Upper Saddle River, NJ: Prentice-Hall, 1963.

Hughes, Sean. "The Philosophy of Science as It Applies to Clinical Psychology." In *Process-Based CBT: The Science and Core Clinical Competencies of Cognitive Behavioral Therapy.* Edited by Steven C. Hayes and Stefan G. Hofmann, 23-42. Oakland, CA: New Harbinger, 2018.

James, William. *The Will to Believe and Other Essays in Popular Philosophy*. New York: Dover, 1956.

Lebowitz, Matthew S., and Paul S. Appelbaum. "Biomedical Explanations of Psychopathology and Their Implications for Attitudes and Beliefs About Mental Disorders." *Annual Review of Clinical Psychology* 15 (2019): 555-577.

Lilienfeld, Scott O. "Public Skepticism of Psychology: Why Many People Perceive the Study of Human Behavior as Unscientific." *American Psychologist* 67, no. 2 (2012): 111-129.

Mead, George Herbert. "The Imagination in Wundt's Treatment of Myth and Religion." *Psychological Bulletin* 3, no. 12 (1906): 393-399.

Molenaar, Peter C. M. "Consequences of the Ergodic Theorems for Classical Test Theory, Factor Analysis, and the Analysis of Developmental Processes." In *Handbook of Cognitive Aging*. Edited by Scott M. Hofer and Duane F. Alvin, 90-104. Thousand Oaks, CA: 2008.

Morf, Martin E. "Agency, Chance, and the Scientific Status of Psychology." *Integrative Psychological and Behavioral Science* 52, no. 4 (2018): 491-507.

O'Neal, John C. *The Authority of the Senses: Sensationist Theory in the French Enlightenment*. University Park, PA: Penn State University Press, 1996.

Pankey, Julieann, and Steven C. Hayes. "Acceptance and Commitment Therapy for Psychosis." *International Journal of Psychology and Psychological Therapy* 3, no. 2 (2003): 311-328.

Paris, Joel. *Overdiagnosis in Psychiatry: How Modern Psychiatry Lost Its Way While Creating a Diagnosis for Almost All of Life's Misfortunes*. 2nd ed. New York: Oxford University Press, 2020.

Rorer, Leonard G. "Some Myths of Science in Psychology." In *Thinking Clearly About Psychology*. Edited by Dante Cicchetti and William M. Grove, 61-87. Minneapolis, MN: University of Minnesota Press, 1991.

Rose, Todd. *The End of Average: How We Succeed in a World That Values Sameness*. New York: Harper Collins, 2015.

Segal, Zindel, Mark Williams, and John Teasdale. *Mindfulness-based Cognitive Therapy for Depression*. New York: Guilford, 2018.

Whitaker, Robert, and Lisa Cosgrove. *Psychiatry Under the Influence: Institutional Corruption, Social Injury, and Prescriptions for Reform*. New York: Palgrave MacMillan, 2015.

A First Person Principle: Philosophical Reflections on Narrative Practice Within a Mainstream Psychiatric Service for Young People

Philippa Byers and David Newman

Abstract: *This paper is a collaboration between David Newman, an experienced narrative therapy practitioner and teacher, and Philippa Byers, at the time of writing a narrative therapy student with an academic background in philosophy. The paper charts ideas developed during Philippa's student placement with David as they discussed narrative practice, other mental health practices, and philosophy. The paper draws on philosophy of language and the philosophy of Paul Ricoeur, applying this to Michael White's injunction to look (and listen) for the experience-near in the words and phrases that are offered to narrative therapists. It offers philosophical reflections on an ethical principle of narrative practice which Philippa and David call a first person principle. The first person principle is elaborated in a discussion of David's narrative practice with young people. This offers philosophical and practical insights to some of the issues and questions that may arise for narrative therapists who, like David, practice within mainstream services, encountering 'neuro' and other professionalised discourses and accompanying expectations.*

Acknowledgment: This chapter was first published in the *International Journal of Narrative Therapy and Community Work* (2019, no. 1). It is included here with permission from Dulwich Centre Publications.

Introduction

This paper is a collaboration between Philippa, a student (at the time of this writing) with a background in philosophy, and David, an experienced narrative therapy practitioner with an interest in developing ideas and resources for narrative practice from new sources. Working with young people in creative ways has been a focus of David's practice over many years. The central theme of the paper is a philosophical and practical investigation of a principle within, or for, narrative practice that we call a *first person principle*. We summarise this practice principle as follows:

> As a narrative therapist speaks with an individual, they attend to what is offered as 'mine' in the first person speech they hear, and they also recognise and respect the distinctive authority that accompanies thoughts, actions, observations, descriptions, hopes and feelings that are offered as 'one's' own or as 'mine'. A narrative therapist then places a practice limit on their own speech, and their own authority: They are guided by the terms and phrases they hear, and do not substitute them with alternative terms and phrases from professional discourses.

The first half of the paper contains Philippa's observations of David's narrative therapy practice, from her perspective as a learner or beginner in narrative practice. This section also explains the first person principle in more detail, arising from philosophical ideas that came to mind as Philippa attempted to make sense of the differences between David's narrative practice and other mental health practices within a hospital setting.

In the second half of the paper, David reflects on the first person principle and describes some practice examples. This includes discussion of a distinction between personal and impersonal discourses, with specific reference to the increasing use of neuroscience discourse within therapeutic settings and in therapeutic conversations.

There is discussion of the first person principle applied in narrative practice with the written word. And a discussion of how the principle assists in bringing distinctive meanings and insights to light in contrast to a focus on types of mental illness and brain disorder as the primary causes of a young person's pain or distress.

David's reflections may be useful for other narrative therapists working within the mainstream psychiatric services where, as this paper suggests, the practice of narrative therapy may appear to lack the professional authority of other approaches. We believe the first person principle can be employed as a form of resistance to professionalised, and at times impersonal, discourses. And, as we hope will be clear to readers of Michael White's work, the paper is also a sustained reflection on his injunction to seek and retrieve words, phrases and meanings that are *experience-near* (White, 2007, p. 40) or *decentred* (White, 1997, p. 200).

Part 1—From Philippa: Developing a philosophical sense of David's practice

I recently undertook a student placement at a mental health service for young people within a hospital and was supervised by David Newman who is an experienced social worker and a dedicated narrative therapy practitioner and teacher. Although the practice of narrative therapy was new to me, philosophical ideas about narrative were not. I've previously studied and taught philosophy, with a focus on moral philosophy and theories of identity and agency. While I observed David's practice and talked with him about narrative therapy and working with young people, ideas from philosophy of language and Paul Ricoeur's seminal work on narrative identity and temporality often came to mind.[1]

I was new to the field of mental health and to hospital settings, and was trying to figure out who was who, and who did what. I attempted to grasp the 'why' of what gets done, and to find out about professional hierarchies and treatment priorities. I was very curious about how a narrative therapy practice fits within a multidisciplinary, mainstream psychiatric service, particularly when diagnostic categories and psychological therapies are given considerable priority. During this time, I also read some of David's work, and some of the early work on narrative therapy by Michael White and others.[2]

As time went on, I noticed that David's therapeutic skills with young people were highly valued by his hospital co-workers. However, I also wondered whether others understood that a distinctive discipline shaped those skills. Perhaps personal gifts are drawn on when working with people who are in pain. And among those with such gifts, my guess is that David would rate very highly. But I did wonder whether his narrative therapy practice was perhaps interpreted in terms of a personal style or a personal gift, and not recognised as a distinctive and disciplined practice with (what seemed to me) an ethical imperative or principle.

I initially wrote a version of this reflection to unpack the differences between David's practice and other mainstream approaches, and as a means to orient myself as a 'would-be' social worker. I was seeking an approach I could endorse in philosophical and ethical terms, and thought that David's narrative practice, specifically its distinction from other approaches, might provide a clue. David and I then discussed and reworked these written ideas and considered how to apply them in practice. This section of the paper is on the preliminary ideas, David's section later in the paper brings them to light in discussions of his practice with young people.

In my view, narrative therapy is not just one more branch of empirically based psychology.[3] I believe it to be a distinctive and disciplined practice, rather than a 'soft' or unscientific version of psychology. As I thought and wrote about the differences between narrative therapy and empirically based mental health practices, I also considered parallels between ideas in philosophy and what I was observing in David's practice.

I claim no expertise here, but it seems to me that psychiatry and clinical psychology claim or acquire legitimacy from their status as empirical sciences and that the two broad fields share some overarching commitments. These are:

1. to identify the possible causes of mental distress
2. to devise therapeutic interventions that counteract the effects of possible antecedent causes
3. to generalise from a number of specific instances to larger populations
4. to make predictions about the likelihood of specific effects arising from specific causes, and the likely efficacy of interventions.

In contrast, it seems to me that narrative therapy does not characterise problems in the same terms, that is, in terms of causes and effects. And it does not draw inferences from small groups to larger populations of human 'subjects.'[4] This is a quick characterisation, and I acknowledge that the idea of 'cause' is not necessarily taken for granted in psychiatry and psychology, nor are the distinctions and interrelations between causes, correlations, influences and consequences.

Nonetheless, these thoughts did raise some questions: If narrative therapy does not identify antecedent causes of mental distress, what is its legitimacy as a therapeutic practice? Without a commitment to antecedent causes, from where, or on what basis, does narrative therapy devise therapeutic interventions? If narrative therapy does not specify norms of health or function, what does narrative therapy aim at in assisting people?

When I posed these questions to David, his usual response was to say that he saw his role within the service as privileging the knowledge of young people by 'retrieving' the words and phrases that they use to convey their own experience, and their quite specific and often unseen efforts to deal with the problems they face.

The retrieval and privileging of first person speech

On a number of occasions, I observed – or heard – the retrieval of distinctive words and phrases as David spoke with young people. Reflecting on what seemed to be David's insistence on retrieving the words and phrases of young people led me to think about ideas concerning first person speech, as discussed in philosophy of language. I then connected these ideas to several ideas in Ricoeur's work and in early phenomenological philosophy.

I'll begin with first person speech. First person speech, involving the first person referent – 'I' – is distinct in a number of ways, some more obvious than others, from second-person speech addressing 'you', and third-person speech in which 'they' are spoken of. Although I won't properly elaborate the point here, these three modes of address are more than convenient ways to identify who is being referred to when someone speaks. I suggest the differences between these modes of address are 'lived' or deeply experienced.[5]

There is a distinct phenomenological quality – a characteristic 'mineness' as Ricoeur would say – that is bound up with first person speech.[6] There is a specific 'something' that it is 'like' to refer to oneself in the first person, to narrate one's actions, experiences, thoughts and feelings with words such as 'I', 'my', 'mine', 'me' and 'myself'.

The phenomenological quality of first person speech – as 'mine' – is connected to a specific kind of authority. This is the authority that goes with being the person who is uniquely placed to narrate actions, experiences, thoughts and feelings as one's own, as 'mine'. Although it is related, the authority of first person speech is not the same as truthfulness. We can be mistaken in our first person claims, say, when memory fails us, and we can intentionally mislead when speaking about our thoughts, intentions, actions and feelings.

The authority of first person speech and, by extension, of first person narratives, is raised in a debate that starts with Wittgenstein, about whether self-referring speech has an 'immunity to error through misidentification'.[7] We have a strong presumption that first person speech is immune to mistakes of identification, and thus of reference. When I speak in the first person, I don't need to check whether or not the person I refer to as 'I' is, in fact, me. When I say 'I', the referent of this term is invariably me.

While the 'immunity to error through misidentification' of self-referring speech is a related philosophical issue, my concern here is the *experience* of first personal authority. This is the experience that accompanies being uniquely placed to narrate one's own actions, experiences, thoughts, hopes and feelings. Others can narrate my actions, experiences, thoughts and feelings, but their words have a different sense and a different form of authority; they do not have first personal authority as they lack the lived experience that first person speech uniquely communicates.[8]

What I observed in David's practice was a stance of accepting and giving priority to the words of young people, and their descriptions of their experience. Their words and their descriptions were accepted and prioritised as uniquely authoritative in the first personal sense I've just described. Reflecting on this brought to mind a foundational idea in early phenomenology, which is that experience is the ground and returning point of philosophical investigation.[9]

To put this another way, experience is not investigated philosophically to get to deeper forms of truth beyond or underlying experience; for phenomenology, the purpose of carefully describing experience is to show how meaning arises for a person out of their experience.[10]

As I observed David's work 'retrieving' and then 'privileging' the words and phrases of young people, I wondered whether the therapeutic effect of such conversations may stem from words and phrases being credited as authoritative, along with the agency and experience of agency that accompany speaking authoritatively about one's experiences. This may seem like a small point, or one so obvious it requires no special skills within a therapeutic setting such as a mainstream psychiatric service. But I think this would be a mistake.

At one point, David commented on his hope for young people: that they leave the psychiatric service having some 'experience of themselves as *knowledged*'. If I understood him correctly, I venture that components of the experience David hopes for young people are:

1. that they experience their own words as authoritative, from their perspective and that of others
2. that they experience their voice as an exercise of first personal agency

This seems particularly important when mental health issues are often experienced as something that is happening *to* 'me' over which there is little control, and when hospitalisation and confinement are overwhelming experiences in and of themselves.

What I observed in David's practice was that rather than focusing directly on gaining control when there seemed to be little, David used conversation and, moreover, listening, to provide opportunities for words to be acknowledged as authoritative and prized as expressions of worth and agency. I suggest that within a mainstream psychiatric service this is no small thing.

A first person principle in narrative practice

On first acquaintance, David's distinctive questioning and listening when talking with young people seemed modest and low key. But what became clear over time, as I became more familiar with it and thus could observe it more closely, was a strict discipline. And although David didn't use the term 'first person', he noticed and pointed out to me whenever I inadvertently reinterpreted a young person's words by using terms that were removed from the words that they had used, particularly where the effect of so doing was to redescribe or reinterpret their words, as if mine were more authoritative. David had a heightened sense of this distinction.

If I were to distil the discipline I observed in David's practice in terms of a single principle, I would say he prioritised first person speech and then limited what he said when speaking to and on behalf of the young people within that service setting to the words and phrases he had heard from them. I suggest this is a first person principle of narrative practice. I will describe it further, hopefully without sounding too prescriptive.

As a narrative therapist speaks with someone, they attend to what is offered as 'mine' in their speech. By asking questions carefully, a narrative therapist acknowledges that particular person's authoritative position with respect to the actions, experiences, thoughts, hopes and feelings that are shared in their words and phrases, and in their descriptions and narratives, as 'mine' or 'my own'.

Acknowledging this authority then places a limit on the therapist's authority. A narrative therapist takes care not to take a meaning that is given and then supply it with a further meaning– one that has not been experienced as 'mine' or 'ours' by the person with whom they are working.[11] As David pointed out to me, supplying a further meaning supplants a young person's own authority with a different kind of authority.

I mentioned above that, unlike psychiatry and psychology, narrative therapy has no specific commitment to identifying underlying causes.[12] The answers that are given in response to a narrative therapist's questions are not interpreted as symptoms or signs of underlying causes that require diagnostic or interpretive expertise by a therapist. Resisting diagnosis and expert interpretation privileges the knowledge and experience of the person with whom a narrative therapist speaks, rather than privileging the interpretive mastery of the expert questioner.

I would also say that interpretive mastery of another's speech presupposes knowledge that the speaker lacks and presupposes superior insight into the causal underpinnings of another's world. In contrast, a narrative therapist only asks questions that can be answered in the first person, in speech that is 'mine' or 'ours'. And, presumably, to an onlooker this may mean that narrative therapy looks a lot like ordinary conversation. Or that when David is working with young people, he and they are just chatting.

I suggest that narrative therapy is not at all like ordinary conversation; it is conversation with the ethical aim of privileging the words and experience of others, by acknowledging their first personal authority. And as such, I believe a first person principle is a principle of ethical practice.[13]

Part 2—From David: Philosophical reflections that build urgency and further critique

During our work together, Philippa presented me with questions and observations that made me think in new ways. I found this to be a rich process and told myself many times during her placement and since, 'I must read more philosophy!' Through the lens of Philippa's philosophical questions and observations, I was returned in new ways to the assumptions of narrative practice, and therefore of my own practice. I would like to share some of this and include some practice stories.

The notion of a first person principle that comes from Philippa's reading of philosophy has a strong resonance with Michael White's concept of decentred practice (1997, pp. 200–214), and his injunction to look for words and phrases that are 'experience-near' (White, 2007, p. 40). Yet it offers a philosophical reflection that emphasises a restraint or limit on what it is possible for us to do with regard to meaning-making and story-building. This philosophical reflection generated a sense of urgency, or an imperative to resist imposing our ideas and our meanings on the lives of those with whom we work.[14]

There was an example of the assistance I received from Philippa's questions and comments that I became most grateful for. I remember talking with her about the explosion of neuroscience and discourses on the brain in many areas, especially in psychiatric services. She spoke about a personal/impersonal distinction from Ricoeur, and how she was employing it to distinguish narrative therapy and social work, on the one hand, from discourses about mental health that draw on brain science, on the other hand.[15]

Her point was not that science is wrong, but that perhaps as narrative practitioners we should pay careful attention to what can and can't be accessed from a first person perspective when we speak with young people. To clarify this point, she showed me a short passage from the French philosopher, Paul Ricoeur:

> The brain, indeed, differs from many other parts of the body, and from the body as a whole in terms of an integral experience, inasmuch as it is stripped of any phenomenological status and thus of the trait of belonging to me, of being my possession ... It is only through the global detour by way of my body, inasmuch as my body is also a body and as the brain is contained in this body, that I can say: 'my brain'. The unsettling nature of this expression is reinforced by the fact that the brain does not fall under the category of objects perceived at a distance from one's body. Its proximity in my head gives it the strange character of nonexperienced interiority. (1990, pp. 132–133)

In this passage, Ricoeur writes that there is something peculiar but also distinctive about the brain. While an expression such as 'my brain' is deeply personal, the brain is a part of a person's body that is not directly experienced, unlike one's hand or, indeed, one's heart.

Ricoeur's phrase is that the brain has a 'strange...nonexperienced interiority' (1990, p. 132). He points out that from a first person perspective, the brain is unsettlingly personal *and* impersonal. Philippa suggested that there may be implications for young people when therapists, doctors and psychiatrists speak to them about their brains and do not take this into consideration.

If a mental health professional speaks to a young person about their brain, nothing could be more personal, but the young person has no access to what is spoken of via their own experience. A young person has no direct experience of their brain, so in this sense, their brain is impersonal. Young people (like all of us) are acquainted with their thoughts, feelings and experiences; it is these that they can talk about with the first personal authority that Philippa describes.

Philippa and I talked about what it might be like for young people when the problems they face are described to them with phrases such as 'your brain gives you the wrong message'. Although we can note dualist or Cartesian assumptions in such phrases, what is unsettling about them is that they are simultaneously personal and highly impersonal. The impersonal character of the brain makes it difficult to resist information about it, especially when the source of that information has professional authority. I intend to fill in this point a little more below, emphasising why it matters: if resistance is unavailable, then the scene is set for domination.

A knowledge discourse that undermines resistance

Philippa's thoughts and Ricoeur's phrase helped me to articulate what I've found troubling about working in a psychiatric context for young people in which 'brain discourses' are more and more in favour. Such brain discourses introduce young people (or anyone else for that matter) to 'scientific' and highly technical knowledge.

If anyone is at the receiving end of scientific, technical knowledge, I suspect it makes it difficult to negotiate or resist the messages that accompany such knowledge for two reasons. As Ricoeur's notion of 'nonexperienced interiority' suggests, there is no personal experience on which to draw when negotiating this knowledge discourse. Even if a person owns their own MRI machine or has advanced skills in interpreting MRI scans, this is still an impersonal or removed perspective. The image thus presented is not an image of one's own experience; it is an impersonal correlate of experience.

Or, to invert Michael White's memorable phrase as a guide here, the image, or information about the image, is *not* experience-near.

The second reason I suspect that discourses about the brain can make it difficult to negotiate or resist professionalised meaning is because this discourse positions a young person as owing gratitude to a mental health professional for sharing their knowledge. In my view, it is extremely difficult for young people to resist the knowledge and attendant meanings of professional workers once they are positioned in this way. This matters because the difficulty in negotiating or resisting meaning and knowledge is so important when knowledge imposition overlaps with identity formation, when a person's very sense of themselves – of their history, their future and their stories – is at stake.

I've subsequently been on the lookout for practices that position young people as owing gratitude to me, brain discourses being a particular and intense example of this.[16] And, as I have suggested above, this is a critique that has been so very clarifying for me.

The first person principle and professional dilemmas

Philippa's proposal that narrative therapy includes a first person principle of practice, and her discussion with me of Ricoeur's phrase 'nonexperienced interiority', has made this hazard of introducing highly technical knowledge and brain discourses, and therefore potentially positioning people as having gratitude, much clearer to me. She has also written that I attempt to privilege the words and meanings that young people use. This is very relevant to my approach when meeting with young people and families at the psychiatric service where I work. It is also relevant when I'm required or invited to speak about young people when they are not present.

I will briefly include just a few of the intricacies of putting such a principle into practice. If I hold the position that I would rather young people speak for themselves than be spoken for, I end up saying less in clinical contexts. Likewise, if I hold a position that young people ought to interpret their own lives rather than having me interpret their lives for them, I can appear to have less professional insight. And if I don't use technical and professional terms, but instead use the language young people use, it can seem like I have less clinical *nous* or *know-how*.

These dilemmas highlight the mismatch between the first person principle applied in practice - limiting words and phrases to those of the young people I work with - and the professionalised skills and terminology of mental health workers, typically valued within psychiatric services. To put this more directly, in the mainstream service where I work, retrieving and privileging the words and phrases of young people can seem less professional than other approaches.

However, the flipside of these dilemmas is that they build a quiet determination on my part to continue privileging the words and phrases of young people and continue to observe or enact a first person principle in my practice. I don't think such dilemmas will evaporate, but naming them and having this quiet determination helps me to stay on track with privileging the words and experiences of young people.

The first person principle and resisting professional language

One way of observing or enacting this principle is by refusing to rename the experiences of those who are admitted to a psychiatric service, by refusing to do what Escher & Romme (2010) describe as a 'moulding' of experience into models and forms of word based on psychiatry's models and forms of words.[17]

The observance or enactment of a first person principle can also include what is required of us when the people we are meeting with are slowly trusting us with words and meanings that are tentatively forming, perhaps for the first time and that we perhaps have never heard before. And it can also include an ethical orientation – of respect and acknowledgement – when we speak to others about the tentative unfolding of such words and meanings.

In response to an invitation from David Denborough,[18] the young people and I have been pulling together a 'dictionary of obscure sorrows/experiences' that is named after a website, The Dictionary of Obscure Sorrows (Koenig,

2009). As the name suggests, this involves creating a compendium of experiences and sorrows that are obscure or hard to find descriptions or words for, then finding descriptions for such experiences, whether they are new words or phrases, images or songs.

For me, this has been one of the most regularly engaging group exercises I have done within the service. The young people can be entranced. They are often keen to contribute their own entry and offer creative and at times hilarious names for experiences that they see as having rarely been offered an airing or given much attention or status.

I introduce the exercise to young people by saying that complex experience, which can be hard to name, often gets reinterpreted and renamed in mental health contexts. And then I say that this exercise will try to simply name an experience that is complex, or hard to name, using language and descriptions that you (the young people) use. In other words, the young people and I work together, and a first person principle of practice is directly shared with them. Of course, I introduce the exercise and explain it, but their discussions about naming experience in their own words and their descriptions become the focus of our time together. And the point is to find first person language, meanings and experiences, as alternatives to professional language.

The first person principle, thinking about influence, and distinguishing meanings from causes

Tied in with and elaborating on the theme of a first person principle, and therefore work that treats seriously and supports first personal authority, was another theme that I started to consider as a result of reflections and conversations with Philippa about meaning-making as influencing or re-influencing the meanings of past events. This pulled my thinking in another generative direction, particularly as I thought about a young person called Beth.[19]

Beth had been admitted to the unit twice; the first time when she spoke about 'being mute', and then six months later with a diagnosis of obsessive-compulsive disorder, among other things. During her second admission, she had been staying up increasingly late at night to perform particular rituals. Beth was quiet on the unit, so when she asked to speak with me one-to-one I was reasonably surprised. Not long into this conversation, Beth told me that she was about to tell me something that she had not told anyone before.

Beth then said in a quietly determined way that she had been sexually abused by her father for many years. And as we delicately sifted through what this meant in terms of who and when to tell this horrid news, as well as what it was like to start speaking of such experience, Beth said something that made me pause. She said 'I don't have a mental illness. This OCD has been a way of dealing with the effects of sexual abuse.'

Beth had turned things upside down and was making a strong claim. From her perspective, there was meaning in her actions that only she could speak of. Her actions were not merely effects of underlying causes that she had no direct access to. Such a change in ascription, from being caused to act to speaking of her actions as having specific meanings for her, brought a radically different life and different commitments to light. In speaking about her past in her own words and defining her actions as meaningful, Beth was establishing her authority with respect to the meanings of those events.

I have subsequently spoken with Beth on a number of occasions. What is striking when she speaks of her experiences in the first person, as described in this paper, is her clarity and her authority. I have also witnessed her generous contributions in conversations with others who have experienced something similar to her, and in these conversations I notice her quiet authority.

I have reflected on Beth's strong stance and renaming of actions and experiences in light of several discussions I have had with Philippa about the notion of cause, of how it can be unpacked in a range of ways in a mental health or psychiatric context. We discussed how care is needed so that young people are not positioned as merely being caused to act or speak in certain ways due to a mental illness, or that their thoughts and feelings are simply caused by what their brains are doing.

On several occasions, Philippa mentioned to me that she is interested in the distinction between causes on the one hand, and meanings as influences on the other. She suggested that some things and some events are strictly causal, but that meanings are better thought of as influential as they are revisable and renewable, hence the potential of telling and re-telling stories.

The influence of the meaning of an event is not one-directional—it is not fixed as an antecedent cause with a determinative effect, as something that is past (and thus unchangeable) that causally determines an effect in the present. Instead, the influence of a meaning can extend from the present to the past, and then from a revisited past to a reconfigured future.[20] Beth was making meaning in the present that revised and reshaped the meaning of events in her past, and also reconfigured her sense of the future and, as such, her meanings and her meaning-making were highly influential.

This idea that meanings are influential (rather than causal) and, as such, are potential sources of renewal and re-influence, has heightened my sense of the importance of a 'light touch' in my choice of words and phrases when working with young people, so as not to impose my meanings on their lives, and to highlight the potential of their own meaning-making to influence and enrich their lives.

I have also considered Philippa's suggestion of a possible over-emphasis on causes, in a strict sense, and subsequently noticed the prevalence of talking to and about young people in terms of causes. I will mention a few: that 'mental illness' causes the actions of young people; that trauma has strictly causal effects; and that chemical imbalances cause mental illness. In the psychiatric service where I work, the brain is regularly laid out as the cause of a young person's mental illness. What can then be overlooked or underestimated are the attempts that young people are already making to respond to and re-visit the meaning of events in their lives.

Returning to Beth, when she talked about her OCD as a way of dealing with abuse, she was talking about the meaning and impact of her life experiences and, crucially, the meaning of her subsequent actions as a response and resistance to abuse. I've reflected on the fact she did not say her actions were caused by her past. I suspect that crediting her actions as meaningful responses rather than effects of antecedent causes is very significant for Beth, as it is through her words that she regains authority and thus resists domination. Privileging her words, phrases and descriptions of her actions and experiences as meaningful and authoritative – observing a first person principle – helps to acknowledge just how significant this is.

Conclusion: From David and Philippa

We both see narrative practice as a rich resource for philosophical reflection, and we have attempted to share this perspective in this paper. We have suggested that a first person principle is a simple but philosophically grounded practice principle that respects and honours what is 'experience-near' for the people we work with. We have highlighted Ricoeur's very suggestive phrase of a 'nonexperienced interiority' which we have considered in the context of therapeutic discussions involving brains and neuroscience.

We have suggested that care and subtlety is needed when language is simultaneously personal and highly impersonal, and noted how knowledge discourses potentially curtail opportunities for resistance, and potentially position others as owing gratitude. We have also suggested a first person principle is a means of carefully limiting a narrative therapist's authority, and highlights the need to do so, and discussed this with some practice examples.

And finally, we have briefly considered how a first person principle highlights meaning and meaning-making as influential, and counters an emphasis on discourses that focus on the ways that people are caused to think, feel and act, and can then fail to credit the words that people use as meaningful and uniquely authoritative.

References

Angus, L., & McCleod, J. (2004). *The handbook of narrative and psychotherapy.* Thousand Oaks, CA: Sage Publications.

Buber, M. (1970). *I and thou* (W. Kaufman, Trans.). New York, NY: Simon & Schuster.

Derrida, J. (2003). *The problem of Genesis in Husserl's philosophy* (M. Hobson, Trans.). Chicago, IL: University of Chicago Press.

Escher, S., & Romme, M. (2010). *Children hearing voices: What you need to know and what you can do*. Herefordshire, England: PCCS.

Evans, G. (1982). *The varieties of reference*. Oxford, England: Clarendon.

Hamilton, A. (2013). *The self in question*. Basingstoke, England: Palgrave Macmillan.

Hamkins, S. (2013). *Art of Narrative Psychiatry*. New York, NY: Oxford University Press.

Koenig, J. (2009). *The dictionary of obscure sorrows*. Retrieved from www.dictionaryofobscuresorrows.com

Morgan, A. (2000). *What is narrative therapy? An easy-to- read introduction*. Adelaide, Australia: Dulwich Centre Publications.

Newman, D. (2008). 'Rescuing the said from the saying of it': Living documentation in narrative therapy. *International Journal of Narrative Therapy and Community Work*, (3). 24–34.

Newman, D. (2012). 'Skills in translating': Using the written word in narrative practice. *Lapidus Journal*, Spring edition.

Newman, D. (2016). Explorations with the written word in an inpatient mental health unit for young people. *International Journal of Narrative Therapy and Community Work*, (4), 45–58.

Ricoeur, P. (1984). *Time and narrative, Vol I*. (K. McLaughlin & D. Pellauer, Trans.). Chicago, IL: University of Chicago Press.

Ricoeur, P. (1985). *Time and narrative, Vol 1*. (K. Blamey & D. Pellauer, Trans.). Chicago, IL: University of Chicago Press.

Ricoeur, P. (1990). *Oneself as another* (K. Blamey, Trans.). Chicago, IL: University of Chicago Press.

White, M. (1997). *Narratives of therapists' lives*. Adelaide, Australia: Dulwich Centre Publications.

White, M. (2004). *Narrative practice and exotic lives: Resurrecting diversity in everyday life*. Adelaide, Australia: Dulwich Centre Publications.

White, M. (2007). *Maps of narrative practice*. New York, NY: Norton.

White, M., & Epston, D. (1989). *Literate means to therapeutic ends*. Adelaide, Australia: Dulwich Centre Publications.

Endnotes

[1] These included Morgan (2000); Newman (2008, 2012, 2016); White, M. (1997, 2004, 2007); White & Epston (1989).

[2] Specific ideas from philosophy of language are discussed below and references are also included below. Some key works on narrative and temporality are Ricoeur (1984, 1985, 1990).

[3] This assertion does not mean that it is not possible to empirically investigate narrative therapy in simple ways, say with the use of pre- and post-intervention measures such as questionnaires. In my view, this kind of 'before and after the fact' empirical investigation has no implications with regard to whether or not a practice is grounded in empirical sciences.

[4] I also acknowledge that psychiatry and clinical psychology include philosophical inquiry and, as practice fields, can also incorporate and engage with narrative practice. See Angus & McCleod (2004) and Hamkins (2013).

[5] An evocative philosophical examination of this point is Martin Buber's (1970) *I and thou*. This is a book about phenomenological modes of being, rather than modes of address.

[6] For elaboration of Ricoeur's use of the term 'mineness' and an elaboration of a personal/impersonal distinction, drawn on later in the paper, see chapter 5 of *Oneself as another* (1990).

[7] See Andy Hamilton (2013, chapter 2), and for a discussion of the issue of 'immunity to error through misidentification', as developed in Wittgenstein's thought and elsewhere. See Gareth Evans (1982, chapter 7) for a broader discussion of the specific characteristics of self-referring speech. Ricoeur was a close reader of analytic philosophy of language, and in this respect unusual for a European philosopher who is steeped in early phenomenology (Husserl), later phenomenology (Heidegger, Merleau-

Ponty, Levinas), and also has what I call 'a critique and a debt' to Derrida's engagement with phenomenology. It is therefore no stretch to bring Ricoeur's thought together with ideas drawn from analytic philosophy of language.

[8] I alternate between 'person' and 'personal' in referring to first person speech and first personal experience to observe the distinction between what is said and what is experienced. Hence with the expression 'first personal authority' I am trying to capture the experience of one's own speech as authoritative, so the emphasis is on experience more so than speech.

[9] Metaphors of retrieval and excavation are not uncommon in phenomenology. Derrida notes that: 'Husserl would have liked to bring back the word "archeology" in the phenomenological sense, which is not that of "wordly" science' (2003, p. 182).

[10] I believe a fruitful parallel can be drawn between the 'in principle' linking of experience and meaning within phenomenology and the 'in principle' linking of experience and meaning within narrative practice, but this task is beyond the scope of this paper.

[11] And by extension, when narrative therapists work with a community or group, they attend to what is claimable as 'ours' and belonging to 'us'. However, this suggestion that there is a direct extension requires qualification. It may be too quick to assume a direct extension from what is 'mine' in the experience of an individual to what is 'theirs' when the experiences of a group or community of people are collectively represented in speech and the written word.

[12] This does not mean that talking to a young person about what they believe has caused something, or what they have been told about the causes of their problems is strictly ruled out.

[13] I mentioned above that narrative therapy is not based on an empirical approach to 'the human subject'. In contrast, I believe it is based on an ethical stance regarding the relationship between a person who speaks and a person who listens.

[14] Our work is informed by our ideas and understandings, as well as our critiques of dominant discourses, but we nonetheless take care not to supplant the authority of the words and phrases of those with whom we work.

[15] This comes from *Oneself as Another* (1990), see chapter 5 in particular.

[16] The point here is not that a brain scan is never useful. If I had an operable brain tumour, I would be grateful that others have expertise in reading scans. To reiterate, the point made here is that, in a therapeutic context, gratitude to those whose knowledge cannot be challenged is potentially dominating.

[17] Escher and Romme are quoting the words of Ron Coleman, who is a voice hearer, who says that 'Psychiatry takes away my experience, moulds it into their model and hands it back to me in a way that is unrecognisable to me.' (2010, p. 32).

[18] David Denborough is a community practitioner and writer at Dulwich Centre.

[19] Beth (not her real name) has given permission to repeat her words and write about her experiences in this paper.

[20] Although meanings can change, there is no implication that meanings are thus 'untied' to what has actually happened. And although meanings are not strictly causal, this does not imply that they are 'free-floating' and can be 'unhinged' from events and actions, or that meanings exist only 'within' the minds of meaning-makers.

Combining Peer Support, Emotional CPR and Open Dialogue Facilitates Recovery from Schizophrenia

Mateusz Biernat, Margaret Zawisza, Magdalena Biernat, and Daniel Fisher

Abstract: *In this study, we illustrate how a combination of peer support, Emotional CPR, and Open Dialogue have enabled a young man to recover from schizophrenia. The client had 15 psychiatric hospitalizations from 2011 through 2017. During that period, traditional clinical practice and medication did not reach him. However, in 2016 during his 13th hospitalization, a peer (Mateusz, the lead author), began a series of meetings with the client. The peer used his lived experience and Emotional CPR to meet the client at a nonverbal level. He developed trust and the client started to talk and engage in Open Dialogue meetings with his family and started to consistently take his medication. He has not been hospitalized for the last six years and he now works.*

Authors' Note: The ongoing peer support, Emotional CPR (eCPR) and Open Dialogue as well as the follow up interviews were all conducted in Polish. Dr. Fisher is very grateful to Ms. Zawisza and Biernat for translation and interpretation.

Introduction

One of the greatest challenges in the mental health field is how to engage persons with severe psychiatric conditions in mental health treatment. Traditional clinical mental health care fails to reach persons with such conditions. The traditional elements of diagnosis, psychotherapy, and medication seem pointless to people dealing with these conditions which shake the foundations of their world. The usual treatments fail to address the most basic need which is to be heard and understood, usually at a nonverbal, emotional level.

Typical mental health care depends on communication at the cognitive and verbal level. The psychiatrist and other mental health professionals are taught to ask a series of questions to pinpoint a diagnosis. But people in acute distress experience direct questions as attacks. Without meaning to, professionals also reinforce a sense of powerlessness by relating in an unemotional manner. Therapists are taught not to show their own feelings. But, in fact, when a person is in acute distress, they want to know there is a human being with them more than anything. Expressing feelings is the most convincing way to assure the person in distress that they are not alone.

The relationships between clients and professionals usually involve the professional problem-solving the client's problems, which is disem-powering. These experiences of powerlessness also diminish hope and motivation. To make matters even worse, clients are blamed for their lack of engagement and are coerced into treatments they feel alienated from. In contrast, people with lived experience have found that they can often more readily communicate with peers than professionals. The vulnerability and authenticity with which peers communicate reduces the power difference they experience with professionals. Instead of feeling hopeless, they are inspired by peers.

In addition, a new training, Emotional CPR (eCPR), is enabling peers and family members to engage with people in severe distress on an emotional level. This approach emphasizes connecting on a heart-to-heart level first, and with words second. People assisted through eCPR experience empowerment because they are encouraged to be equal partners in their care. The people assisting share their own feelings in a manner that makes their relating more authentic. The CPR in eCPR stands for Connecting, emPowering, and Revitalizing.

In addition, a group of Finnish psychologists realized that typical family therapy was not helping people with severe emotional issues. They have developed a highly respectful approach called Open Dialogue in which every voice is valued. Open dialogue was greatly enhanced by a combination of peer support and eCPR with a young man and his family, in Poland, as will be shown below. This combination of three approaches helped the person in acute distress to have a voice in their family meetings, thereby enabling them to emerge from their monologue and enter the polyphonous community.

In summary, the unifying principles underlying peer support, Emotional CPR and Open Dialogue are compassion, love, understanding and hope. The person in distress and their family feel the team cares, they regain motivation to live, and they are revitalized.

D and His Family History

We share here the story of a young man "D" (we will use this initial to protect his identity) in his late 30s in Poland who has shown significant recovery from schizophrenia through the synergistic effect of peer support, eCPR, and Open Dialogue.

According to his twin sister "C", D was a very shy child. He had one friend in primary school. Teachers commented on his absenteeism, isolation from classmates, and lack of interest in meeting with peers. His condition worsened significantly after his older brother and sister moved out of the house. In high school, he began meeting with a psychologist once a week. Those meetings lasted for 2.5 years.

After a while, he stopped drinking liquids, eating, and lost a lot of weight. His hair was falling out. He didn't sleep. He sat in front of the computer. He was inattentive to self-care. D's mother asked to see the attending psychologist. The psychologist did not want to talk to the family. To the mother's concerns about weight loss and starvation, the psychologist responded: "Do you want a fat person in the house? My children don't eat either."

D did not socialize during high school and only attended the school prom for an hour. At age 18, D began studies at a university with a major in environmental protection. In January, he began to come home very sad, constantly lying in bed. He stopped eating again, and his hair began to fall out. In May, he came home announcing that he would not return to his studies. At the age of 20, he received a call to enlist in the army. After tests in the army, an initial opinion came out suggesting "schizophrenic behavior." However, it was not a diagnosis but a description—and an opinion that none of the family paid attention to.

At age 21, D went to a psychologist who administered the MMPI and a Rorschach. Here are some of the results: D had a

> sense of psychological discomfort, inner restlessness, persistent repetition of "proven" routines in behavior, inward-directed aggression, inhibition of activity, uncertain testing of reality, tendency toward social introversion, increased deep anxiety, low self-esteem, low self-acceptance, sense of low position in the social hierarchy, predominance of anxiety-based defense mechanisms, significant disruption of social contacts, strong internal normative conflict, sense of loss of control.

At age 22, a psychiatrist diagnosed depression and prescribed him his first medication. He did not experience any positive change. Another psychiatrist, Dr. H, concluded, "I have no doubt that this is simple schizophrenia. It develops very slowly, and it is the worst type of schizophrenia. You will have to take medication for the rest of your life because this disease lasts for the rest of your life." The doctor prescribed Solian, an antipsychotic medication. He discontinued the medication after about 2 years.

At age 24, upon recommendation by friends, D began day treatment. There were meetings with actors, cooking classes, and other activities. He was supposed to go there every day. One day, in the evening during a huge storm, he said he was going for a walk. He returned at 5 AM soaking wet. When asked where he had been, he replied that he had been for a walk—then left again. His older brother tried to stop him but to no avail. They found D in just his shorts three days later in the stairwell of a neighboring town. He was hospitalized for the first time at age 27 for 12.5 weeks.

This was the first of 15 hospitalizations during the next six years. During that time, he would stabilize in the hospital with support and medication but would never follow up with treatment in the community. D's sister, C, was desperate. She could see that traditional mental health care was not working. She was losing hope. C looked everywhere for a therapist, but they only wanted to give him drugs—nobody wanted to try to reach D without drugs. D was hopeless, he was afraid of people.

Then, in 2015, C heard Daniel Fisher give a talk describing his own recovery from schizophrenia and his journey to become a psychiatrist. This talk gave her hope that D could recover. In the talk, Daniel described that peer support, Emotional CPR, and Open Dialogue can facilitate recovery.

Peer Support, eCPR and Open Dialogue

C encouraged Mateusz, a peer, with lived experience of recovery to meet with D during his 13th hospitalization. Mateusz could see himself in D—he, too, had felt oppressed by the system. He saw a person in pain who was nonverbal. His mother spoke for him. Mateusz decided he would be D's voice. Mateusz was the first person to connect with D. Daniel became curious. He wanted to discover how Mateusz was able to connect with D when no other mental health worker had been able to do so. So, Daniel asked C, "How did Mateusz connect with D?" C said:

> Mateusz saw D as a human being. He treated him as a normal person who could speak. Mateusz's approach was different from traditional clinicians. Mateusz looked at D as a person in distress, because he looked beyond D's diagnosis. He was not hopeless. Mateusz did not judge D. He was not afraid of him. Mateusz saw D as a normal person in an abnormal environment.

C felt hopeful when she met Mateusz because she could feel Mateusz's hope. C felt that Mateusz understood D's family situation. D did not want to live in the hospital and Mateusz supported that impulse. Mateusz was D's megaphone. D was not talking when they met. Then he started to use words and, eventually, whole sentences. Peer support created an understanding and connection on an emotional level.

Once he felt connected to Mateusz, D joined the family in Open Dialogue meetings. These were conducted by Mateusz. Everyone was on an equal level, which allowed for a polyphony—that is, for all voices to be heard. Mateusz was available whenever the family wanted to talk. He was reliable. It was very important that Mateusz heard and valued every voice in the family including D's mother who had been excluded in previous meetings conducted by professionals. In Mateusz's eyes, everyone was of equal importance. Mateusz never took sides—he walked in the middle.

To find ways that she could connect with D, C took the eCPR workshop. She said, "eCPR helped me to open up to my emotions, and it allowed me to start to talk about my emotions." Mateusz also took the eCPR class. Daniel asked Mateusz what about his approach resembled eCPR. Mateusz said that the emphasis in eCPR on nonverbal communication was consistent with his way of connecting with D. He said eCPR helped him to put into words what he had intuitively used to reach D.

Mateusz said, "When I first met D, I met him as a person. I started with eye contact. I empathized with D. I could feel his sadness. I wanted to cry." When Daniel asked Mateusz how he reached D, Mateusz said:

> D actually reached me. I felt a tightness in my stomach and chest. When I shared this feeling, D said he also felt a tightness in his stomach. I felt D was telling people one thing but feeling something else. When D could not speak, I felt a tightness in my throat.

In sharing this bodily feeling, Mateusz formed a tight bond with D. Mateusz also used a religious metaphor to reach D. He suggested to D that he was a lost human trying to find himself. Then D started to comment on another patient's tattoos. He was especially moved by a tattoo of a bleeding heart. D could feel it.

Once Mateusz had formed a trusting relationship with D, he felt he could conduct Open Dialogue meetings with D, C, and their mother. D's mother wanted D to return to the hospital, but he did not want to go. C said that taking eCPR helped her to open up and express her feelings in the Open Dialogue meetings. So, when her mother wanted D to be back in the hospital, C could more readily express her anger and sided with D. She argued that he did not need to return to the hospital. C was also angry that her mother did not listen to what her children wanted.

Mateusz believes you have to have gone through a period of losing hope in order to connect with a person with D's degree of distress. It is difficult for the doctors to feel that degree of empathy because they often have not suffered to that degree. D met with Mateusz several times while he was in the hospital, and then the family met with Mateusz every two weeks for several years while D was living at home.

D has not been hospitalized since 2017. He has been working during the last several years, first doing cleaning then working at a sawmill with his father. He is attending a peer support group. D's posture is better, and he is speaking up more. D is now better able to make important decisions in his life.

D and C respond to a series of follow-up questions

1. What did D experience during the first family meeting with professionals at the Centre for Neurology and Psychiatry before he met Mateusz? What feelings made it difficult for him to attend any other meetings with the following doctor?

In commenting on his first Open Dialogue meeting at the Centre for Neurology and Psychiatry in Warsaw, D said, "I felt judged. There was no ordinary conversation or dialogue. The facilitators were poorly prepared. They didn't want to listen. C cried a lot." D was not able to stay there. After this meeting, D didn't want to attend the meetings with Dr. E because he anticipated that it would be the same—that there would be no conversation on an equal level; that they would not understand him. D felt anxious.

2. What feelings did D experience that allowed him to meet and connect with Mateusz? Did D notice any sensations in his body? Was it helpful that Mateusz was a person with similar experiences of hospitalization, medication, and psychiatric diagnosis?

The first meeting with Mateusz was organized by C during D's 13th hospitalization. D stated that,

> Mateusz and I started with a short, normal conversation as equals. I could see that Mateusz could easily communicate with the other patients and staff. Mateusz told me that I did not need to take medication. I felt that Mateusz knew my perspective. There was a

sense of understanding from another person that someone was on my side. I felt he understood me.

They made contact because Mateusz understood the perspective of a hospitalized patient such as being ambivalent about taking medication, constantly returning to the hospital, and experiencing a revolving door. D admired that Mateusz defied the psychiatric system.

3. What allowed D to stay and engage in Open Dialogue meetings with his family and Mateusz?

D said, "[in the Open Dialogue meetings conducted by Mateusz] there was dialogue, there was no judgment." The relationship that was established, the simple conversation, and the lack of judgement were very important. D also saw that his sister and his mum were changing due to these meetings. They were starting to understand him. They understood that the whole system that D was locked into was sick.

The family understood that things could no longer be the way they were before—that the way of treatment had to be changed to a more social, people-friendly way. The meetings were also necessary for D because they changed the routine of D's ordinary grey day, his boredom, and overreliance on medication.

4. Did D's relationship with Mateusz help D stay in the family meetings run by Mateusz?

D experienced a change and an alternative, different approach during meetings with Mateusz. He no longer left the meetings. He accepted them because Mateusz was taking his side and feeling what he was feeling. Mateusz wanted D to be able to negotiate his way of taking medication. Even though everyone around D was pushing him to take the medication, Mateusz understood what it meant to take medication. Mateusz understood his perspective.

D felt Mateusz wanted to help him and was his voice in his relationship with his family. D felt he could finally say something. They could talk freely. There was dialogue. The family started to hear him, and they stopped pushing for medication as the only treatment. They realized they didn't have to worry about D being sick and could go about their business.

They understood that it was not him who was sick, but the whole community that was making him sick. They understood that it was not an illness in the narrow medical sense. Instead, it was the result of difficult experiences with his family, school, university, and psychiatrist. It's not an illness—it's the result of traumatic experiences.

5. Did being with C help D when she spoke up more often at family gatherings? Did he feel that C and Mateusz were his allies?

At first, C made him very nervous because she, herself, was very nervous. Then she started to understand. C didn't want D to go back to hospital and that was important to him.

6. What is D 's daily life like now and what has changed after his meetings with Mateusz?

D is living in harmony with each member of his family and community. He continues to meet with Mateusz and feels that he will be fine.

Conclusion

Here is the case of a young Polish man who was diagnosed with schizophrenia and hospitalized 15 times in a six-year period. Traditionally trained professionals were unable to engage him in individual therapy, case management, family therapy, or medication. He described the professional treatment as dehumanizing and disempowering.

However, through a recovery-based approach embodied in peer support, eCPR and Open Dialogue, the young man engaged in treatment. He has been free of hospitalizations and has cooperated with psychiatric treatment. He is working and free from delusions or hallucinations.

The young man and his family identify the more egalitarian relationships in these recovery-based approaches as crucial. They identified the conversational, personal approach of peer support as important in building trust. By learning eCPR, the peer and the person's sister were able to reach the young man on an emotional level. Emotional expression was also important in allowing the peer and his sister to encourage the young man to speak up to his parents.

The goal of Open Dialogue is to make sure that every member of a family's voice is heard. When the "person of focus" (Open Dialogue term for the person with the most severe problem) has difficulty speaking, as was the case here, a combination of peer support and eCPR can be an excellent complement to Open Dialogue. Peer support and eCPR empower the person of focus and thereby ensure that their voice is as important as other members of the family. We recommend that Open Dialogue meetings be facilitated by peers, and that peers and family members learn eCPR as a unifying set of intentions.

Additional Resources

Information on peer support, ECPR and Open Dialogue can be found on the National Empowerment Center website: www.power2U.org

Awareness - rising information and examples of recovery on the Human Foundation website: https://human-foundation.eu/

A Contemplative Phenomenological Approach to Psychodiagnosis

G. Kenneth Bradford

Abstract: *Psychological diagnosis informed by the DSM and the approach of empirical science misdirects experientially-based psychotherapies and undermines core principles of Humanistic, Transpersonal and Holistic Psychologies. This chapter presents a mindfulness-based, phenomenologically-informed contemplative approach to psychodiagnosis that more appropriately grounds practices of experiential therapies favoring holistic orientations. Recognizing that the diagnosing of other minds occurs within an inter-subjective field, calculative, objectifying and concept-driven thinking is contrasted with meditative, non-conceptual, relational cognizance. A distinction is made between experience-distant systems of interpretation and the experience-near process of explication. A case study exemplifying the differences between empirical and contemplative diagnosis is folded into the discussion.*

Acknowledgement: "A Contemplative Phenomenological Approach to Psychodiagnosis" was first published in *The Journal of Transpersonal Psychology, 2009, 41(2), 121-138,* and appeared in rewritten form in Bradford, G. K. (2013). *The I of the Other: Mindfulness-based Diagnosis and the Question of Sanity,* Paragon House.

If our science of mental health is to become more effective, psychotherapists will have to balance their knowledge of psychological concepts and techniques with a contemplative awareness...that exercises itself day after day in quiet openness.
   – Medard Boss, 1978, p. 191

From the Buddhist point of view, there is a problem with any attempt to pinpoint, categorize, and pigeonhole mind and its contents very neatly. This method could be called psychological materialism. The problem with this approach is that it does not leave enough room for spontaneity or openness. It overlooks basic healthiness.
   - Chogyam Trungpa, 2005, pp. 137-138

Psychological diagnosis strives to make valid knowledge claims regarding the pathology and normative status of other minds. In addition, experience-near therapies and spiritual disciplines go beyond merely distinguishing between normal and abnormal mental states by discerning subtle, complex, and exceptional states of mind that may be neither conventionally "normal" nor categorically "pathological."

Whether making a clinical distinction between normal and abnormal or making a more nuanced assessment of the subtleties and complexities of a non-normative experiential process, it is incumbent upon psychologists and spiritual guides to consider how truly and thoroughly it is possible to know the mind of an Other. This is especially important as a psychological diagnosis exercises formidable power both in terms of dictating medical treatment and in shaping a person's identity in their own eyes and in the eyes of others.

Diagnosis as conventionally practiced is particularly problematic for Humanistic and Holistically-inclined therapies. As codified in the medical model of the *DSM* (*Diagnostic and Statistical Manual of Mental Disorders*), psychodiagnosis tends to be dehumanizing and/or compartmentalizing. Due to its objectifying (thus dehumanizing) discourse in which clusters of symptoms are reified into mental disorders and attributed to a discrete self, the *DSM* violates fundamental tenets of both humanistic and holistic thought—and misdirects practices of experientially-based therapies in general.

Although the *DSM* may be the dominant and most flagrantly objectivizing psycho-diagnostic system—privileging as it does the *content* of objective categories over the *process* of a living subjectivity—the tendency to assess others according to preconceived categories is not limited to the *DSM*. Humanistic, Holistic and Transpersonal diagnostic systems which are tacitly based on empirical scientific assumptions[i] likewise posit delimited categories into which people are conformed. Categorical ways of thinking about others and encouraging them to think about themselves clash with experience-near therapies that emphasize the open-ended flow of inner sensing, the search for authenticity, and thinking outside of boxes.

The Meaning of *Dia-gnosis*

Yet, if we understand "diagnosis" in its originary sense, unconfined by its practice according to the priorities of the medical model and scientific empiricism, it is possible to diagnose with fidelity to core humanistic, holistic and transpersonal values that inform a wide range of experientially-rigorous therapies. The word *diagnosis* is a combination of *gnosis*, which means to know; and *dia*, which means through or thorough.

So, in its basic sense, *diagnosis* simply refers to a thorough knowing. In regard to other minds, what kind of knowing grants a thorough kind of access? Echoing the meaning of *gnosis* in Christian mysticism and *prajna* in Buddhist psychology, to know someone thoroughly involves knowledge that is non-conceptual, inclusive, and unmediated.

In particular, experientially-keyed — rather than concept-driven — therapies attend to psychic and somatic subtleties in order to surface the implicit complexities, inner contradictions and unrealized potentialities that are often embedded and hidden in psychological depths. An in-depth, inclusive diagnosis requires a nuanced assessment in order to gauge therapeutic responses that more closely accord to the actuality of an Other's experience, and to what that person is ready and able to hear at a particular time.

Responses that are better keyed to a client's readiness to face difficult truths arise from a knowing that is more empathic than conceptual, more open-ended than categorical, and more intuitive than discursive. Attending to the holistic immediacy of experience rather than conceptual constructs about experience, an intuitive and felt knowing arises through a co-presence that is inclusive (*dia*) as well as unmediated (*gnosis*). So, how does one *diagnosis* another person in this holistic, experiential sense?

A Matter of Approach

Since *how* we see a person influences *what* we see in that person, it is important to consider the theoretical assumptions which form and inform our diagnostic vision. We must also consider the practical challenge of how to gain access to an Other's subjectivity — including its hidden recesses —

and through that access, come to understand the implicit complexities of that other mind. This is essentially a question of *approach* (Giorgi, 1970).

In psychology, the matter of approach often remains unquestioned or only tentatively questioned since the dominant approach of Empirical Science is either taken for granted or grudgingly accepted as the de facto paradigm of the field. However, as has been thoroughly discussed by eminent philosophers and psychologists for over a century (e.g., Boss, 1983; Ferrer, 2002; Gadamer, 1960/1982; Giorgi, 1970; Husserl, 1954/1970; James, 1912/1922; Merleau-Ponty, 1942/1963; Szasz, 1974; and Van den Berg, 1972), the Cartesian-Newtonian approach of Empirical Science is inadequate for understanding the complexities and subtleties of human experience.

As its starting point, empiricism assumes the existence of an objective, external world separate and distinct from the subjective, internal observer of that world. It presumes that the minds of human beings exist as do other observable objects. This dualistic vision does not recognize that the division it introduces and the knowledge it produces is constructed (Berger & Luckmann, 1967). Instead, it takes the apparently sharp split between self and world—and self and other—as pregiven.

In construing an external world of objects—thus objectifying the world, including others—empiricism cannot do justice to the subject matter of psychology understood as human subjectivity and intersubjectivity. Even less is it able to comprehend the holistic eco-intelligence in which a human being is a part of—rather than apart from—existence as such. Yet, it remains psychology's principal approach and dictates the epistemological terms of diagnostic formulations.

There have been a number of constructive efforts in recent years to soften the pathological edge of objectivizing diagnoses, in general, and the *DSM*, in particular. Several critiques (Hutchins, 2002; Ingersoll, 2002; Jerry, 2003; Lukoff, 1985, 1988) have sought to minimize the *DSM*'s overtly pathologizing character by emphasizing positive characteristics and transpersonal potentialities of the human condition.

However, as constructive as these and related revisions are, they continue to categorize others according to logical-categorical landscapes of objectively posited criteria such as DSM V-codes, personality types, or discrete levels within a spectrum of consciousness. They remain expressions of a thinking which does not fully succeed in liberating the knowing of others from a discourse of reification, a *knowing about*, which posits an Other—and Otherness—as external to the conceiving subject. To this extent, they fall short of more radically holistic *trans*-personal and *inter*-subjective forms of knowing.

Psychodynamic, Humanistic, and Transpersonal diagnostics have not yet fully taken to heart the epistemological implications arising from the understanding that observed behavior does not exist apart from the observer of that behavior. To more fully comprehend the *inter-ness* of subjective experience, it is necessary to make a leap of cognition from a conceptual to a contemplative (a non-conceptual or trans-conceptual) kind of cognition.

If one does not make this leap (this *trans*-), then one winds up thinking and talking about intersubjective and transpersonal experiences *as if* they were objective, self-existing realities. Among others, Jorge Ferrer (2002) and Peter Fenner (2002) describe how the emphasis on reifying and personalizing spiritual experience limits the development of transpersonal theory and the potentialities for *trans*personal realization.

It seems to me that the ontological and epistemological basis for both mature Intersubjective and Transpersonal Psychologies must be the recognition that human experience is quintessentially *trans*-, impermanent, and a phenomenon of *inter*-ness and motility that cannot be captured within the notion of a fixed, static Self (or Other) as an encapsulated entity. To maintain fidelity to *trans*personal experience and experientially-based therapies, selfhood is best understood as a process that is both *intersubjective* (embedded in and inseparable from the world of others and otherness) and *intentional* (a meaning-seeking project hurtling through a time that it co-creates). Rather than assuming an observer/observed split as the beginning of inquiry and proceeding on that basis, contemplative attention turns back on itself, folding the observer into the field of observation.[ii]

This reorientation requires a double shift in terms of how we consider human subjectivity (being) and time. In terms of subjectivity, it requires a shift from thinking conceptually *about* others as self-existing, empirically observable entities (who can then be inserted into preconceived categories) to an emphasis on felt experiencing that is intersubjective in the sense that it thinks *with* otherness. It also requires, as Husserl (1928/1964) noted, a shift in conceiving of time as something that exists objectively and is external to the experiencer—like a river one is passively floating on—to a recognition that time is a subjective flow. That is, the river of time is not other than the being moving through it.

Time is internal to a consciousness engaged in the passing moment and that passage does not occur apart from one's participation in it. For instance, lived time is not static like clock time, but can "drag on" or "fly by" depending on how one is engaged in living it. This shifts the focus from what has happened or what might yet happen to a focus on what *is* happening just now within and between us. This does not mean that we attend inflexibly to the present moment to the exclusion of the past or future, but that we notice—when something arises to notice—how the momentum of the past and lure or threat of the future create a living present through our (perhaps unwitting) participation in it.

To flesh out this shift in approach, I will draw upon two well-established and complementary traditions: Buddhist psychology with its core method of mindfulness meditation and Phenomenology with its emphasis on contemplative attention will intertwine to form an alternative diagnostic approach. This approach is in accord with William James understanding of "Radical Empiricism" (James, 1912/1922). Empirical in the ("radical") sense of being experience-near and subjectively rigorous rather than experience-distant and objectivizing (conventional). The discussion proceeds by following Heidegger's (1959/1966) rough distinction between "calculative thinking" and "meditative thinking," and considers how the psychological knowing of other minds can proceed as a mindfulness practice of interpersonal meditation.

Recognizing that the intersubjective field is the actual locus in which any psychological diagnosis is made, we need to acknowledge straight away that in "my" getting to know "you"—your "youness"—is mediated through "my" seeing of you and all the influences that form the contours of my vision. Thus, fundamental questions for psychodiagnosis become,

- Is it possible for me to see you as you are or only as I conjure you through my personal projections and theoretical constructs?
- To the extent that I see you as I conjure you, who is it I am actually diagnosing?
- To the extent I see you as you are, how is it that I am able to do that?

We will consider the questions through an examination of calculative thinking and conventional empirically-informed diagnosis followed by a consideration of meditative thinking and phenomenological inquiry. Contemplative diagnosis as discussed here is offered to serve psycho-therapies and psychospiritual disciplines which seek to facilitate existential reckoning and transpersonal awakening. This approach may not be necessary for therapies and spiritual direction which have more modest goals in the service of social adaptation.

Calculative Thinking and Empirical Diagnosis

The mind strives to make sense of things. It forms *gestalts*, imposing an order on the apparent chaos of experience. We are compelled to wrap the immensity of *being* into a coherent picture, into constructs within which we feel oriented and secure. In this way we construct an inhabitable world, create "myths to live by" that give meaning and purpose to our lives and the lives of others.

However, the orientation and mastery we gain comes at a price. We become captivated within our intentional thought processes and live inside boxes in which we do not recognize, and tend to forget that it is our own calculating minds (reinforced by those around us) that have constructed our self-limited, provisional world. Calculative thought is at constant risk of taking its relative constructs, including diagnostic formulations, as absolute givens and losing itself in the process.

As Heidegger (1959/1966) put it, "Calculative thinking computes....[It] races from one prospect to the next...never stops, never collects itself" (p. 46). Moving from project to project, concept to concept, the calculating mind always looks outward. Thus, we remain hidden to ourselves. Self-hiddenness and the processes of projection it begets give rise to experience that is chronically anxious and incomplete.[iii]

Whether in our personal lives or in working with others, the calculating mind is either going after this or running away from that—and lost to itself. This lostness gives rise to the feeling it (I) is lacking something, which elicits an urgency to fill the sense of inner lack with some outer thing, experience, or knowledge (Loy, 1996; Bradford, 2021). All the while we are perpetuating the split between self and world/other, but without awareness that we are doing so.

Psychodiagnosis inadvertently reinforces this estrangement when it succumbs to the anxiety of the striving mind—including the wanting-to-help mind—and focuses solely on the pursuit of something (a diagnosis) out there and then rather than the open-ended presence that is here and now. In terms of psychotherapy, how much favor do we wish to grant calculative thinking and the influence such thought is likely to have over our clients and our psychotherapy? As Germer, Seigel and Fulton (2005) have put it:

> Problems arise when we take our descriptive clinical categories to be natural representations of an objective world of disorders, conveniently provided in a treatment manual...A diagnostic label used as a kind of shorthand can come to replace a more nuanced appraisal of the whole person. In the process, we stop looking, convinced that we know enough. It becomes a cover for our ignorance, masquerading as knowledge and certainty. (p. 69)

Calculative thought tends to reify opinions and ideas which it then clings to as armor against the inherently unsettled, impermanent, open-ended nature of existence. The positing of objective diagnoses, including personality typologies, may be just another way of defending ourselves— as therapists and clients alike—against the immensity of the mind and unpredictability of life by imposing a schematic order upon it. To the extent we cling to a reified view of Self and Other, regardless of the nosological reference system defining those categories, we introduce fixation into the exchange:

> To hold any fixed view, including a fixed view of our patients or ourselves, leads to suffering. Fixed positions are snapshots, arrested moments sampled from an unfolding flux, instantly out of date. The desire to find something stable is natural; we seek certainty to bind the anxiety of the unknown. Once we take up a position, we begin to defend it and attempt to shape our view of reality to fit our concepts. (ibid. p. 71)

Unwilling to tolerate the anxiety and tensions within transient experiencing, the risk of psychodiagnosis is that we latch onto a fixed view of the Other, thus partitioning them and distancing ourselves from them. This may temporarily reduce our anxiety, but only by risking a reification and freezing of the relational field between us. A calculating mindset is keyed to ignoring its own (inter-)subjectivity by focusing on identifying, labeling, and categorizing an Other (even if that other is oneself).

The psychological impact diagnosis can have on a patient, quite apart from the diagnostic value it may hold for a clinician, will be exemplified in the following vignettes of a client I will call Beatrice. Her story is pertinent in that she was diagnosed both empirically and contemplatively.

The Story of Beatrice, Take 1: Conventional Empirical Diagnosis

In her early twenties, Beatrice ("Bea") began suffering bouts of terror which would briefly incapacitate her. She had grown up in a family culture of withering criticism and bruising disavowal, especially from her mother who would occasionally tell Bea that she wished she would never have been born.

In college, Bea consulted a counselor who referred her to a psychiatrist who diagnosed her as having panic disorder coupled with clinical depression. Medication was prescribed and psychotherapy attempted, but these were of little help. In fact, Bea wound up regretting reaching out for help since the diagnosis of her pathology seemed to confirm her mother's accusations that she was fundamentally flawed; only this time it was a credible medical authority who indicted her. Beatrice carried this assessment of herself as a shameful weight for the next twenty years.

Through various psychological consultations, meditation practices, and her own reading and research during this period, she discovered some behavioral techniques for managing the panic attacks and was able to get by. "Getting by" meant living in fear of being incapacitated by an anxiety attack at any moment. Although she secretly sensed there might be some legitimate meaning to her anxiety—something that was not merely a confirmation of her disorderedness—she was afraid of opening herself to a psychologist for fear of again being pathologized.

Beatrice Take 2: Transpersonal-Empirical Diagnosis

While stretching conventional psychology to include spiritual potentials, humanistic and transpersonal thought have not yet thoroughly challenged the dualistic assumptions of empirical science (Ferrer, 2002). Accepting the empiricist principles of the DSM and working within that context, theorists such as Lukoff, Lu and Turner (1998) and Jerry (2003) worked to revise the DSM to include "religious and spiritual problems" as V-codes.

Others, such as Hutchins (2002) and Ingersoll (2002), worked to complement the standard differential diagnosis of the DSM by envisioning axes that include alternative and/or non-pathological criteria. Sympathetic to the principles of "positive psychology," Hutchins proposed a 5 axis "gnosis model" to complement the pathologically-skewed DSM with an assessment of gifts, callings, and abilities. Ingersoll, who accepts DSM diagnoses as a "necessary evil," complemented this with a broader "integral differential diagnosis" based on Ken Wilber's work.

In addition to providing refreshing alternatives to the DSM, these kinds of innovative diagnostic calculi deserve no small merit insofar as they authorize a focus on humanistic, holistic, and transpersonal potentialities—and are valuable in reducing anxiety and despair by helping to mitigate negative self-assessments. For instance, identifying my fixation point on the Enneagram may lessen the anxiety and self-criticism I feel as I realize that I am not a mutant, but belong to whole class of kindred spirits who are similarly fixated. This knowledge may well allow me to be more self-accepting.

In addition, once I Ennea-type you and see that the disturbing way in which you relate to me is less about me than about your own fixation style, I may be able to take your "attitude" less personally, be more understanding and forgiving. Nevertheless, let us not mistake a calculative project that helps us get along better in samsara with a contemplative undertaking which aims at freeing us from samsara.[iv] It seems to me that any genuine transpersonal psychology and spiritual path ought not take its eye off this big freedom.[v]

It is important to respect that Holistic, psycho-spiritual and Transpersonal Psychologies (as well as much psychotherapy in general these days) are "big tent" disciplines, making space for myriad meditative and psychological approaches. The particular understanding of "trans-personal" sketched in this article is but one of several understandings. In fact, no fewer than forty definitions of transpersonal psychology were catalogued over 30 years ago (Lajoie & Shapiro, 1992). I imagine things have only metastasized further since then.

While a contemplative approach recognizing the non-dual nature of existence and aiming toward awakening from samsara—the illusion of separate selfhood—is surely within the purview of Transpersonal and Holistic fields, it does not follow that all Transpersonal and Holistic approaches are "contemplative" in this sense. Much holistic, integrative, and psycho-spiritual psychology remain empirically and dualistically informed, as Bea discovered.

During the years following her initial diagnosis, Bea was a student of spirituality and occasional Zen practitioner, and at the end of this period found the courage to seek guidance from a popular psychospiritual organization that included individual consultations as part of a comprehensive program of psychospiritual development. Although the individual sessions were often conducted by licensed therapists who were themselves advanced students in the program, the organization was careful to distinguish what it did as "education" rather than "psychotherapy," at least partially to sidestep professional liability issues.

It, therefore, screened new students to ascertain their readiness to engage in what could be evocative and psychologically challenging work. To assess a student's readiness, program counselors relied heavily on psychoanalytic developmental theory. This is ostensibly done for the sake of the student—to make sure they have enough "ego strength" to handle the rigors of in-depth experiential work.

As with other such programs, the screening process is based on the conventional assumption that there is an observable and valid difference between psychopathology (including weak ego strength) and spiritual readiness (strong ego strength). The thing is: How do you accurately assess ego strength? If we are honest about it, this is a measure which turns out to be impossible to objectively ascertain. Where does an ego-entity appear which can be identified, much less measured, as to its relative strength? In adopting a conventional empiricist reference system to assess its students, even an unabashedly holistic program resorts to an objectivistic, categorical form of assessment which undermines the non-dual foundation upon which its holistic program is based.

In Bea's case, following a nearly year-long screening period while awaiting the start of new training group (in which she was candid and forthcoming about her psychological issues), it was decided that she was not a candidate for the deep work the program offered. Her individual teacher/counselor decided that she lacked readiness due to her ongoing anxieties and potential of having further panic attacks, as well as her inability to develop a sufficiently "trusting relationship" with the counselor.

Although a few of her positive qualities were reflected to her, Bea was rejected from the program and advised to seek remedial psychotherapy to address her unreadiness for "deeper work." This second diagnosis and the rejection it occasioned hit Bea quite hard confirming once again that she was seriously flawed—this time not by a cruel mother or random psychiatrist, but by a spiritual authority whose judgment she respected. Worse, this diagnosis felt still more entrapping than the earlier one since at this point, she was in mid-life and more aware that her time was limited. Her anxiety, hopelessness, and desperation escalated. It was at this point that she sought me out.

Meditative Thinking and Phenomenological Diagnosis

Heidegger (1959/1966) describes meditative thinking as an "openness to the mystery" in which our normal habit of dualistic thinking is loosened, allowing for unmediated awareness (*gnosis, prajna*) to function spontaneously. The meditative openness of which Heidegger speaks is informed by a phenomenological epistemology and method of inquiry.

Whereas conventional empirical science proceeds by isolating variables and privileging objectivity, phenomenology is inclusive of the complexity of experience, privileging subjectivity, and the exercise of intuition (rather than logical deduction) as the primary cognizant function. To see another person as a phenomenon, or mystery, is both to invite the Other to reveal themself as they are and to be willing to be awe-struck by their otherness. Adapted to clinical inquiry, phenomenology can serve as a bridge between calculative, sharply dualistic thinking and non-dualistic contemplative knowing.

Within calculative thought, psychological reference systems mediate experience through the conceptual lens of their theories. Depending on the priorities of the system, some elements of experience come into sharper focus while other elements remain fuzzy or are ignored. Without rejecting the value that may come from seeing the Other through the lens of any particular system or through multiple lenses of several systems (as in Integral approaches), phenomenology endeavors to encounter other minds as they reveal (and conceal) themselves—as free as possible from the mediating concepts of any theoretical reference system.

Phenomenological inquiry proceeds by intentionally "bracketing" the filtering constructs of the therapist's reference systems in order to discover how the client is tacitly constructing their own self-world.[vi] This method presents us with the challenge of engaging in meditative attention, which as Heidegger (1959/1966) observed, "At times requires a greater effort. It demands more practice. It is in need of even more delicate care than any other genuine craft. But it must also be able to bide its time, to await as does the farmer, whether the seed will come up and ripen" (p. 47).

Within calculative thought, diagnosis is an orienting function conducted prior to a treatment function based upon it. But for experientially-based meditative awareness, the separation between these functions does not hold as diagnosis is always already part of the treatment. In getting to know a person, the way in which we approach an Other is already making an impression on that person. In diagnosing someone, we are already "treating" the person in a particular way and with a particular attitude, which may, for instance, encourage or discourage the person's trust and self-disclosure, as it did for Bea.

Since we can only gain access to the mind of an Other through *participating* with that mind, phenomenological diagnosis requires from the outset that we take into consideration how we are seeing, and perhaps distorting, the Other through our own constructs. In order to minimize distortion and open our field of vision, it is of primary importance to bracket any assumptions of belief or disbelief we have in regard to the other person and what they say.

A phenomenologically-oriented therapist neither confirms nor disconfirms the truth of a person's story, but listens as unconditionally as possible with what Freud called "neutrality" accomplished via "evenly-suspending attention." This is similar to the Buddhist mindfulness practice of *bare attention*: moment to moment sensory awareness.[vii] Whereas our usual tendency is to get caught up in calculative thoughts and react emotionally in regard to them, meditative attention temporarily suspends the striving of discursive thought. Without trying to keep anything in mind or to push anything away, the therapist can more fully enter into and participate in the intersubjective exchange allowing for increasingly subtle, complex and contradictory perceptions to arise.

As Heidegger notes, "Meditative thinking demands of us not to cling one-sidedly to a single idea, nor to run down a one-track course of ideas. Meditative thinking demands of us that we engage ourselves with what at first sight does not go together at all" (1959/1966, p. 53). This invites us to attune to the "felt sense" (Gendlin, 1978) that opens to the totality of an experience, even though we may not be able to say what that totality is. Effectively, this practice is a rudimentary form of interpersonal meditation and, as such, is a unique contribution of Western psychology to traditional Eastern forms of solo meditation practices.

Beatrice Take 3: Phenomenological-Contemplative Diagnosis

By being present within the felt saturation of an intersubjective field, knowledge arises intuitively and empathically through noticing and explicating what is implicit within that field. For example, when Bea told me how her mother ruthlessly belittled her as a child, I was less drawn to what happened to her than with how she took, and continued to take, what happened to her (this being what was happening as we spoke).

In our conversations, she spoke of what struck me as horrible experiences with a wan smile. But the smile did not correspond to the humiliation I was empathically feeling in listening to her story. Being moved by the tragedy, yet without either validating her as being a victim or invalidating the gravity of what happened, I was able to observe what I felt as the incongruity of her smile in conjunction with the horror I was feeling by what she was saying.

As I shared this observation with her, she blanched, paused, looked me in the eye, and said in a shaky voice, "*I know. That nervous smile. I think I do that a lot.*" In this exchange, I described something that was still largely implicit for her and for me. Yet my reflection did not rise to the level of an objective diagnosis or even an interpretation, since I did not grant it any meaning beyond the transient exchange we were having. However, that Bea noticed this incongruity as a habitual reaction on her part did mean something to her, and potentially it could mean that she was flawed and could be taken as yet another proof of her unworthiness. Or not.

Bea's emotional incongruity reveals something of her *self and world construct* system (Bugental, 1978). Identifying a self-structure is a typical purpose of psychodiagnosis, including one phenomenologically derived. It is not sufficient in phenomenology to describe various elements of subjective experience without intuiting the coherence of those elements.

Phenomenological knowing seeks to comprehend how the various dimensions, inner tensions, contradictions, and potentialities of a person coalesce into an integral, *invariant organization* of subjectivity.

As Idhe (1977) writes, the phenomenological method, *"Seek[s] out structural or invariant features of the phenomena"* (p. 39). Phenomenologically, there is no problem considering the complexities and interactive constructs of multiple theoretical reference systems. Since the constructs of any reference system are already bracketed by an evenly-suspended attention, one is less tempted to cling to the knowledge they delimit. Indeed, the formulations of any particular reference system(s) might fruitfully illuminate something of a person's self-organization. However, such a formulation is to arise intuitively-empathically out of a meditative involvement with the Other rather than logically in deference to a preferred theory or nosological category.

Nevertheless, even this more open, intuitive understanding of a self-structure tends toward a subtle reification of that person. In seeking to discover "structural and invariant features," phenomenology presumes to arrive at a knowledge that is not conditioned by its method of questioning. In presuming to know an Other apart from the Self doing the knowing, phenomenology is emboldened to make a claim of absolute (invariant) knowledge.

In doing so, it is at risk of reverting to a form of dualistic, calculative thinking. As helpful as it is, the meditative method of bracketing by evenly suspending judgment is an intentional act of holding biases and distractions at bay. This holding-back introduces a subtle separation into the relational field. Awareness of the Other is still being managed from a distance; thus, it is not fully *inter*-subjective, experience-near and true to the transient nature of experience.

Identifying a structure of subjectivity does not reveal *who* a person is. It reveals *how* a person is construing their world and the self they are taking themselves to be. A self-world structure is a composition of psychological tendencies which are intentional (even if unconscious) practices one tends to repeat and so perpetuate. For experiential therapies, it is not enough to identify a self (-world) organizing structure since merely identifying a fixation or construct is rarely enough to release it.

Remaining on a conceptual level does not penetrate the depths of conditioning. To more thoroughly liberate a constricting construct of subjectivity, it is necessary to open to *how* one is intending (constructing) that self-world in order to not intend (construe) it into the future. The challenge is this: to experientially discover that one's (constructed) self is not something (someone) one *is*, but is something (someone) one *practices*.[viii]

Recognizing how I am (and have been) unconsciously participating in a particular, habitual way of being in the world opens the door for me to release that (structuring) participation. A more thorough self-liberation requires that I see—experience—that the self is not an entity but a set of practices, a kind of play that I have—and still am—unwittingly performing. Experientially-keyed therapy focuses attention on the moment-to-moment participation of how one is engaged in construing and perpetuating a particular self-world. Such attention is meditative in the sense that it attends to what is ordinarily pre-reflective, below or outside everyday conscious awareness. Thus, it is more conducive to empathic, energetic, somatic and relationally-robust forms of cognizance.

Of course, it is also possible, and often desirable, to proceed from pre-reflective, non-conceptual openness to conceptual reflection and constructive self-understanding. But we ought not lose sight that moving into self-understanding and conceptual reflection will likely shift the therapeutic exchange from a meditative to a calculative (reifying) mindset.

Certainly, there are many instances where moving from unintegrated feeling states into more conceptually-bound states is called for. This is especially true when a person is at risk of being swamped by overwhelming emotion which may trigger a re-traumatization of some kind. But stepping back into conceptual reflection also makes sense as one strives to better understand one's hidden motives and unconscious reactions in order to integrate one's self-sense in a less hypocritical or reactive direction. The challenge for an experience-near therapist is to move back and forth between unintegrated states including the openness of simply being and constructive understandings without unnecessarily reifying those constructions by lending the weight of professional authority to them.

In psychological knowledge, it is all too easy to think or speak about an insight into self or other as if that insight were something that exists in reality rather than as that which it is: something that exists only in a conception of reality. For instance, it would be easy to speak of Bea's "critical superego," "negative maternal introject," or "inner critic" as if the critic, introject, or superego existed independent of our construction and her practice of it. Of course, naming this kind of thing is often a vital step toward releasing it, but only if it remains a step and is not reified into an identity.

While Bea did take her insight as yet another indictment against herself, I was struck by the conviction of her self-indictment—and said so. This gave her another pause. In this pause, Bea did not know what to think and neither did I, dropping us both into a kind of freefall. For my part, practicing the best I could within a meditative awareness, I let myself fall, relaxing in her presence without knowing what to say and without succumbing to the impulse to fill in this gap and relieve us from having to bear the unknowing.

Sitting together in the openness of silent attunement, I soon sensed Bea's mind starting to cogitate again and wondered what she was thinking. So, I ventured, "What do you notice as we sit here?" This opened an exchange during which she oscillated between affirming the old self-construct of being flawed and opening to the possibility—which she experienced as "groundless"—that this might not be the case.

This therapeutic traverse was nothing short of an identity crisis for her. If she was not fundamentally flawed, then fundamentally, who was she? In the oscillating play of this inquiry, each of us describing what we were noticing and noticing what we were describing, Bea and I were practicing an experience-near *explication* of meaning.

Explication Versus Interpretation

Whereas an *interpretation* makes meaning based on the concepts of a reference system that filter and funnel raw experience into the categories of its particular constructs, an *explication* arises within the field of intersubjective experiencing and does not disengage from the felt complexity of that field. The meaning that arises through an open-ended process of explication is unique and unpredictable unlike the calculated meanings that are interpreted according to preconceived categories within a circumscribed theoretical system. Interpretations are content-based and serve utilitarian goals of expedience, proceeding in a single direction from chaos to order, from raw experience to conceptual understanding, from (following Freud) unconsciousness to consciousness.

On the other hand, explications arise through meditative attunement, are process-based, serving the lucency of opening as such and sense of wonder. They remain transitory and proceed dialectically, oscillating between the mysterious implications of felt experience and the explicit understandings which emerge from it. *In contemplative cognizance, diagnosis is no-thing*. It is neither the conceptual understanding, such as would be carried in words like "depression" or "incongruent," nor is it the mute, raw experience to which the words refer.

Rather, diagnosis takes place in the to-and-fro between experience being understood and understanding being experienced, checked as to its felt accuracy, and then either released (if accurate) or re-understood (more accurately). In this sense, diagnosis is not a *noun* identifying some psychological content, but a *verb* identifying a treatment process that entails a clarifying of understanding along with a deepening of experience.

True to the transient nature of experience, the process of explication aims not to nail down a meaning, but to free up meaningfulness by allowing for the emergence of deepening understandings. Since (as long as we live) there is no end to experience, there is no end to the meaning we may discover through opening to it.

It turns out to be impossible, as Gendlin (1973) observes, to arrive at any invariant structure of subjectivity or any final meaning regarding who or what or how we are. Experience being endlessly variable, understanding is also endlessly variable. Facing the way things actually are reveals there is no fixed psychological structure, no self-ground, to be found, as Beatrice noticed in her brief, but exhilarating experience of "groundlessness."

For some moments, she found no constructs—and in those open, free-floating moments, there was no panic or anxiety, but an unfamiliar peace of mind. Her open-ended experience closed rather soon as worrisome thoughts started up again, but the gap of those moments left an impression. We noticed together that when she let herself be, groundlessness—that is, not knowing or being able to identify where she stood—need not be feared. On the contrary, it offers a fertile avenue of buoyant experiencing she had not previously permitted.

Beatrice Take 4: Contemplative Diagnosing

Bea's initial guardedness, porcelain smile and the shakiness of her voice revealed to me why her previous counselor may have concluded she was too brittle for in-depth work. In the early weeks of our work together, I, too, felt uncomfortable in her nervous presence. Yet I could also sense in her shaky voice, speaking as it did at times with direct eye contact, a fount of relational courage and self-honesty. For a while, I did not know how to address this—and rather than force something, I decided to linger in the silence of my unknowing.

Very soon, she revealed that she experienced my silence as terrifying in the sense that she was populating it with her own fears that I might be judging her critically. Yet, she found the nerve to share this experience and ask me about it, which facilitated my responding to her in a way that observed both her fear and her courage in daring to open and speak candidly about herself.

Repeated exchanges like this led her to feel a steadiness with me, and so with herself, allowing her to take in that she could be both terrified and brave. She eventually disclosed that it was my simply being with her, more than any particular sense I made during that time, that allowed her to relax and more deeply trust me and herself.

From a calculative perspective, Bea's previous counselor and I would probably have agreed on her psychodynamic diagnosis. However, we came to exactly opposite conclusions regarding what that meant for her readiness to engage in deep work. I found Bea to have enough courage, candor and capacity for relational openness required for such an inner journey. The crux of the difference was less what we each saw in Bea (since we saw some of the same things) than how we each saw her. Again, whereas a contemplative approach accents the *how* of the *what*, a calculative approach emphasizes the *what* over the *how*, thus tending toward reification of the Other.

Within a predominantly calculative attitude, the program counselor saw and reflected Bea back to herself as an anxious and rather difficult person with whom to relate. Seeing herself through the eyes of a scrutinizing Other and lacking the strength to shake off this gaze, Bea displayed herself as the object she was (yet again) being seen to be. Thus, she confirmed the counselor's (and her own) vision of her as seriously flawed.

Caught in a dualistic vision, the counselor was not able to see the whole picture of what was happening. She did not see that it was not Bea, in herself, who was anxious and difficult to connect with, but that it was Bea in relation to the counselor that evoked anxiety. The difficulty did not lie solely with Bea and the intrapsychic dynamics of her separate mind—as Object Relations theory (which mediated the counselor's vision) affirms— but lay between the two of them. Bea was experienced as difficult for the counselor, but the counselor's difficulty was left out of the equation.

In contrast, by adopting a contemplatively relational attitude, I was more able to remain aware of the subjective tensions influencing my own seeing as well as the tensions I was noticing in Bea. Remaining within the intersubjective field, I allowed that Bea's anxieties were not fixed inside her separate mind but existed in the *inter-being*[ix] between us. Within this less-divided, more holistic vision, I did not assume that the relational problem belonged to either Bea or to me alone, but was (in an experiential sense) somehow *ours*.

The sense of relatedness Bea felt in this approach allowed her to relax her guard, and with the immediacy of the relational contact permitting little room for distraction, pressed her to open herself and to be seen/see herself as she was in relationship (here and now) rather than in isolation. Thus, we came to see potentialities in Bea her previous counselor missed.

While it is true that I did not have to screen Bea for admission to a psychospiritual program, I did need to screen her as a psychotherapy client whom I could treat within the scope of my competence. Since an Other can only be known and treated through one's own knowing and treatment of them, it makes no sense to screen the readiness of a supposedly isolated "I," but only the *compatibility* of the other person and oneself (or the program one represents).

It was unfortunate for Bea that she was identified as inadequate in herself when the truth was that the inadequacy was in the incompatibility between her and the approach—the psychospiritual vision and skillful means at the disposal—of the program. It would have been both more honest and more humble for the program's counselor to have admitted that she herself was unable to establish a good enough working relationship with Bea, and that perhaps the program also lacked the support and relational means she felt were necessary for Bea to benefit from it.

Understanding this, it also did not escape our attention that it was due to her dismissal from that program and the advice of her teacher/counselor to seek therapy that Bea did seek out a therapy that enabled her to engage a more vital, integrative process. This is ironic on two counts. On one point, it shows that Bea actually did trust her counselor and her advice, even though the counselor partly dismissed her for having a lack of trust. Secondly, the dismissal and advice for remedial therapy actually did work in Bea's favor as intended.

There is a temptation to judge the program counselor as either wrong for not diagnosing Bea in a more holistic, intersubjective manner or as right for referring her out for personal psychotherapy. However, from a contemplative perspective, both of these judgments miss the point. While the point of calculative diagnosing may indeed focus on distinguishing between what treatment is right and wrong in the sense of either/or, contemplative diagnosing seeks to open the mind and heart to the free play of awareness and the potentiality of *ands*.

Within an open field of inter-being, the play of discrimination intertwines with that of empathic resonance and is oriented toward strengthening the capacity of self and other to more deeply open to the spontaneous responsivity of unconditional presence.

Going Forward: Inter-Being and the Challenge of Non-Doing

Recognizing that others do not exist independently of our consciousness of them but only appear within an intersubjective field of consciousness, the meditative attention of phenomenology opens the door to a more saturated contemplative awareness. Rather than emphasizing conceptual under-standing and elaboration of a particular emotional fixation or self-world construct, contemplative knowing emphasizes being present to the ambiguous and paradoxical otherness of self-fixations and self-constructs.

This process- and awe-based approach proceeds by letting beings be the beings they are. By offering an Other a relational field and way of knowing that does not cling to any particular position or content, the natural emergence and release of fixations is facilitated. In this, there is nothing special we need to do. In fact, letting be presents us with the challenge of non-doing.

Contemplative letting be does not neglect fixations by drifting into distraction or psychic numbness. Neither is it a discursive thinking about them. Rather, it involves taking the time to let the open awareness in which fixations and insights arise remain open. Whatever understandings or misunderstandings arise within an inquiry, they need not be separated from the open-ended field of awareness within which they emerge. Privileging the groundlessness of awareness by remaining open as understandings and misunderstandings emerge, clarify, and pass helps us not lose touch with the incomprehensible mystery of being and impermanent nature of existence.

Daring to be true to what is in this way, knowing is direct (*gnosis*). Since knowledge of an Other is not separated from its essentially open nature, it is not limited in any fundamental way. Thus, it is thorough (*dia*). So, a diagnosis that is true to the transience and inter-ness of the subjective field in which it arises does not finally mean anything in particular, nor does it lack any particular meaning. Since this is the case, the knowing of other minds can be practiced as a kind of humble, loosening play. I have found that just this way of knowing and being with an Other is the essence of what heals in psychotherapy.

References

Adams, W. (1995). Revelatory openness wedded with the clarity of unknowing Psychoanalytic evenly suspended attention, the phenomenological attitude, and meditative awareness. *Psychoanalysis and Contemporary Thought, 18*(4), 463-494.

Berger, P., & Luckmann, T. (1967). *The social construction of reality: A treatise in the sociology of knowledge.* New York, NY: Doubleday.

Boss, M. (1978). Eastern and Western therapy. In J. Welwood (Ed.), *The meeting of the ways* (pp. 183-191). New York, NY: Schocken.

Bradford, K. (2021). *Opening Yourself: The psychology and yoga of self-liberation.* Manotick, ON: Sumeru Press.

Bradford, K. (2023). On the essence of freedom. *The Journal of Existential Analysis, 34(1),* 376-392.

Bugental, J. (1978). *Psychotherapy and process.* New York, NY: Addison-Wesley.

Fenner, P. (2002). *The edge of certainty: Dilemmas on the Buddhist path.* York Beach, Maine, USA: Nicolas-Hays.

Ferrer, J. N. (2002). *Revisioning transpersonal theory.* Albany, NY: SUNY Press.

Gadamer, H.G. (1982). *Truth and method.* (G. Barden & J. Cumming, Trans.). New York, NY: Crossroad. (Original work published in 1960)

Gendlin, E. T. (1973). Experiential phenomenology. In M. Natanson (Ed.), *Phenomenology and the social sciences* (pp. 281-319). Evanston, IL: Northwestern University Press.

Gendlin, E. T. (1978). *Focusing*. New York, NY: Bantam.

Giorgi, A. (1970). *Psychology as a human science: A phenomenologically based approach*. New York, NY: Harper & Row.

Giorgi, A. (1985). *Phenomenological and psychological research*. Pittsburgh, PA: Duquense University Press.

Germer, C. K., Siegel, R. D., & Fulton, P. R. (2005). *Mindfulness and psychotherapy*. New York, NY: Guilford.

Heidegger, M. (1966). *Discourse on thinking*. (J. Anderson & E. H. Freund, Trans.). New York, NY: Harper Colophon. (Original work published 1959)

Husserl, E. (1964). *The phenomenology of internal time-consciousness*. (M. Heidegger, Ed., J. Churchill, Trans.). Bloomington: Indiana University Press. (Original work published 1928)

Husserl, E. (1970). *The crisis of European sciences and Transcendental Phenomenology* (D. Carr, Trans.). Evanston, IL: Northwestern University Press. (Original work published 1954)

Hutchins, R. (2002). Gnosis: Beyond disease and disorder to a diagnosis inclusive of gifts and challenges. *Journal of Transpersonal Psychology, 34*(2), 101-114.

Idhe, D. (1977). *Experimental phenomenology: An introduction*. New York, NY: Capricorn.

Ingersoll, E. (2002). An integral approach for teaching and practicing diagnosis. *Journal of Transpersonal Psychology, 34*(2), 115-128.

James, W. (1922). *Essays in radical empiricism*. New York, NY: Longmans, Green & Co. (Original word published in 1912)

Jerry, P. A. (2003). Challenges in transpersonal diagnosis. *Journal of Transpersonal Psychology, 35*(1), 43-59.

Lajoie, D. H., & Shapiro, S. I. (1992). Definitions of transpersonal psychology: The first twenty-three years. *Journal of Transpersonal Psychology, 24*(1), 79-98.

Loy, D. (1996). *Lack and transcendence: The problem of death and life in psychotherapy, existentialism, and Buddhism*. Atlantic Highlands, NJ: Humanities Press.

Lukoff, D., Lu, F., & Turner, R. (1998). From spiritual emergency to spiritual problem: The transpersonal roots of the new DSM-IV category. *Journal of Transpersonal Psychology, 38*(2), 21-50.

Merleau-Ponty, M. (1963). *The structure of behavior* (A. L. Fisher, Trans.). Boston: Beacon. (Original work published 1942)

Namkhai Norbu, C. (1994). *Buddhism and psychology*. Arcidosso, Italy: Shang Shung Edizioni.

Schneider, K. (2008). *Existential-integrative psychotherapy: Guideposts to the core of practice*. New York, NY: Routledge.

Spinelli, E. (1989). *The interpreted world: An introduction to phenomenological psychology*. London: Sage.

Szasz, T. S. (1974). *The myth of mental illness: Foundations of a theory of personal conduct*. Revised Edition. New York, NY: Harper & Row.

Trungpa, C. (2005). *The sanity we are born with: A Buddhist approach to psychology*. Boston: Shambhala.

Van den Berg, J. H. (1972). *A different existence: Principles of phenomenological psychopathology*. Pittsburgh: Duquesne University Press.

Endnotes

[i] Empirical scientific assumptions include an insistence on objectivity, involving a strict separation between observer and observed as well as a presumption of neutrality on the part of the researcher/therapist; the exclusion of extraneous ("contaminating") variables, involving a decontextualizing of the research subject and a focus on discrete parts or aspects rather than on interactive wholes; the privileging of logical deduction as the primary cognizant capacity (as distinct from intuition or empathic attunement for instance), with statistical indices being the arbiter of meaning; and the prime scientific directive being that of prediction and control of nature.

[ii] A more thorough discussion of the subject/object split and phenomenology of self as an imaginal artifact of dualistic consciousness is undertaken in Bradford, 2021.

iii Sitting down to meditate for even a few minutes to quiet our mind makes apparent how dominated we are by discursive proliferation we mistakenly think we are in control of.

iv This is a paraphrase of Chogyal Namkhai Norbu (1994, p. 13)

v For a discussion on the essence of freedom as distinct from existential and psychological kinds of freedom, see Bradford, 2023.

vi See Giorgi, 1985, pp. 8-22; Idhe, 1977, pp. 29-54; and Spinelli, 1989, pp. 16-31, for elaboration of the phenomenological method applied to the Human Sciences.

vii See Adams, 1995, for a discussion of the congruencies between Phenomenological, Psychoanalytic and Buddhist meditative attitudes.

viii The psychodynamics of the phenomenology of self as described in Buddhist Psychology is discussed in Bradford, 2021, pp. 53-79.

ix Thich Nhat Hanh deserves credit for having coined this excellent term.

Social and Emotional Wellbeing: Ancient Wisdom from Australia's Aboriginal and Torres Strait Islander People as a Valuable Alternative to Western Biomedical Models of Mental Health

Kathleen Martin and Timothy A. Carey

Abstract: *Understandings of mental health from a Western biomedical perspective have not served as well. Problems with our diagnostic systems are well-articulated in the literature. Rates of mental health problems continue to rise and problems, such as increased stigma and reduced life-expectancy, are potent indicators of a system that is failing. Aboriginal and Torres Strait Islander Australians' framework of social and emotional wellbeing (SEWB) offers a viable alternative to how we conceptualise and promote contentment, wellbeing, and social harmony. From this perspective, living contentedly involves achieving balance and connectedness across the seven domains of: body; mind and emotions; family and kinship; community; culture; country; and spirit, spirituality, and ancestors. Life from an SEWB perspective is a dynamic process of achieving and maintaining balance or stability across important domains of intra and inter connectedness. The SEWB approach is strengths-based rather than being a deficit or illness model and is holistic in the sense of considering the individual within the social and physical context in which they live their life. By shaping our approaches to helping from the position of SEWB we can provide compassionate and respectful assistance that is based on the perspective of the person seeking help rather than being determined by the person providing the help.*

To make programs and services as effective and efficient as possible, we think it's important to be clear about the problem being addressed. Without adequate definitions, it's not possible to tell whether something even is a problem. Currently, in health, generally, and mental health, more specifically, we are hampered by a lack of helpful definitions (Carey, 2022).

The problem with a lack of suitable definitions is that, in the absence of being clear about what is and is not a problem, we could be providing treatments and other interventions unnecessarily. Treating things that don't need to be treated wastes limited financial resources and can even result in harm. In fact, inappropriate healthcare is already a global phenomenon that results in billions of wasted dollars each year along with people suffering the effects of treatments they should never have received (Carey, 2017).

The ancient wisdom of Australia's First Nations peoples can be harnessed to develop services that are more effective and efficient. From the teachings of Aboriginal and Torres Strait Islander Australians, we can understand both health and mental health more clearly and holistically. A holistic perspective is crucial for promoting an understanding of health and healthcare as a means to an end, not the end in itself (Carey, 2017). The "end" that should always be at the front of our minds is living a life one has reason to value (Marmot, 2006).

Being healthy is only important because it enables us to live as we would wish. Poor health compromises the way we live our lives. At the same time, it is important to remember that wellbeing ≠ being well (Carey, 2013). Again, this is an important reminder to consider people holistically within the contexts in which they are situated whenever any "helping" is being considered.

In the Western biomedical healthcare industry, health is often treated as an end in itself with people's goals, priorities, and preferences with regard to the life they want to live being of less or no importance. Adopting perspectives from Aboriginal and Torres Strait Islander Australians could be very helpful in correcting this means-end imbalance.

We have written this chapter because we thought the combination of our different perspectives would provide people with some practical and applicable alternatives to the current Western biomedical system of diagnosis and treatment. I (KM) am a proud Aboriginal woman from the Arrernte language group in central Australia. I am a Traditional Owner of land around Alice Springs and am regarded as an Elder in family. I work as an academic at Flinders University where I teach about cultural Safety and Aboriginal Health to medical and other health students.

I (TAC), on the other hand, am a non-Indigenous man. I have a background in education, statistics, and clinical psychology and had the privilege of living in Alice Springs for 10 years. When I began to learn about Aboriginal and Torres Strait Islander knowledge systems, I recognised the benefits they could bring to Western ideas and conventional ways of working.

Understandings of health for Aboriginal and Torres Strait Islander Australians are influenced by nine guiding principles. These principles provide important direction for the development of health services and programs. Swan and Raphael (1995) provide a full description of the principles which we summarise here:

1. Aboriginal and Torres Strait Islander health is viewed in a holistic context that encompasses mental health and physical, cultural, and spiritual health.
2. Self-determination is central to the provision of Aboriginal and Torres Strait Islander health services.
3. Culturally valid understandings must shape the provision of services.
4. The experiences of trauma and loss are a direct outcome of disruptions to cultural wellbeing and have inter-generational effects.
5. The human rights of Aboriginal and Torres Strait Islander peoples must be recognised and respected.
6. Racism, stigma, environmental adversity, and social disadvantage must be appreciated as ongoing stressors.
7. Family and kinship are of central importance as well as bonds of reciprocal affection, responsibility, and sharing.
8. There is no single Aboriginal or Torres Strait Islander culture or group, but numerous groupings, languages, kinships, and tribes, as well as ways of living.
9. It is important to recognise the great strengths, creativity, and endurance of Aboriginal and Torres Strait Islander peoples as well

as their deep understanding of the relationships between human beings and the environment.

These principles are woven through Aboriginal and Torres Strait Islander concepts of health and mental health. Importantly, they also provide valuable information for people who are developing services and other programs to ensure that interventions are effective, efficient, relevant, and meaningful to the people who are accessing them.

Health From an Aboriginal and Torres Strait Islander Perspective

It can be difficult to appreciate the fact that the things we think we know a lot about can be considered very differently in other cultures. Health is one of those things. These words from the National Aboriginal Health Strategy (National Aboriginal Health Strategy Working Party, 1989, p. ix) give a sense of the gulf between Western and Aboriginal and Torres Strait Islander views of health:

> "Health" to Aboriginal peoples is a matter of determining all aspects of their life, including control over their physical environment, of dignity, of community self-esteem, and of justice. It is not merely a matter of the provision of doctors, hospitals, medicines or the absence of disease and incapacity. … In Aboriginal society there was no word, term or expression for 'health' as it is understood in western society. It would be difficult from the Aboriginal perception to conceptualise 'health' as one aspect of life. The word as it is used in Western society almost defies translation but the nearest translation in an Aboriginal context would probably be a term such as "life is health is life."

These words are profound in their implications for effective, efficient, relevant, and meaningful healthcare. From this Aboriginal and Torres Strait Islander perspective, to be healthy people need to be able to control important aspects of their life.

While treating tumours, fevers, and other problems will always be important, it is just as crucial for people to live in a safe environment, to have adequate shelter, and so on. It is also essential that people have reasonable decision-making scope regarding their daily activities.

Mental Health from An Aboriginal and Torres Strait Islander Perspective

While considering health from an Aboriginal and Torres Strait Islander point of view is refreshing and empowering, it is perhaps not as dramatic a shift in perspective as the way mental health is understood by Aboriginal and Torres Strait Islander peoples. The term "social and emotional wellbeing" (SEWB) is used rather than "mental health" (Gee, Dudgeon, Schultz, Hart, & Kelly, 2014).

SEWB can incorporate constructs related to mental health, but it is much broader than the Western biomedical approach to psychological wellbeing. Crucially, SEWB is a strengths-based, holistic approach to understanding social and psychological functioning rather than an illness focussed model.

Central to the SEWB approach is the concept of connectedness (Gee et al., 2014). Seven domains are specified and ideal SEWB arises when a person's connections with each of these domains are balanced the way they want them to be. From a SEWB perspective, "connection" refers "to the diverse ways in which people experience and express these various domains of SEWB throughout their lives" (Gee et al., 2014, p. 58). The SEWB domains are: body; mind and emotions; family and kinship; community; culture; country; and spirit, spirituality, and ancestors (Gee et al., 2014).

It is essential to appreciate the way in which a person's unique individuality is honoured and respected in this approach. Not everyone will place the same importance on each domain. In fact, domains can take on different importance at different times of a person's life—and with changing circumstances and conditions.

Furthermore, people will vary in the ways they consider connectedness in each domain. Connection strength that is best in one domain won't necessarily be the right level of connection for another domain. Domain connectedness can also vary over time depending on a person's age and other circumstances. The SEWB model, therefore, demands that the perspective of the person accessing services is the perspective that informs and guides all aspects of decision-making with regard to the provision of services (Carey, 2017).

Another strength of this model is that it can be usefully applied cross-culturally with people who have different beliefs, norms, and values. A sense of community, for example, might not be such a high priority for a person from a more individualistic culture. However, there may be community, social, or, perhaps, even sporting groups to which a person likes to feel connected. Similarly, for some people the domain of spirit, spirituality, and ancestors might not immediately resonate with them, yet they might like to have a sense of meaning and purpose in their life. Learning to think broadly about these domains can help with the applicability of the model.

For me (KM), knowing where you come from and knowledge of who your ancestors were, their dreams, totems, and dances (their spirituality) is about identity. Not being able to connect to this important aspect of your identity can lead to feelings of emptiness, loss, and no connection. I (TAC) can also relate to the importance of identity. My son is named after my father, and I enjoy finding out about where my family's origins were and how they came to be in Australia. I like doing things that have meaning for me (like writing this chapter) and give me a sense that I'm contributing in some small way.

Connection to body

Being physically able to navigate the demands of daily living can be important for a person's peace of mind. Achieving contentment and satisfaction is more difficult if one is in pain, tired, or otherwise finds it a burden to move around in their environments. Physical markers such as weight, blood pressure, urine albumin-to-creatinine ration, and blood glucose levels can all signal areas where changes could help to improve a person's ability to achieve the goals that are important them.

While indicators of functioning can tell a story, in my (KM) culture an illness is often seen as coming from an external source such as when another person has wronged an individual. We always think about the person as a whole, not just the separate systems such as cardiovascular, neurological, and renal systems. When things are internal and can't be seen, we often look for the external causes of the illness. Lifestyle choices are also important.

Coincidentally, I (TAC) also think that markers of internal functioning need to be considered within the context of the whole individual and the life they are living. I have often had blood test results which some medical practitioners interpret as me having high cholesterol, so they have offered me medication. I have no other signs of heart disease, however, and I know the cholesterol story is not as simple as it is often portrayed—so I tend to be a lot less concerned about my cholesterol "score" than some of the medical practitioners with whom I have consulted.

Connection to mind and emotions

Equally important to a person's physical integrity is their psychological functioning. We're using the term "psychological functioning" in a broad sense here to cover both thinking and feeling. The longer one spends with these concepts, the more blurred they can become.

If a person thinks they're sad, is that a thought or a feeling? Similarly, if someone feels like they're in a reflective, observing state of mind, is that a feeling or a thought? Finally, when someone stubs their toe, where is the pain experienced? Although it seems logical that the pain must be in the toe, the sensation or experience of the pain occurs in the brain. It is just as important, then, for people to be aware of and in tune with their mental activity as it is for them to connect with their physical toing and froing.

Although the mind and emotions are about the individual in my (KM) culture, it is important to recognise that they are heavily influenced by what is happening around us. For example, I (KM) remember an interpreter being called to speak with a young woman in a hospital ward because she was hallucinating and not making any sense. The interpreter was able to talk to her and found that a friend of hers had died, but she hadn't attended the funeral and wasn't able to express her grief.

Because she hadn't been able to pay her respects to the friend and the friend's family, she didn't sleep or eat for several days. With this new information, the medical practitioners were able to re-assess the woman's situation. They came to appreciate that all she needed was some sleep and to be able to grieve for her friend, so they changed their treatment plan.

Emotions are important to Aboriginal people, and we are generally very open about expressing them. For example, if we cry and wail when a person dies, we are showing respect for the deceased—and once we have grieved, we can then move on to the healing process.

I (TAC) think our Western approaches to helping could benefit a lot by genuinely adopting a more holistic and contextualised understanding of people and their problems. For example, it doesn't make any sense to me that we would place arbitrary time limits on the length of time someone should grieve for the death of someone to whom they were very close. Everyone has their own story and their own way of making sense of their experiences.

Connection to family and kinship

Family relationships can be critically important in both positive and negative ways to a person's ability to live a life they value. From our very first breath, our family influences the experiences we have and the learnings we accumulate. Without really knowing it, we can develop preferences for certain things or dislikes for other things based on the activities and interactions we have with our family members.

From this perspective, "family" doesn't only refer to those with whom people are genetically or legally related. Family groupings can comprise members who would otherwise be unrelated, but who have a great deal of involvement and influence in a person's life. Finding the right balance in connections with family and kinship is essential for contented living. Sometimes, connections can be too strong and may need to be softened or separated a little. At other times, connections are too weak and distant, and the person's wellbeing would benefit from strengthening those connections.

For Aboriginal and Torres Strait Islander peoples, knowing your kinship in relation to others gives individuals a purpose because these kinship relationships involve responsibilities to others—especially during events such as special ceremonies and funerals. When kinship connections are too distant and weak, people may not be aware of the roles they and others have which can result in them being perceived as an outsider with no purpose or responsibilities.

As a white Western male, family connections are important to me (TAC) as well, although roles and responsibilities aren't as clearly defined in my family as they are in Aboriginal and Torres Strait Islander cultures. When I finished my PhD, I travelled with my wife to Scotland where we lived and worked for five years. My maternal grandfather had emigrated from Scotland to Australia, so I wanted to spend some time connecting with that part of my family. Knowing where my family comes from and the ways in which I am connecting to my extended family gives me a sense of place and position in a kind of relational community.

Connection to community

Community is another important contributing factor to a person's sense of wellbeing. Many people build a sense of identity through the community groups they are embedded in (Gee et al., 2014). There is perhaps no greater illustration of our design as social animals than our propensity to seek out and form groups.

The internet has created a multitude of additional ways that we can connect and commune. Some people prefer face-to-face interactions and other people get more out of a virtual environment. Whatever an individual's tastes are, seeking out others with similar interests and beliefs seems to be important to us.

My (KM) connections within and throughout my community is, once again, related to identity. For Aboriginal and Torres Strait Islander people, it is important to know where they are from and who their "mob" is. Being accepted by the community provides someone with a sense of purpose as well as different responsibilities within the community. When someone from outside is accepted by the community, they are "adopted" by giving them a "skin" name. A skin name gives them a position within the community which allows others in the community to interact with them. A skin name is also accompanied by certain rules of avoidance related to their place in the community which they must obey.

I (TAC) also like to create a sense of community through various groups but, once again, the rules and roles of the communities within which I participate are not as clearly specified or delineated as they are with Aboriginal and Torres Strait Islander cultures. It may also be easier to move in and out of various Western types of communities than it is with Aboriginal and Torres Strait Islander cultures. Perhaps some of our Western problems, such as addictions and crime, are related to a lack of connectedness people feel within the communities in which they are embedded.

Connection to culture

A culture can be thought of as the system of beliefs a person has, the customs and rituals they engage in, and the people they spend their time with. Culture can influence the foods we eat and the clothes we wear. Behaving in ways that are at odds with your culture can create psychological unrest and turmoil. Sometimes experiencing another culture, such as through travel or forming a relationship with a person from that culture, can be unsettling and confusing. It can also be enriching and enlivening, too, but it all depends on the person and their circumstances.

Because culture can have such a pervasive impact, it is important to become more familiar with your own culture and how it shapes your life. Being connected to my (KM) culture comes in many forms, from partaking in ceremonies to attending community meetings, having input into decision making, attending funerals, acknowledging and respecting our elders and others in the community, as well as living on country and caring for country.

Culture is an area in which I (TAC) must admit to feeling a little envious people from other cultures such as Aboriginal and Torres Strait Islander cultures. As a white Western male, I don't really have a strong sense of Western "culture." I wouldn't really know how to describe such a thing if

I was asked. I have always liked growing up and living in Australia, but I don't really think of that as "culture" in the same way that I see Aboriginal and Torres Strait Islander people and others enjoying their cultures. Nevertheless, people have systems of beliefs that can be explored whenever they are less content than they would like to be.

Connection to country

Not everyone can immediately relate to the need to be connected to country, but for some cultures—such as the Aboriginal and Torres Strait Islander cultures—connection to country is pivotal (Gee et al., 2014). For Aboriginal and Torres Strait Islander people, being connected to country is a deeply spiritual sense of belonging (Dudgeon, Wright, Paradies, Garvey, & Walker, 2014).

For other people from different cultures, the connection may not be the same, but they might still relate to a sense of belonging to a certain place or area. Many people have particular locations they like to return to when they need to recharge or rejuvenate. The SEWB models help us to understand the importance of this sense of connection.

From my (KM) people's perspective, being connected to country is another aspect of day-to-day living that gives Aboriginal people a sense of belonging. It is used when we are introducing ourselves to others, it is part of our identity, and, at times, we use it to "prove" our Aboriginality.

Once again, I (TAC) don't have the same sense of connection to country that Aboriginal and Torres Strait Islander people describe, although my first visit to Scotland was very emotional. I felt like I'd "come home."

Connection to spirit, spirituality, and ancestors

Many people have beliefs about where they came from and what will happen to them when they die that transcend the birth and death of a physical body. In different belief systems, one can find concepts such as a soul or an atman. Some people involve themselves in organised religions whereas other people prefer a more private approach.

Even people who don't subscribe to a cyclical view of life and death, the self may still pursue a sense of meaning and purpose in life. For Aboriginal and Torres Strait Islander peoples, spirituality can be a pervasive component of their life affecting many different aspects including their sense of time and the interconnectedness between the past, present, and future in their journey. In Aboriginal spirituality, a concept of "everywhen" has been described to capture this interconnectedness (Grieves, 2008). Whichever way people construct their views of themselves, a narrative of a connection to a higher being or greater purpose is often common and can be one of the important factors in living a valued life.

In the stories of creation in my (KM) culture, where mythical beings formed the landscapes and animals, these spiritual beings could transform into human life forms to explain where the people came from. To honour the spirits and ancestors, people sing and dance and tell stories of their journeys across the lands. These songs and dances are passed on from generation to generation. Teaching the next generation is how we have kept our history, stories, song, and dance lines alive with no deviation from the original stories. These ancient stories connected our ancestors to the spirit world. The spirit world is often used to explain things that we don't know about—it is how we put it into a concept that we Aboriginal people understand.

In my (KM) culture, we consider that it's important to make sure we heal our spiritual side, and we use traditional healers for this purpose. It is not uncommon for Aboriginal and Torres Strait Islander people to ask for an Anangkerre (An-ung-oo-ra) before they are treated with Western medicine and other approaches. We believe that, by healing the spirit and then using other approaches, there is a better outcome for patients. Smoking ceremonies are also an important way of clearing negative energy.

In Western society there seem to be many ways of expressing beliefs about who we are and why we are here. I (TAC) don't participate in formal religious groups and ceremonies, but ideas of purpose and meaning are important to me. It seems to me that people like to have a sense of what life is all about, although they search for that in different ways.

SEWB For Improved Contentment and Daily Living

The seven SEWB domains provide a framework or structure for people to examine their lives and identify areas they can change, adjust, or modify to help them live more as they would wish to. These domains are not a prescriptive recipe but, instead, provide the map of a territory that matches the landscape of each individual's life and can help people navigate the path they would most like to travel.

Rather than considering psychological distress to be an indicator of illness or that an individual is somehow deficient or otherwise broken, the SEWB model considers these seven interconnected domains to be a web that can be stretched and relaxed with the ebb and flow of life. The SEWB model puts lasting contentment and wellbeing within everyone's grasp.

Concluding Comments

The Western biomedical model of mental illness has not served us well. In fact, there is evidence that our current diagnostic systems increase rather than decrease stigma and do not lead to better treatment outcomes (Timimi, 2014). The Aboriginal and Torres Strait Islander SEWB model, on the other hand, provides a blueprint for a more holistic, strengths-based, respectful, and compassionate approach to helping people live lives they value.

For me (KM), it is important to acknowledge that ill health, including what might be described as mental health problems, can be brought on when an individual does not have these connections. Even when people live in areas where the cultural practices are quite strong, not having the appropriate connection in any one of these domains can affect the health of an individual. If an individual, for example, is not connected to country or community in the way that is right for them, they can become unwell.

Considering our travels through life in terms of the seven SEWB domains can help us identify areas of strength that nourish us and areas where there are opportunities for learning and improvement. By using the ancient wisdom of Australia's First Nations peoples, we can have greater control and steer a course of our own design through the ups and downs of modern life.

People in the helping professions may find the SEWB model of enormous assistance in providing flexible, responsive, and targeted support effectively and efficiently. And people who require support from time to time might benefit from a model that recognises and honours their unique characteristics within a framework of social and emotional wellbeing. Through the widespread understanding and application of the SEWB model, our global village could become a more contented and harmonious neighbourhood.

References

Carey, T. A. (2013). Defining Australian Indigenous wellbeing: Do we *really* want the answer? Implications for policy and practice. *Psychotherapy and Politics International, 11*(3), 182-194.

Carey, T. A. (2017). *Patient-perspective care: A new paradigm for health systems and services.* London: Routledge. https://doi.org/10.4324/9781351227988

Carey, T. A. (2022). Finding normal: Let's start at the very beginning. In E. Maisel, & C. Ruby (Eds.), *Critiquing the psychiatric model: The Ethics International Press Critical Psychology and Critical Psychiatry series* (pp. 106-115). Bury St Edmunds, United Kingdom: Ethics International Press.

Dudgeon, P., Wright, M., Paradies, Y., Garvey, D., & Walker, I. (2014). Aboriginal social, cultural and historical contexts. In P. Dudgeon, H. Milroy, and R. Walker (Eds.), *Working together: Aboriginal and Torres Strait Islander mental health and wellbeing principles and practice* (2nd ed., pp. 3-24). Canberra: Commonwealth of Australia.

Gee, G., Dudgeon, P., Schultz, C., Hart, A., & Kelly, K. (2014). Aboriginal and Torres Strait Islander social and emotional wellbeing. In P. Dudgeon, H. Milroy, and R. Walker (Eds.), *Working together: Aboriginal and Torres Strait Islander mental health and wellbeing principles and practice* (2nd ed., pp. 55-68). Canberra: Commonwealth of Australia.

Grieves, V. (2009). *Aboriginal spirituality: Aboriginal philosophy the basis of Aboriginal social and emotional wellbeing. Discussion paper No. 9.* Darwin: Cooperative Research Centre for Aboriginal Health. Accessed 20

September 2023 from DP_9_text_2-libre.pdf (d1wqtxts1xzle7.cloudfront.net)

Marmot, M. (2006). Health in an unequal world: Social circumstances, biology and disease. *Clinical Medicine, 6*(6), 559-72.

National Aboriginal Health Strategy Working Party. (1989). *A national Aboriginal health strategy*. Canberra: National Aboriginal Health Strategy Working Party.

Social Health Reference Group. (2004). *A national strategic framework for Aboriginal and Torres Straits Islander People's Mental Health and Social and Emotional Well Being 2004-09*. National Aboriginal and Torres Straits Islander Health Council and National Mental Health Working Group. 2004. Canberra: Department of Health and Ageing.

Swan, P., & Raphael, B. (1995). *Ways forward: National Aboriginal and Torres Strait Islander mental health policy national consultancy report*. Canberra: Commonwealth of Australia.

Timimi, S. (2014). No more psychiatric labels: Why formal psychiatric diagnostic systems should be abolished. *International Journal of Clinical and Health Psychology, 14*(3), 208-15.

That was Then, This is Now, Part 1: Psychodynamic Psychotherapy for the Rest of Us

Jonathan Shedler

Abstract: *Psychoanalytic therapy has an image problem. The dominant narrative in the mental health professions is that psychoanalytic approaches are outmoded and discredited. What most people know of them are pejorative stereotypes and caricatures dating to the horse and buggy era. The stereotypes are fueled by misinformation from external sources, including managed care companies and proponents of other therapies who treat psychoanalysis as a foil or whipping boy. But psychoanalysis also bears responsibility. Historically, psychoanalytic communities have been insular and inward facing. People who might otherwise be drawn to psychodynamic approaches encounter impenetrable jargon and confusing infighting between rival theoretical schools. This chapter and the next (Parts 1 and 2) provide an accessible, jargon free, non-partisan introduction to psychoanalytic thinking and therapy for trainees, clinicians trained in other therapy approaches, and the public.*

Author's note: This chapter is a jargon-free introduction to contemporary psychodynamic thought. I wrote it because existing books did not meet my students' needs. Many classic introductions to psychoanalytic therapy are dated. They describe the psychoanalytic thinking of decades ago, not today. Others contain too much jargon to be accessible, or they assume prior knowledge few contemporary readers possess. Still others have a partisan agenda to promote one psychoanalytic school of thought over others, but trainees are ill-served by treating them as pawns in internecine theoretical disputes. Finally, some otherwise excellent books assume an interested and sympathetic reader—an assumption that is often unwarranted. Students today are exposed to considerable disinformation about psychoanalytic thought and often approach it with pejorative preconceptions.

The title is a double *entendre*. "That was then, this is now" alludes to a central aim of psychoanalytic therapy, which is to help free people from the bonds of past experience in order to live more fully in the present. People tend to react to what *was* rather than what *is*, and psychoanalytic therapy aims to help with this. The title also alludes to sea changes in psychoanalytic thinking that have occurred over the past decades. For too many, the term *psychoanalysis* conjures up century-old stereotypes that bear little resemblance to what contemporary practitioners think and do.

This chapter was intended as the beginning of a book. I may finish it one day, but the project is on the back burner. For the moment, this is it.

A version of this chapter originally appeared in *Contemporary Psychoanalysis* (Shedler, 2022).

Roots of Misunderstanding

Psychoanalytic psychotherapy may be the most misunderstood of all therapies. I teach a course in psychoanalytic therapy for clinical psychology doctoral students, many of whom would not be there if it were not required. I begin by asking the students to write down their beliefs about psychoanalytic therapy. Most express highly inaccurate preconceptions. The preconceptions come not from first-hand encounters with psychoanalytic practitioners but from media depictions, from undergraduate psychology professors who refer to psychoanalytic concepts in their courses but understand little about them, and from textbooks that present caricatures of psychoanalytic theories that were out of date half a century ago.

Some of the more memorable misconceptions are: that psychoanalytic concepts apply only to the privileged or wealthy; that psychoanalytic concepts and treatments lacks scientific support (for a review of empirical evidence, see Shedler, 2010; Leichsenring et al., 2023); that psychoanalytic therapists "reduce everything" to sex and aggression; that they keep patients in lengthy treatments merely for financial gain; that psychoanalytic theories are sexist, racist, classist, etc. (insert your preferred condemnation); that Sigmund Freud, the originator of psychoanalysis, was a cocaine addict who developed his theories under the influence; that he was a child molester (a graduate of an Ivy League university had gotten this bizarre notion from one of her professors); and that the terms "psychoanalytic" and "Freudian" are synonyms—as if psychoanalytic knowledge has not evolved since the horse and buggy era.

Most psychoanalytic therapists have no idea how to respond to the question (all too common at social gatherings), "Are you a 'Freudian?'" The question has no meaningful answer, and I fear that *any* answer I give could lead only to misunderstanding. In a basic sense, *all* mental health professionals are "Freudian" because so many of Freud's concepts have simply been assimilated into the broader culture of psychotherapy. They now seem so commonplace, commonsense, and taken-for-granted that people do not recognize they originated with Freud and were radical at the time.

For example, most people take it for granted that trauma can cause emotional and physical symptoms, that our care in the early years shapes our adult lives, that people have complex and often contradictory motives, that sexual abuse of children occurs and can have disastrous consequences, that emotional difficulties can be treated by talking, that we sometimes find fault with others for the very things we do not wish to see in ourselves, that it is exploitive and destructive for therapists to have sexual relations with patients, and so on. These and many more ideas that are commonplace in the culture of psychotherapy are "Freudian." In this sense, *every* contemporary psychotherapist is a (gasp) Freudian, like it or not. Even the practice of meeting with patients for regularly scheduled appointment hours originated with Freud.

In another sense, the question "Are you a Freudian?" is unanswerable because *no* contemporary psychoanalytic therapist is a "Freudian." What I mean is that psychoanalytic thinking has evolved radically since Freud's day—not that you would know this from reading psychology textbooks. In the past decades, there have been sea changes in theory and practice. The field has grown in diverse directions, far from Freud's historical writings. In this sense, *no one* is a "Freudian." Psychoanalysis is continually evolving new models and paradigms. The development of psychoanalytic knowledge did not end with Freud any more than physics ended with

Newton, astronomy with Copernicus, or the development of the behavioral tradition in psychology ended with John Watson.

There are multiple schools of thought within psychoanalysis with different and sometimes bitterly divisive views, and the notion that someone could tell you "the" psychoanalytic view of something is quaint and naïve. There may be greater diversity of viewpoints within psychoanalysis than within any other school of psychotherapy, if only because psychoanalysis is the oldest of the therapy traditions. Asking a psychoanalytic therapist for "the" psychoanalytic perspective may be as meaningful as asking a philosophy professor "the" philosophical answer to a question.

I imagine the poor professor could only shake her head in bemusement and wonder where to begin. So it is with psychoanalysis. Psychoanalysis is not one theory but a diverse collection of theories, each of which represents an attempt to shed light on one or another facet of human functioning.

What it isn't

It may be easier to say what psychoanalysis is *not* than what it is. For starters, contemporary psychoanalysis is not a theory about id, ego, and superego (terms, incidentally, that Freud did not use; they were introduced by a translator). Nor is it a theory about fixations, or sexual and aggressive instincts, or repressed memories, or the Oedipus complex, or penis envy, or castration anxiety. One can dispense with every one of these ideas, and the essence of psychoanalytic thinking and therapy would remain intact. There are psychoanalysts who reject every one of them.

If you learned in university that psychoanalysis is a theory about id, ego, and superego, your professors did you a disservice. Please don't shoot the messenger for telling you that you may be less prepared to understand psychoanalytic thought than if you had never taken a psychology course at all. Interest in that particular model of the mind (called the "structural theory") has long since given way to other theories and models (cf. Person et al., 2005). There is virtually no mention of it in contemporary psychoanalytic writings other than in historical contexts. In the late 20th century, the theory's strongest proponent eventually concluded it is no longer relevant to psychoanalysis (Brenner, 1994). When psychology textbooks present the theory of id, ego, and superego as if it were synonymous with psychoanalysis, I don't know whether to laugh or to cry.

It is fair to ask how so many textbooks could be so out of date and get it all so wrong. Students have every reason to expect their textbooks to be accurate and authoritative. The answer, in brief, is that psychoanalysis developed outside the academic world, mostly in freestanding institutes. For complex historical reasons, these institutes tended to be insular, and psychoanalysts did little to make their ideas accessible to people outside their own closed circles.

Some of the psychoanalytic institutes were also arrogant and exclusive in the worst sense of the word and did an admirable job of alienating other mental health professionals. This occurred at a time when American psychoanalytic institutes were dominated by a hierarchical medical establishment (for a historical perspective, see McWilliams, 2004). Psychoanalytic institutes have evolved, but the hostility they engendered in other mental health professions is likely to persist for years to come. It has been transmitted across multiple generations of trainees, with each generation modeling the attitudes of its own teachers.

Academic psychology played a major role in perpetuating widespread misunderstanding of psychoanalytic psychotherapy. A culture developed within academic psychology that disparaged psychoanalytic ideas—or, more correctly, the stereotypes and caricatures it *mistook* for psychoanalytic ideas—and made little effort to learn how psychoanalytic therapists really thought and practiced. Many academic psychologists were content to use psychoanalysis as a foil or straw man. They'd regularly win debates with dead theorists who were not present to explain their views (it is fairly easy to win arguments with dead people). Many academic psychologists still critique caricatures of psychoanalysis and outdated theories that psychoanalysis has long since left behind (cf. Bornstein, 1995, 2001; Hansell, 2005). Sadly, most academic psychologists have been clueless about developments in psychoanalysis for the better part of a century.

Much the same situation exists in psychiatry departments which in recent decades saw wholesale purges of psychoanalytically oriented faculty members and have become so pharmacologically oriented that many psychiatrists no longer know how to help patients in any way that does not involve a prescription. Interestingly, being an effective psychopharmacologist involves many of the same skills that psychoanalytic therapy requires—for example, the ability to build rapport, create a working alliance, make sound inferences about things patients cannot express directly, and understand conscious and unconscious fantasies that almost invariably get stirred up around taking psychiatric medication. There seems to be a hunger among psychiatry trainees for more comprehensive ways of understanding patients and for alternatives to biologically reductionistic treatment approaches.

It may be disillusioning to realize your teachers misled you, especially if you admired those teachers. You may even be experiencing some cognitive dissonance just now (and dissonance theory predicts that you might be tempted to dismiss the information here, to help resolve the dissonance). I remember my own struggle to come to terms with the realization that professors I admired had led me astray. I *wanted* to look up to these professors, to share their views, to be one of them. It also made me feel bigger and more important to think like they did and believe what they believed, and I felt personally diminished when they seemed diminished in my eyes.

I suspect I am not alone in this reaction. I have often wondered whether this is one reason otherwise thoughtful and open-minded students sometimes turn a deaf ear to any ideas labeled "psychoanalytic" (although they readily embrace them when they are repackaged as something new and described with different terminology).

A comment on terminology

I use the terms "psychoanalytic" and "psychodynamic" interchangeably. The term *psychodynamic* gained traction after World War II when it was introduced at a conference on medical education and used as a synonym for *psychoanalytic*. I am told the intent was to secure a place for psychoanalysis in psychiatry residency training without unduly alarming training directors who may have regarded "psychoanalysis" with some apprehension (R. Wallerstein, personal communication; Whitehorn et al.,

1953). In short, the term *psychodynamic* was something of a ruse. The term has evolved over time to refer to a range of treatments based on psychoanalytic concepts and methods where meetings do not necessarily occur five days per week or involve lying on a couch.

At the risk of offending some psychoanalysts, a few words are also in order about psychoanalysis versus psychoanalytic (or psychodynamic) psycho-therapy. In psychoanalysis proper, sessions take place three to five days per week and the patient often lies on a couch. In psychoanalytic or psychodynamic psychotherapy, sessions typically take place once or twice per week and the patient sits in a chair. Beyond this, the differences are murky.

Psychoanalysis is an interpersonal process, not an anatomical position. It refers to a special kind of interaction between patient and therapist. It can facilitate this interaction if the patient comes often and lies down, but this is neither necessary nor sufficient. Frequent meetings facilitate, in part because patients who come often tend to develop more intense feelings toward the therapist, and these feelings can be utilized constructively in the service of understanding and change. Lying down can also facilitate for some patients because lying down (rather than staring at another person) encourages a state of reverie in which thoughts can wander and flow more freely. I will take up these topics in the next section.

However, lying down and meeting frequently are only trappings of psychoanalysis, not its essence (cf. Gill, 1983). With respect to the couch, psychoanalysts now recognize that lying down can impede as well as facilitate psychoanalytic work (e.g., Goldberger, 1995; Schachter & Kächele, 2013). With respect to frequency of meetings, it is silly to maintain that someone who attends four appointments per week is "in psychoanalysis" but someone who attends three cannot be.

Generally, the more frequently a patient comes, the richer and deeper the experience. But there are patients who attend five sessions per week, lie on a couch, and nothing goes on that remotely resembles a psychoanalytic process. Others attend sessions once or twice per week and sit in a chair and there is no question a psychoanalytic process is taking place. It really has to do with who the therapist is, who the patient is, and what happens between them. For these reasons, I will use the terms psychoanalysis, psychoanalytic psychotherapy, and psychodynamic psychotherapy interchangeably.

Finally, I generally use the term *patient* rather than *client*. In truth, both words are problematic, but *patient* seems to me the lesser of evils. The etymology of *patient* is "one who suffers." But for some, the word has come to connote a hierarchical power dynamic or conjure images of medical authoritarianism. These connotations are dismaying because psychoanalytic therapy is a shared, collaborative endeavor between two human beings, neither of whom has privileged access to the truth of another's experience.

On the other hand, the term *client* does not seem to do justice to the dire, sometimes life-and-death seriousness of psychotherapy or the enormity of the responsibility psychotherapists assume. My hairdresser, accountant, and yoga teacher all have clients but none, to my knowledge, have accepted professional responsibility for caring for an acutely suicidal person, received a desperate phone call from a terrified family member of a person decompensating into psychosis, or struggled to help someone make meaning of being raped by her own father.

Neither word is ideal and some colleagues I respect prefer one word and some the other. I have tried to explain the reasons for my personal preference. Readers with an aversion to *patient* may substitute the word *client* where they wish. The choice of terminology is less important than reflecting on the meanings and implications of our choice.[1]

Foundations

If psychoanalysis is not a theory about id, ego, and superego or about fixations, or about repressed memories, what *is* it about? The following ideas play a central role in the thinking of most psychoanalytic

---

[1] Nancy McWilliams (personal communication) has commented on the irony that many people have come to associate the mercantile rather than the medical metaphor with greater compassion and humanity.

practitioners. These ideas are intertwined and overlapping; I present them separately only as a matter of didactic convenience.

Unconscious mental life

We do not fully know our own hearts and minds, and many important things take place outside awareness. This observation is no longer controversial to anyone, even the most hard-nosed empiricist. Research in cognitive science has shown repeatedly that much thinking and feeling goes on outside conscious awareness (e.g., Bargh & Barndollar, 1996; Kahneman, 2011; Nisbett & Wilson, 1977; Weinberger & Stoycheva, 2019; Westen, 1998; Wilson et al., 2000).

Usually, cognitive scientists do not use the word "unconscious" but refer instead to "implicit" mental processes, "procedural" memory, and so on. The terminology is not important. What matters is the concept—that crucial memory, perceptual, judgmental, affective, and motivational processes are not consciously accessible. Psychoanalytic discussions of unconscious mental life do, however, emphasize something that cognitive scientists tend not to emphasize: It is not just that we do not fully know our own minds, but there are things we seem not to *want* to know. There are things that are threatening or dissonant or make us feel vulnerable in some way, so we tend to look away.

I came across a poignant example early in my career. I was interviewing participants in a research project on personality development and my job was to learn as much as I could about each participant's personal history. In general, these were easy interviews to conduct. Most people, with a little encouragement, enjoy talking about themselves to someone respectful, sympathetic, genuinely interested in what they have to say, and sworn to confidentiality. But one interview was puzzlingly tedious. Although the interviewee, whom I will call "Jill," was attractive and intelligent, and although she seemed to answer all my questions cheerfully and cooperatively, I did not feel engaged at all. Slowly, I began to recognize that Jill's answers to my questions amounted to a string of abstractions, clichés, and platitudes. I simply could not get a sense of Jill or the people important to her.

Our conversation went something like this:

> "Can you tell me some more about your sister? What sort of person
> is she and what sort of relationship have you had?"
> "She is neurotic."
> "In what way is she neurotic?"
> "You know, just neurotic in the usual way."
> "I'm not sure what 'the usual way' is. Can you help me understand
> how she is neurotic?"
> "You're a psychologist, you know what 'neurotic' means. That's the
> best word to describe her. I'm sure you've seen a lot of people like
> her."

After much questioning, Jill eventually told me that her sister was spiteful
and said mean things about their father just to embarrass him. Jill described
her father as a kind, caring man who had done nothing to deserve such a
hostile, ungrateful daughter. I had to ask Jill repeatedly for a specific
example of the kind of thing her sister complained about.

Eventually, Jill described an incident that occurred when Jill was five and
her sister was seven. The family was at the beach and her sister was being
"bitchy and provocative." Her kind, caring father lost his temper and held
his seven-year-old daughter underwater until she nearly drowned. As Jill
told this story, the emphasis was entirely on how provocative her sister had
been. Jill seemed completely unaware that she had just described an
incident of child abuse. Jill told me other examples of how her sister was
"neurotic," all of which ended with her father violently out of control.

I did not have the sense that Jill was trying to mislead me or hide the truth.
What was striking was that Jill seemed unaware that there were any
conclusions to draw from the events except that her sister was neurotic.
This is a stark example of the kind of thing I mean when I say there are
things we seem not to want to know.

Please note this vignette has nothing to do with "repressed memories,"
which get a lot of attention in undergraduate textbooks and the media—
and have virtually nothing to do with contemporary psychoanalytic
therapy. The goal of psychoanalytic treatment is *not* to uncover repressed

memories, nor has it been since the early 1900s. It is to expand freedom and choice by helping people to become more mindful of their experience in the here and now. To my knowledge, *none* of the therapists involved in widely-publicized controversies about "false memories" were psychoanalysts.

Jill's difficulty was not that she did not remember. On the contrary, her memories were crystal clear. Rather, Jill was fixed on one interpretation of events and had not allowed herself to consider alternate interpretations of her experience. This rigidly-held view doubtless once served a purpose for Jill. For example, it may have allowed her, as a small child, to preserve a desperately needed sense of safety and security in a family that was terrifyingly unsafe.

This touches on an important concept in psychoanalytic psychotherapy: most psychological difficulties were once adaptive solutions to life challenges. They may have been costly solutions, but they were solutions, nevertheless. Difficulties arise when circumstances change and old solutions no longer work or become self-defeating, but we continue to apply them anyway.

The mind in conflict

Another central recognition is that humans can be of two (or more) minds about things. We can have loving feelings and hateful feelings toward the same person, we can desire something and also fear it, and we can desire things that are mutually contradictory. There is nothing mysterious in the recognition that people have complex and often contradictory feelings and motives.

Poets, writers, and reflective people in general have always known this. Psychoanalysis has contributed a vocabulary with which to talk about inner contradiction, and techniques for working with contradictions in ways that can help alleviate suffering. To paraphrase F. Scott Fitzgerald, wisdom is the ability to hold two contradictory ideas in mind at the same time and still continue to function. Psychoanalytic psychotherapy seeks to cultivate this form of wisdom.

The terms *ambivalence* and *conflict* refer to inner contradiction. *Conflict* in this context refers not to opposition between people, but to contradiction or dissonance within our own minds. We may seek to resolve contradiction by disavowing one or another aspect of our feelings—that is, excluding it from conscious awareness—but the disavowed feelings have a way of "leaking out" all the same. One result is that we may work at cross-purposes with ourselves. An analogy I sometimes use with my patients is driving a car with one foot on the gas and one foot on the brake. We may eventually get somewhere but not without a lot of unnecessary friction and wear and tear.

Many people experience conflict around intimacy. We all seem to know someone who desires an intimate relationship but repeatedly develops romantic attractions to people who are unavailable. These attractions may represent an unconscious compromise between a desire for closeness and a fear of dependency. A friend of mine always seemed to become romantically interested in more than one person at a time. He agonized about which person was right for him, but his simultaneous involvement with multiple people ensured that he did not develop a deeper relationship with any.

One of my first patients could not allow himself to recognize or acknowledge his desire for caring and nurturing. He equated these desires with weakness and chose women who were cold, detached, and even hostile. These women did not stir up his discomfiting longings for nurturing. Not surprisingly, he was dissatisfied with his intimate relationships. Through therapy, he came to recognize his desire for emotional warmth. Only then was he able to choose a loving and caring partner.

When both members of a couple struggle with conflict around intimacy, we often see a dance in which the partners draw together and pull apart in an unending cycle. As one pursues, the other withdraws and vice-versa. Deborah Luepnitz (2002) has written a moving book on psychoanalytic therapy that emphasizes just this dilemma titled *Schopenhauer's Porcupines*. The title refers to a story told by Schopenhauer about porcupines trying to keep warm on a cold night. Seeking warmth, they huddle together, but when they do they prick each other with their quills. They are forced to move apart but soon find themselves cold and needing warmth. They draw together again, prick each other again, and the cycle begins anew.[2]

Conflicts involving anger are also commonplace. Some people, especially those with a certain kind of depressive personality, seem unable to acknowledge or express anger toward others but instead treat themselves in punitive and self-destructive ways. In his first-person account of depression, *Darkness Visible: A Memoir of Madness*, William Styron described winning a $25,000 literary prize and promptly losing the check. He realized afterward that the accident of losing the check was not so accidental but reflected his deep self-criticism and feeling of unworthiness.

There are many reasons why people disavow angry feelings. We may fear retribution or retaliation, we may fear that our anger will harm someone we love, we may fear that it will lead to rejection or abandonment, the angry feelings may be inconsistent with our self-image as a loving person, we may feel guilt or shame for having hostile feelings toward someone who has cared for us, and so on.

I once treated a man whose parents were holocaust survivors, who sacrificed greatly so their son could have a better life. They worked long hours at menial jobs so he could go to medical school and become a prosperous person. Under the circumstances, anger toward either parent would have evoked crushing guilt. My patient could not allow himself angry feelings toward either parent, but he treated his friends and colleagues—and *himself*—quite badly. It took considerable work before he could recognize his angry feelings and recognize that love and gratitude can coexist with anger and resentment. He came to understand that anger toward his parents did not diminish his love for them, his grief for the suffering they had endured, or his gratitude for their sacrifices.

---

[2] For readers who may have been taught that psychoanalytic approaches are relevant only to the privileged or wealthy, Luepnitz's book also provides moving examples of psychoanalytic therapy with economically disadvantaged and culturally marginalized patients.

Some people express disavowed anger through passive-aggressive behavior (yet another psychoanalytic term that has been assimilated into the broader vocabulary of therapy). For example, someone who regularly burns the family dinner may be expressing, in the same act, their devotion to their family and their resentment. Preparing the dinner expresses love and devotion; making it unpalatable expresses anger.

My mother often expressed anger passive-aggressively by making people wait for her. She'd arrange to pick me up at the airport when I came home from college, but she'd show up two hours late. In her mind, meeting me at the airport was an act of devotion, consistent with her view of herself as a loving, self-sacrificing mother. Being late was circumstantial. Unfortunately, the same "circumstances" arose time and again. The sources of my mother's resentment were no doubt manifold, but I believe one source of resentment was that I had gone away in the first place.

A charming example of ambivalence occurred while I was editing this chapter, working on my laptop computer at a sidewalk café. A fifteen-month-old girl toddled over from an adjacent table, picked up a pretty leaf from the ground, and offered it to me with a huge smile. Just as I said "thank you" and reached to take it, she snatched it away with obvious delight. I encounter similar behavior in adults, but it is generally less charming.

A last and more obviously "clinical" example of conflict can be seen in certain patients who suffer from bulimia. On the one hand, binge eating may express a desperate wish to devour everything, perhaps to fill an inner void. The symptom seems to say, "I am so needy and desperate that I can never be filled." Purging expresses the other side of the conflict and seems to say, "I have no needs. I am in control and require nothing."

Of course, things are generally more complicated, and inner (or intrapsychic) conflict can have many sides, not just two. The example illustrates just two of many possible meanings that may underlie bingeing and purging behavior. Psychological symptoms often have multiple causes and serve multiple purposes. We use the terms *overdetermination* and *multiple function* to describe this multiplicity of meanings. We will revisit these terms shortly.

Psychoanalytic therapists were the first to explicitly address the role of inner conflict or contradiction in creating psychological difficulties, but it is noteworthy that *every* therapy tradition addresses conflict in one way or another. Cognitive therapists may speak of contradictory beliefs or schemas, behaviorists may speak of approach/avoidance conflict or responsiveness to short-term versus long-term reinforcers, humanistic therapists may speak of competing value systems, and systems-oriented theorists may refer to role conflict. There is universal recognition that inner dissonance is part of the human condition.

Cognitive scientist Daniel Kahneman won the Nobel Prize for empirical research describing competing cognitive decision processes which he called "System 1" and "System 2" (Kahneman, 2003, 2011). System 1 works intuitively and automatically and is relatively unresponsive to new information or changing circumstances. Its operations "are typically fast, automatic, effortless, associative, *implicit (not available to introspection)*, and often emotionally charged" (Kahneman, 2003, p. 698, emphasis added). In contrast, "the operations of System 2 are slower, serial, effortful, more likely to be consciously monitored and deliberately controlled" (Kahneman, 2003, p. 698). These cognitive systems work in tandem and often produce disparate results. Such contradictions may be rooted in the structure of the brain, with the different decision systems reflecting activity of the basal ganglia and prefrontal cortex, respectively.

These findings from cognitive science, based on rigorously controlled experiments, have striking parallels with Freud's descriptions, many decades ago, of conscious and unconscious mental processes. *Far from discrediting core psychoanalytic assumptions, research in cognitive science and neuroscience has provided an empirical foundation for many of those assumptions.* It is also helping psychoanalytic thinkers refine their understanding of mental processes and effective intervention (e.g., Gabbard & Westen, 2003; Weinberger & Stoycheva, 2019; Westen & Gabbard, 2002a, 2002b).

The past lives on in the present

Through our earliest experiences, we learn certain templates or scripts about how the world works (a cognitive therapist would call them schemas). We learn, for example, what to expect of others, how to behave in relationships, how to elicit caring and attention, how to act when someone is angry with us, how to express ourselves when we are angry, how to make people proud of us, what it feels like to succeed, what it feels like to fail, what it means to love, and on and on. We continue to apply these templates or scripts to new situations as we proceed through life, often when they no longer apply. Another way of saying this is that *we view the present through the lens of past experience* and, therefore, tend to repeat and recreate aspects of the past. In the words of William Wordsworth, the child is father to the man.

Examples of how we recreate the past abound. A little girl's father is emotionally distant. As a result, her early experiences of love come packaged with a subtle sense of emotional deprivation. In adulthood she finds herself drawn to men who are emotionally unresponsive, and the men who are emotionally available do not interest or excite her. She may recreate this pattern in therapy. When her male therapist seems distracted or bored, she perceives him as powerful and important. When he seems caring and attentive, she perceives him as bland, boring, and of little use to her.

Consider a child who receives her mother's undivided attention only when she is physically ill. At these times, her mother dotes on her and comforts her. In adult life she develops physical symptoms when she feels neglected by her husband—an unconscious effort to elicit his loving attention. (Unfortunately, her husband does not respond with doting attention, leaving her feeling confused and betrayed in ways she cannot begin to put into words.) In therapy she talks about her physical symptoms and does not seem to have language for feelings. She assumes her therapist is interested primarily in her aches and pains and seems confused by her invitation to talk about her feelings.

Another person is a victim of childhood physical and sexual abuse. The *dramatis personae* in her life are abusers, victims, and rescuers. In adulthood she recreates these role patterns by getting into situations in which she feels betrayed and victimized, looks for rescuers to extricate her, and then recreates the roles of victim and abuser with her would-be rescuer. In therapy, she initially idealizes her therapist and treats him as a savior. The therapist responds to her idealization and her intense need by scheduling extra appointments, allowing sessions to run over time, accepting late night phone calls, and reluctantly acquiescing to her demands for hugs at the end of therapy sessions.

Eventually the therapist feels overwhelmed and depleted and attempts to reestablish limits. The patient then feels abandoned, betrayed, and enraged. She files an ethics complaint against the therapist, pointedly noting his lack of professional boundaries (thereby becoming the abuser and turning the therapist into a victim) and finds another naïve therapist to rescue her from the harm done by the first. This scenario may sound extreme, but the seasoned therapist will recognize a familiar pattern (e.g., Davies & Frawley, 1992; Gabbard, 1992). It is a pattern characteristic of certain patients we describe as having borderline personality organization.

It is impossible *not* to perceive and interpret events through the lenses of past experience. There is simply no other way to function. Past experience contextualizes present-day experience and shapes our perceptions, interpretations, and reactions. A person who felt loved, valued, and nurtured in childhood experiences the death of a spouse. He is profoundly sad for a time, goes through a period of mourning, but eventually goes on to love again. A person who experienced his childhood as a string of failures, rejections, and losses also experiences the death of a spouse. For him, the loss becomes a recapitulation of earlier losses and proof that his efforts in life can lead only to pain. He sinks into a bitter, angry depression and does not recover. In both cases, the "objective" external experience of loss is the same, but the psychological meanings of the event are very different.

Every school of therapy addresses the impact of the past on the present. Cognitive therapists may discuss the assimilation of new experiences into existing schemas, systems-oriented therapists may note the repetition of family dynamics across generations, behaviorists may speak of conditioning history and stimulus generalization. *The goal of psychoanalytic psychotherapy is to loosen the bonds of past experience to create new life possibilities.*

Transference

A person starting therapy is entering an unfamiliar situation and a new relationship and necessarily applies his previously formed templates, scripts, or schemas to organize his perceptions of this new person—the therapist—and make sense of the new situation. There is no alternative other than to view this new relationship through the lens of past relationships; it is not a matter of choice. Thus, different patients show dazzlingly different reactions to the same therapist.

I begin therapy with all new patients in much the same way. I greet the patient, offer him a seat, and invite him to tell me why he has come. But I am *not* the same person in the eyes of the patients. Some see me as a benevolent authority who will advise and comfort them, some see me as an omniscient being who will instantly know their innermost secrets, some see me as a rival or competitor to impress or defeat, some see me as an incompetent bungler, some see me as a dangerous adversary, some see me as a disapproving parent to appease, some see me as sexy and alluring, some as cold and unresponsive, and on and on.

These and a thousand other configurations emerge as therapy unfolds. Anyone who has practiced therapy for any length of time cannot help but be struck by the diversity of reactions we elicit from our patients and by how far our patients' perceptions can diverge from our self-perceptions and the perceptions of others who know us in other contexts. (The opposite is also true and often far more disconcerting. Some patients seem to have an uncanny sixth sense that enables them to home in on our very real limitations, vulnerabilities, and insecurities with laser-like precision. But that is a topic for another time.)

When I was in graduate school, a friend of mine began therapy with a man whose last name sounded something like "Hiller." In the eyes of virtually everyone, Dr. Hiller was a gentle and compassionate man who was rather meek and self-effacing. For a significant period in her therapy, however, my friend perceived him as an aggressive tormenter and referred to him, only half-jokingly, as "Hitler." My friend's perception changed over time, but I believe it was important for her to go through this phase, and essential that her therapist was able to tolerate this perception of him. Instead of trying to convince her otherwise, he allowed her to have her own perception and patiently explored the thoughts, feelings, and memories that lay behind it.

The term *transference* refers specifically to the activation of preexisting expectations, templates, scripts, fears, and desires in the context of the therapy relationship, with the patient viewing the therapist through the lenses of early important relationships. In psychoanalytic psychotherapy, our patients' perceptions of us are not incidental to treatment and they are not interferences or distractions from the work. They are at the heart of therapy. *It is specifically because old patterns, scripts, expectations, desires, schemas (call them what you will) become active and "alive" in the therapy sessions that we are able to help patients examine, understand, and rework them.*

Not long ago, I treated a patient whose alcoholic (and probably bipolar) father had abused him emotionally and physically. His father had castigated him, shamed him, and beat him with little provocation. It was one thing for my patient to tell me that he viewed people with distrust and suspicion. It was another when this relationship template came alive in treatment, and he began responding to *me* as if I were an unpredictable, angry adversary. Consciously, he viewed me as an ally who had his welfare at heart (and he was paying me good money for my help). At the same time, he seemed to do everything in his power to "protect" himself from me by shutting me out and fending me off, acting as though I would use whatever he told me as a weapon to hurt him. He responded this way automatically and reflexively; his responses were so ingrained that he did not recognize that they were at all out of the ordinary.

I did not regard my patient's attitude toward me as an obstacle to therapy. On the contrary, reliving and reworking this relationship pattern was central to his recovery. Repeatedly I would point out, as gently as I could, that he was responding to me as if I were a dangerous adversary. I would say, "When you turned to your father for help, he humiliated you. Given your experiences, it's understandable that you would now expect the same treatment from me." Or "You are letting me know that our work means nothing to you, and you couldn't care less if you never saw me again. Perhaps you are convinced I will disappoint and hurt you and are rejecting me first to protect yourself."

Over time he came to understand—not in an intellectual way, but in a way that truly sunk in emotionally—that he was treating me (and other important people in his life) in ways that were more applicable to another person in another time and another place. Gradually, he began to call into question his expectations, reactions, and interpretations of events. Additionally, I weathered his suspicions, accusations, and rage without retaliating and without withdrawing (at least most of the time). Our relationship, therefore, served as a template for a new and different kind of relationship. Over time he came to view relationships through different lenses. The world began to feel less dangerous, and his relationships became more fulfilling.

In psychoanalytic therapy, we deliberately arrange things so that our patients' interpersonal expectations, templates, or schemas are cast in high relief in the treatment. In other words, we do our best to allow transferences to unfold and to become palpable. It is the hallmark of psychoanalytic therapy that we *utilize* the transference (and the countertransference—that is, our own emotional reactions to our patients) as a means of understanding the patient and effecting change. *It is a central premise of psychoanalytic psychotherapy that problematic relationship patterns reemerge in the relationship with the therapist.* This is how we come to know our patients and where we ultimately target our interventions.

Empirical research shows that the most effective therapists are those who recognize transference and utilize it therapeutically, regardless of the kind of therapy they *think* they are practicing. Enrico Jones and his colleagues (Ablon & Jones, 1998; Jones & Pulos, 1993) studied recordings of psychotherapy sessions from the NIMH *Treatment of Depression Collaborative Research Program*, rated the sessions on 100 variables that assessed the kinds of interventions the therapists employed. The therapists with the best outcomes were those who consistently noted their patient's emotional responses to *them* in the therapy sessions, and drew links between these responses and their responses to other important people in their lives. This was true even for therapists providing manualized cognitive-behavioral therapy (CBT), which did not officially acknowledge transference as a mechanism of change. The therapists were effective because they *departed* from the interventions specified in the treatment manual.

It is fair to ask whether something unique about therapy evokes strong transference reactions or whether transference is ubiquitous in all relationships. The answer is both. We view all relationships through the lenses of early important relationships. At the same time, therapy can elicit especially raw feelings. This is because therapy is not just another relationship. It is an ongoing relationship between a person who may be in desperate need and a person who is there to provide help. The situation inherently stirs up powerful longings and dependency.

In fact, the therapy situation psychologically recapitulates our relationships with our earliest caregivers and, therefore, exerts an especially regressive pull. The therapist becomes a magnet for unresolved desires and fears. Therapy can evoke any and all of the untamed feelings we once experienced toward our early caregivers, including expectations of omnipotence, powerful yearnings, love, and hate. Woe to the therapist who fails to recognize the power inherent in the therapist role.

Other aspects of the therapy situation also exert a regressive pull. More frequent meetings intensify transference feelings. (This is one reason why psychoanalytic therapy can accomplish more when meetings occur several times per week. By the same token, some more troubled patients cannot tolerate the intensity and do better in once or twice per week therapy.) The fact that communication in therapy is largely one-sided also encourages regressive fantasies. In ordinary social interaction, people take turns sharing information, but in therapy the patient does most of the talking. The therapist learns a great deal about the patient's life, but the patient may know little about the therapist's life. In the absence of information, people tend to fill in the gaps with their own desires, fears, and expectations (much as the shapes we perceive in Rorschach cards reveal as much about us as they do about the actual inkblots).

Many schools of therapy are now converging on the recognition that people recreate problematic relationship patterns in their relationship with their therapists and that this can be used for therapeutic ends. Cognitive therapists are increasingly attending to patients' emotional reactions to the therapist rather than treating them as distractions from the work (Safran, 1998; Safran & Segal, 1990), and I was a bit surprised when I heard my students who identify themselves as "radical behaviorists" discussing something called a "CRB," an acronym for Clinically Relevant Behavior). A CRB is defined as an instance of symptomatic behavior expressed in the therapy session toward the therapist—in other words, *transference*. From the point of view of radical behaviorism, effective intervention involves helping patients recognize CRBs and develop new ways of relating (Kohlenberg & Tsai, 1991).

Such convergences among schools of therapy are not surprising. It makes sense that thoughtful professionals, struggling to understand the same psychological dilemmas, would eventually converge on similar ideas. However, I confess I find it disconcerting when adherents of other therapy traditions invent new names for phenomena that psychoanalytic practitioners have recognized for generations and proceed to discuss them as if they were new discoveries.

I would be remiss in concluding this section on transference without emphasizing that transference takes two. Psychoanalysis has long since abandoned the notion that transference is created solely by the patient. Our experience of the therapist is necessarily a blend of old and new, reflecting preexisting templates and new experiences in the present, as is the case in all relationships. Contemporary theorists emphasize that transference is co-created by two people, mutually shaping and influencing their experience of one another on an ongoing basis.

There were once tempests in the psychoanalytic literature about the influence of the role of the therapist's real characteristics on transference, but they need not concern us here. It seems undeniable that patients bring their personal histories into the therapeutic interaction, that their early relationship templates become reactivated and replayed, and that unresolved hurts and longings get directed toward the therapist.

It also seems undeniable that the therapist's personality and patterns of responding shape the therapeutic interaction and influences which templates come into play and how. It is not only patients but also therapists who bring their past into the consulting room.

Bibliography

Ablon, J.S. & Jones, E.E. (1998). How expert clinicians' prototypes of an ideal treatment correlate with outcome in psychodynamic and cognitive-behavioral therapy. *Psychotherapy Research*, 8(1), 71-83.

Bargh, J., & Barndollar, K. (1996). Automaticity in action: The unconscious as repository of chronic goals and motives. In P.M. Gollwitzer & J. Bargh (Eds.), *The Psychology of Action: Linking Cognition and Motivation to Behavior* (pp. 457-481). New York: Guilford Press.

Bornstein, R. (1995). Psychoanalysis in the undergraduate curriculum: An agenda for the psychoanalytic researcher. Electronic publishing: http://www.columbia.edu/~hc137/prs/v4n1/v4n1!2.htm

Bornstein, R. (2001). The impending death of psychoanalysis. *Psychoanalytic Psychology*, 18, 3-20.

Brenner, C. (1994). The mind as conflict and compromise formation. *Journal of Clinical Psychoanalysis*, 3 (4), 473-488.

Davies, J.M. & Frawley, M.G. (1992). Dissociative processes and transference-countertransference paradigms in the psychoanalytically oriented treatment of adult survivors of childhood sexual abuse. *Psychoanalytic Dialogues*, 2, 1, 5-36.

Gabbard G.O. (1992). Commentary on "Dissociative processes and transference-countertransference paradigms" by Jody Messler Davies and Mary Gail Frawley. *Psychoanalytic Dialogues*, 2, 1, 37-47.

Gabbard, G., & Westen, D. (2003). Rethinking therapeutic action. *International Journal of Psycho-Analysis*. 84: 823-841.

Gill, M. (1983). Psychoanalysis and psychotherapy: a revision. *International Review of Psychoanalysis*, 11, 161-179.

Goldberger, M. (1995). The couch as defense and as potential for enactment. *Psychoanalytic Quarterly*, 64, 1, 23-42.

Hansell, J. (2005). Writing an undergraduate textbook: An analyst's strange journey. *Psychologist-Psychoanalyst*, 24, 4, 37-38. (Electronic publishing: http://www.apadivisions.org/division-39/publications/newsletters/psychologist/2004/10/issue.pdf)

Jones, E.E. & Pulos, S.M. (1993). Comparing the process in psychodynamic and cognitive-behavioral therapies. *Journal of Consulting and Clinical Psychology*, 61(2), 306 316.

Kahneman, D. (2011). *Thinking, Fast and Slow*. NY: Farrar, Straus & Giroux.

Kahneman, D. (2003). A Perspective on Judgment and Choice: Mapping Bounded Rationality. *American Psychologist*, 58, 9, 697-720.

Kohlenberg, R. J. & Tsai, M. (1991). *Functional Analytic Psychotherapy: A guide for creating intense and curative therapeutic relationships*. New York: Plenum.

Leichsenring, F., Abbass, A., Heim, N., Keefer, J.R., Kisely, F. Luyten, P., Rabung, S., Steinert, C. (2023). The status of psychodynamic psychotherapy as an empirically supported treatment for common mental disorders—an umbrella review based on updated criteria. *World Psychiatry*, 22, 286–304.

Luepnitz, D. (2002). *Schopenhauer's Porcupines*. NY: Basic Books.

McWilliams, N. (2004). *Psychoanalytic Psychotherapy: A Practitioner's Guide*. NY: Guilford.

Nisbett, R., & Wilson, T. (1977). Telling more than we can know: Verbal reports on mental processes. *Psychological Review*, 84, 231-259.

Persons, E.S, Cooper, A.M, & Gabbard, G.O. (2005). *Textbook of Psychoanalysis*. Washington, D.C.: American Psychiatric Publishing.

Safran, J.D. & Segal, Z.V. (1990). *Interpersonal Process in Cognitive Therapy*. NY: Basic Books

Safran, J.D. (1998). *Widening the Scope of Cognitive Therapy: The Therapeutic Relationship, Emotion, and the Process of Change*. Northvale, NJ: Jason Aronson.

Schachter, J. & Kächele, H. (2013). The couch in psychoanalysis. *Contemporary Psychoanalysis*, 46, 3, 439-459.

Shedler, J. (2010). The Efficacy of Psychodynamic Psychotherapy. *American Psychologist*, 65, 98-109.

Shedler, J. (2022). That Was Then, This Is Now: Psychoanalytic Psychotherapy for The Rest of Us. *Contemporary Psychoanalysis*, 58:2-3, 405-437. https://doi.org/10.1080/00107530.2022.2149038

Weinberger, J. & Stoycheva, V. (2019). The Unconscious. Guilford Press.

Westen, D. (1998). The scientific legacy of Sigmund Freud: Toward a psychodynamically informed psychological science. *Psychological Bulletin*, 124, 333-371.

Westen, D., & Gabbard, G. (2002a). Developments in cognitive neuroscience, 1: Conflict, compromise, and connectionism. *Journal of the American Psychoanalytic Association*, 50, 54-98.

Westen, D., & Gabbard, G. (2002b). Developments in cognitive neuroscience, 2: Implications for the concept of transference. *Journal of the American Psychoanalytic Association*, 50, 99-133.

Whitehorn, J.C., Braceland, F.J., Lippard, V.W., Malamud, W. (Eds.) (1953). *The Psychiatrist: His Training and Development*. Washington, DC: American Psychiatric Association.

Wilson, T. D., Lindsey, S., & Schooler, T. Y. (2000). A model of dual attitudes. *Psychological Review*, 107, 101–126.

That Was Then, This is Now, Part 2: Psychodynamic Psychotherapy for the Rest of Us

Jonathan Shedler

Abstract: *This chapter is Part 2 of That Was Then, This is Now. The chapters (Parts 1 and 2) provide an accessible, jargon free, non-partisan introduction to psychoanalytic thinking and therapy for trainees, clinicians trained in other therapy approaches, and the public.*

Author's note: A version of this chapter originally appeared in *Contemporary Psychoanalysis* (Shedler, 2022).

Defense

Once we recognize there are things we prefer not to know, we find ourselves thinking about how it is that we avoid knowing. *Anything* a person does that serves to distract his or her attention from something unsettling or dissonant can be said to serve a defensive function. There is nothing at all mysterious about defensive processes. Defense is as simple as not noticing something, not thinking about something, not putting two and two together, or simply distracting ourselves with something else.

The psychoanalyst Herbert Schlesinger (2003) described defense in the context of systems theory. Systems (biological and psychological) regulate themselves to maintain equilibrium or homeostasis (for example, biological regulatory processes work to keep our body temperature near 98.6 degrees Fahrenheit despite large variations in outside temperature). When something is sufficiently dissonant with our habitual ways of thinking, feeling, and perceiving that it would disrupt psychological equilibrium, we tend to avoid, deny, disregard, minimize, or otherwise disavow it. Family systems therapists work to disrupt homeostatic processes that maintain dysfunctional family patterns, expecting that the system will reorganize in a more adaptive way. Analogously, psychoanalytic therapists work to disrupt homeostatic processes that maintain problems in living.

Older psychoanalytic writings refer to *repression* of thoughts and feelings, but I no longer find the term particularly helpful, and it is my impression that other contemporary psychoanalytic writers also struggle for better words. I believe the word contributes to mystification of something simple, ordinary, and commonplace. Bruno Bettelheim (1982) has argued that the word "repress" may be a poor translation of the German word Freud "used," and has suggested "disavow" as a more helpful translation. My dictionary's definition of "disavow" is "to disclaim knowledge of, responsibility for, or association with; disown; repudiate."

Disavowal of experience is commonplace. Jill, whom I used as an example in the section on "unconscious mental life" (Part 1 chapter, this volume), disavowed knowledge that her father had been abusive. She defended against this recognition by keeping thoughts about her family members at the level of generalities and not focusing on details. People often think and speak in generalities when attention to specifics would call into question cherished beliefs. Jill did not make a conscious decision to think and speak in generalities. She did this habitually and reflexively, without realizing it. It had become a part of her character. Later in our interview, it began to dawn on Jill that her father had been violently out of control. Even with the ugly truth out in the open, Jill sought to preserve psychological homeostasis by downplaying its meaning. Noting my grave reaction when she told me her father had nearly drowned her sister, Jill quickly sought to reassure herself and me that the event held no special significance. Emphasizing again how ill-behaved her sister had been, she added, "Anyone's father would have done that, right?"

Earlier in the prior chapter, I mentioned a patient who had difficulty recognizing and acknowledging his desire for caring and nurturing, who repeatedly chose cold, detached women. His choice of partners served a defensive function because it helped him avoid the difficult feelings stirred up in him by kind, loving women. He worked to see himself as strong, rugged, and independent, and he disavowed his gentler, more tender side.

He liked me as a therapist because he perceived me as rational and tough-minded, unlike the "mushy" and "touchy feely" therapist he had seen previously and from whom he had fled.

Any thought or feeling can be used to defend against any other. Angry feelings can defend against feelings of abandonment or rejection, depression can defend against anger, haughtiness can defend against self-contempt, confusion can help us avoid facing painful truths, and relentless clinging to logic (like Spock in the original Star Trek) can help us ignore feelings of rage or humiliation.

We can be dismayingly unaware of an undesirable trait in ourselves and quick to attribute it to someone else instead (projection). We can mask an attitude by emphasizing its opposite, like the anti-pornography crusader who reveals his own fascination with pornography by constantly seeking out pornographic material to condemn (reaction formation). We can blandly disregard information that is right in front of our noses, like the parent who fails to notice that her anorexic daughter is starving, or the therapist who doesn't hear her patient's references to a suicide plan (denial).

We can think about emotionally charged topics in coldly abstract ways, like a patient of mine who tried to decide whether or not he was in love by doing a cost-benefit analysis (intellectualization). We can convince ourselves that we are unafraid by plunging recklessly into the situation that frightens us (counterphobic behavior). We can direct our feelings toward the wrong person, like the woman who is oblivious to her husband's infidelity but becomes enraged when she learns his friend is having an affair (displacement). We can induce feelings in another person that we cannot tolerate in ourselves, then try to manage them in the other person (projective identification). We can disclaim responsibility for our behavior by attributing it to circumstances outside our control (externalization). We are infinitely creative in finding ways to avoid or disavow what is distressing.

Certain defenses receive considerable external reinforcement. From time to time, a depressed patient will tell me during an initial consultation that his difficulties are due to a "chemical imbalance." This often means the patient does not want to consider the possibility that his perceptions, expectations, choices, conflicts, relationship patterns, or anything else that is within his power to understand and change might be causing, maintaining, or exacerbating his suffering. In insisting that their difficulties are due entirely to "chemical imbalance," such patients are often letting us know that they do not wish to examine themselves. This is a particularly pernicious defense because it is bolstered by messages from pharmaceutical companies (which have an obvious financial incentive to portray emotional suffering as a biological illness) and often by trusted doctors (who receive information from those same pharmaceutical companies).

Such patients may regard any acknowledgment of a psychological component to their suffering as an intolerable admission of weakness or personal failure. The harsh self-judgment and self-condemnation that lies just beneath the surface of this attitude may be precisely what is perpetuating the depression, but their reluctance to examine themselves may preclude the kind of therapy that would lead to change. In such cases, I have found it best not to challenge patients' convictions directly, but to try to stimulate their curiosity and self-reflection in other ways. (For the record, I am *not* suggesting that we can ignore biological factors or should not avail ourselves of pharmacological treatment options. I am suggesting that an appreciation of biology should not make us deaf and blind to psychology.)

Undergraduate psychology textbooks generally catalog *defense mechanisms*, but these presentations rarely foster a deeper understanding of psychoanalytic therapy. One problem with the term *defense mechanism* is that it sounds, well, mechanistic, and the life of the mind is anything but mechanistic. Also, the term *mechanism*, a noun, makes it sound like a defense is a *thing*. It is more helpful to think of *defending*, a verb, as something people *do*. Another problem is that *defense mechanism* implies a discrete process or event, which is also not quite right. Rather than being discrete events, ways of defending are woven into the fabric of our lives and reflected in our characteristic ways of thinking, feeling, acting, coping, and relating. Our ways of defending become part of our enduring personality or character.

For example, some people characteristically immerse themselves in detail and miss the forest for the trees. The focus on concrete details takes the focus off difficult emotions. Other people seem unable to focus on details at all. Their perceptions of self and others seem glib and superficial. This defensive style may deflect attention from troubling facts. Some people feel superior and act self-important to help banish from awareness painful feelings of emptiness or inadequacy. Some people are chronically inattentive to their own needs but lavish care on others instead (a common pattern in mental health professionals). Defense and personality are inseparable.

Psychoanalytic psychotherapy helps us recognize the ways we disavow aspects of our experience, with the goal of helping us to claim or reclaim what is ours. This has the effect of expanding freedom and choice. Things that previously seemed automatic or obligatory become volitional and life options expand. Of course, freedom and choice bring their own dilemmas. With choice comes responsibility, which can sometimes be terrifying. The desire to deny responsibility can therefore be a significant impediment to change.

Perhaps Erica Jong had this dilemma in mind when she wrote:

> No one to blame!... That was why most people led lives they hated, with people they hated… How wonderful to have someone to blame! How wonderful to live with one's nemesis! You may be miserable, but you feel forever in the right. You may be fragmented, but you feel absolved of all the blame for it. Take your life in your own hands, and what happens? A terrible thing: no one to blame. (Jong, 1977)

In the section on *transference*, I described research showing that the most effective therapists address transference in psychotherapy (Ablon & Jones, 1998; Jones & Pulos, 1993). The same research found that the most effective therapists also help patients recognize defenses by calling attention to them as they arise in treatment. Both types of interventions are empirically linked to good treatment outcome.

If we think of defense in systemic terms, as an effort to preserve equilibrium and homeostasis, then psychotherapy poses a paradox. People come to therapy to change, but change necessarily represents a threat to equilibrium and homeostasis. Thus, every patient is ambivalent about treatment, oscillating between the desire to change and the desire to preserve the status quo. This ambivalence can be palpable at the start of therapy. Among patients who schedule appointments at our university clinic, roughly half do not keep their first appointment. I believe this is typical for many clinics. When patients telephone the clinic, they are expressing one side of an inner conflict, the side that seeks change. When they fail to keep their appointments, they are expressing the other side of the conflict, the side that seeks to maintain homeostasis.

I recall starting my own psychoanalysis. I scheduled my first appointment two weeks in advance. I thought about the upcoming appointment day and night throughout the two weeks. On the day of the actual appointment, however, it completely slipped my mind. When the analyst and I eventually managed to meet, he asked if it was like me to forget appointments. I told him with embarrassment that it was not. He shrugged and said, "So, it seems you have an unconscious too."

Psychotherapy is an ongoing tug-of-war between a part of us that seeks change and a part of us that strives to preserve the known and familiar, however painful that may be. As therapists, we side with the forces seeking growth. I believe Freud (1912) had this paradox in mind when he wrote: "The resistance accompanies the treatment step by step. Every single association, every act of the person under treatment must reckon with the resistance and represents a compromise between the forces that are striving for recovery and the opposing ones" (p. 103).

The terms *defense* and *resistance* are closely related. They refer to efforts to disavow or disclaim thoughts, feelings, or responsibility. More technically, resistance refers to defensive processes that emerge within the therapy relationship itself, that impede the shared task of exploration and inquiry. It is not particularly helpful to think of resistance as opposition between therapist and patient. Rather, resistance arises out of conflict or discord *within the patient*. This can be difficult to keep in mind when resistance takes forms therapists find unpleasant such as when patients arrive late, miss appointments, fall silent, fill sessions with small talk, ignore the therapist's comments, and so on.

However frustrating for therapists, such behavior reflects the patient's efforts to maintain equilibrium. The therapist's best approach is alliance with the parts of the patient that seek growth and change. Ideally, patient and therapist develop a shared sense of curiosity regarding defensive processes, viewing them non-judgmentally with a desire simply to examine and understand.

The concepts of defense, conflict, and unconscious mental life are intertwined. The word *unconscious* is merely a form of shorthand, referring to the thoughts, feelings, and behaviors we disavow, repudiate, or defend against. We often see an active push and pull between defensive processes and the thoughts and feelings they defend against. As hard as we work to push them away, so hard do they seem to push back, seeking some form of outlet or expression. Thus, there is conflict or dynamic tension between those parts of us that repudiate and those parts of us that get repudiated. Psychoanalytic theorists use the term *dynamic unconscious* to remind us that unconscious thoughts and feelings are not dormant or inert, but actively seek expression. They influence our thoughts, feelings, and actions in indirect ways.[1]

Psychological Causation

Psychological symptoms often seem senseless. They serve no apparent purpose and often feel alien to the person suffering from them. Many depressed patients have told me that feelings of despair and sadness come on "out of the blue." Feelings of anxiety or even panic can also come on unpredictably. In fact, the DSM diagnostic criteria for panic disorder specify that the panic attacks come on "unexpectedly," that is, with no apparent cause.

---

[1] Note that the word *unconscious* has a specific meaning in psychoanalytic theory. Many mental processes take place outside of awareness, but we generally reserve the term *unconscious* for thoughts, feelings, and behaviors that we *actively* repudiate and that *actively* seek expression. Thus, the word *unconscious* really means *dynamic unconscious*. Psychoanalytic theorists generally use other terms (such as *non*-conscious) to refer to mental processes that take place outside of awareness, but that are not conflictual or actively defended against.

However random or meaningless symptoms may seem, it is our working assumption that symptoms have meaning, serve psychological functions, and occur in a psychological context. Because the psychological circumstances that contextualize a symptom may not be consciously accessible, a symptom may *appear* senseless or random. As a person's scope of awareness expands and she becomes better able to recognize and articulate a broader range of experience, the meaning and function of the symptom may become clear. Generally, as this occurs, the person is able to find new solutions to old problems and the symptom fades.

The more we are strangers to ourselves, the more random, accidental, and fragmented our experience may seem. Psychoanalytic therapy helps us recognize the connections that exist between thoughts, feelings, actions, and events. For example, if a patient says to me, "I don't know why I did that," I may respond by saying, "Let's see if we can look beyond 'I don't know.' Let's examine what happened before that." What happened before could be an external event or internal events like thoughts and feelings.

A patient recovering from a heart attack kept "forgetting" to take his medication. I put "forgetting" in quotation marks because the patient, whom I will call Steve, was an intelligent person and his memory for other things was just fine. Steve's doctors responded with "patient education," explaining why the medication was necessary. Steve wanted to take care of his health and tried to follow his doctors' treatment plan. Still, he kept forgetting.

I suggested to Steve that there might be more to his forgetting than meets the eye, and asked if he had any ideas about this. Steve eventually said that something about taking the medication gave him a bad feeling, but he could not say what. He genuinely did not know. I asked him to tell me any thoughts or feelings that occurred to him, whether or not they seemed relevant or made sense to him. Steve said he did not know why it came to mind just then, but he found himself thinking about his younger brother. As a child, Steve had been popular, athletic, and a good student. In contrast, his brother had been sickly and weak, and was always taking pills for one thing or another. He did poorly in school and was no good at sports. He was a disappointment to his parents.

Note the *sequence* of Steve's thoughts. His first thought was about taking medication. His next associations were to his sickly younger brother. We call the thoughts "associations" because we assume they are in some way linked to, or associated with, the preceding thoughts. On the surface the two topics seem unrelated, but our working assumption is that they are connected.

In this case, the sequence of thoughts suggests a hypothesis: in Steve's mind, taking pills means being like his younger brother—that is, weak, sickly, and less loved. If the hypothesis is correct, no amount of "patient education" would have sufficed, despite his doctor's best efforts. In fact, Steve stopped forgetting his medication only after we were able to discuss his fear of being weak and a failure, and his related fear of losing the love of the people who mattered to him. More specifically, Steve recognized that taking medication would not turn him into his brother. That was an irrational fantasy. The fantasy operated outside awareness, but it influenced Steve's behavior and could have cost him his life.

Another patient, who was a bit overweight, had periodic eating binges. She'd sneak to the McDonald's drive-through and order cheeseburgers and milkshakes. Afterward, she'd hate herself for it. She had tried for years to control her eating binges with little success. After an eating binge, I asked her to notice any thoughts that occurred to her, whether or not they seemed related to the eating binge. Her thoughts ran to her husband. She said he was self-centered, controlling, and disregarded her needs. She said he treated her as a trophy to display, not as a human being with needs and feelings of her own. Her additional associations were that her husband was happy when she was thin because she was a better trophy, that she felt emotionally deprived and unloved, and that she felt dependent on her husband and trapped.

"Could it be," I wondered aloud, "that your eating binge was a way of getting back at your husband?" My comment was aimed at making explicit or conscious a potential link between thoughts, feelings, and actions that had thus far been implicit or unconscious. My patient had great difficulty acknowledging anger toward her husband despite the fact that she complained about him constantly, and it was a struggle for her to give my comment serious consideration. Eventually, she began to put into words her anger, her revenge fantasies, and the thought that her husband was "such a prick that he doesn't deserve a thin wife."

My patient's eating binge was embedded in a complex web of associations and meanings. As it turned out, her behavior served simultaneously to punish her husband, to compensate for her emotional deprivation (because she associated food with love), to reassure herself that she was not under his control, to help suppress fantasies about leaving him (because being overweight would make her less desirable to other men), and to punish herself for her vindictive thoughts (because she hated being overweight).

This multiplicity of causes and meanings illustrates the concepts of *overdetermination* and *multiple function* that I mentioned earlier. In the life of the mind, we do not necessarily find simple, one-to-one cause and effect. A symptom or behavior may have multiple causes (overdetermination) and can serve multiple purposes (multiple function). All competent psychoanalytic therapists share a deep appreciation of the complexity of mental life. For this reason, psychoanalytic psychotherapy is not "cookie-cutter" therapy. It is not a collection of standardized techniques, nor can it be reduced to a step-by-step manual. It relies on empathically attuned inquiry into the most private, personal, and deeply subjective aspects of inner experience. In this sense, no two treatments can ever be alike.[2]

My patient did not experience a sudden insight or dramatic cure, and she had not come to treatment because of her secret visits to McDonald's. Nevertheless, over time we were able to trace out some of the links in the complex web of meanings that gave rise to her binge eating. She slowly became more comfortable acknowledging and expressing anger, more aware of her own emotional needs, and better able to communicate them to her husband and others. Her relationship with her husband improved and her eating binges subsided. Eventually she reported that for the first

---

[2] There are academic researchers who would have us believe that only "manualized" therapies (conducted by following an instruction manual) are scientifically sound and "evidence based." I will deal with these claims later. Such therapies—tidy, standardized, and time-limited—are also favored by health insurance companies which are in the business of enhancing profit, not patients' lives.

time in years, she was able to lose weight and keep it off, and it did not feel like a constant struggle. She never won the battle absolutely. Over the ensuing years she did have the occasional binge—always when she was furious with her husband.

These examples are meant to illustrate how psychological symptoms are embedded in organized networks of thoughts, feelings, perceptions, and memories that contextualize them and give them meaning. This applies not only to symptoms but to *all* mental events. It is a working assumption of psychoanalysis that *nothing in the life of the mind is random*. The mind is an elaborate associative network, with mental events linked to one another in meaningful, albeit complex, ways.

Within certain broad parameters, all mental activity follows the logic of the associative network, whether or not the connecting links are explicit or conscious. This applies not only to thoughts, feelings, and memories, but also to dreams, daydreams, mistakes, and slips of the tongue (the infamous "Freudian slip"). It is possible to start with any seemingly random mental event and trace the multiple associations linked to it. Often, the event makes sense when the larger associative network becomes explicit.

An analogy to an associative network is the internet, where web pages are linked in intricately interconnected networks (Peebles-Kleiger, 2002). We can call up a web page, follow a link to another page, and then another and another. Within a few clicks we can get far indeed from our starting point. We could start on a page about global warming and end up, a few clicks away, on a page about Shakespearean sonnets. Somebody who looked at our computer screen at that moment might never have guessed how we got there. If we wanted, however, we could re-trace the sequence of links that brought us from where we started to where we ended, and we could explain why we followed those links.

Missing from the internet analogy is the role of affect. Unlike the web, where links are based mostly on content, mental associative networks are organized along affective lines. That is, things are connected that bring up similar feelings. *Associative pathways tend to lead to what is emotionally charged or problematic.* This has profound implications for therapeutic technique: if we allow ourselves to observe our thoughts without editing or censoring them, and we follow them where they lead, they often lead to what is troubling.

Contemporary research in cognitive science and neuroscience is based on the concept of mind as associative network, and cognitive researchers have developed experimental methods to study associative linkages (for example, priming experiments and reaction time experiments). Interestingly, the concept of associative pathways has *always* been central to psychoanalytic theory and practice. Freud was a master at tracing associative links to discover psychological meanings, untangling associative connections with a detective's precision.

Freud's thinking is most accessible and compelling in his 1904 monograph, *The Psychopathology of Everyday Life*, which I recommend to all students and therapists. Certainly, there were instances where Freud was carried away by his own cleverness and guilty of reading questionable meanings into patients' associations. Those with an agenda to criticize will find ample ammunition in Freud's writings but they would miss the point.

To help trace associative linkages, we ask our patients to say whatever comes to mind without editing or censoring their thoughts, encouraging them to observe their thoughts non-judgmentally (as in some forms of Buddhist meditation), without regard for whether or not the thoughts make sense or seem socially appropriate. This is called *free association*. Its purpose is to help make explicit associative linkages that are otherwise implicit. Every psychoanalytic therapist has a collection of phrases aimed at encouraging the free flow of thought and communication. We are constantly saying things like, "Can you say more about that?" and "What comes to mind?" and "What more occurs to you?" and "Where do your thoughts go from there?" and sometimes just "go on" and "uh huh."

In everyday social conversation, we automatically edit and censor our thoughts. We try to stay on topic, structure our thoughts to make coherent sentences, and edit out things that may embarrass or offend. Free association means suspending the usual editing and censoring and it often leads us places we could not have anticipated. Free association is therefore especially difficult for people who like to feel composed, collected, and in control.

When patients describe therapy as "venting" or liken it to conversing with a friend (descriptions that have always struck me as deeply devaluing of psychotherapy), it is a sure sign that they are *not* involved in a meaningful therapeutic process. No one who has engaged in genuine free association would ever liken therapy to ordinary conversation. Psychoanalytic therapy takes place at the edge, on the precipice of the abyss, at the border between the known and the unknown. There is nothing ordinary about it.

A male patient of mine, who was gay, made a slip of the tongue and called me by another person's name—let's say James. I asked him what occurred to him about the slip, and he responded with the usual protestations that it was a random occurrence and meant nothing. I suggested we find out by seeing where his thoughts led. What did the name "James" bring to mind? He recalled a friend of a friend who was named James, and he hastened to assure me this person meant nothing to him. "Okay," I said. "Perhaps he means nothing. All the same, where do your thoughts go next?" My patient paused, then blushed. James, he said, had been attracted to him and had wanted to seduce him. I asked, "Why does that embarrass you?"

It was not James's attempted seduction that embarrassed him. Rather, my patient had been working hard to push something out of his mind. That something was that *I* might be gay and might want to seduce him. In fact, he had had a graphic daydream about it, and he had discussed it with his partner, who found the possibility intriguing. My patient had resolved not to think about it again and not to mention it, yet here it was. His associations to his "random" slip of the tongue ran directly to what was most emotionally charged for him at that moment—as is so often the case.

To the reader who thinks this example sounds implausible, contrived, or biased by theoretical preconceptions, I say: try it. Next time you make a mistake, a slip of the tongue, or forget a word or a name, try free associating and follow your thoughts where they lead. It helps to write your thoughts down. At the point when you feel you are done and want to stop, ask yourself what comes to mind *next*. And after that, ask yourself what comes to mind *next*. Force yourself to push past the inner resistance you will encounter (e.g., "this exercise is stupid," "this is boring," "my thoughts aren't leading anywhere") and follow the chain of associations where it leads. Humor me, if need be, but try it. You will never see the data if you do not conduct the experiment.

Officially, this non-randomness of mental processes is called *psychic determinism*. The term refers to the recognition that thoughts, feelings, behavior, and symptoms are not random or accidental, but are influenced or determined by the mental events preceding them. I prefer the term *psychic continuity* to psychic determinism. It reminds us that there is continuity from one thought to the next, and that thoughts and feelings are chained in meaningful associative sequences, even when they seem unrelated or discontinuous.

The term *determinism* has its roots in the mechanistic, materialist scientific zeitgeist of the 19th century, and I am not sure its connotations are as helpful in our time. I have encountered students who reject psychoanalytic approaches because they think, mistakenly, that psychoanalysis rejects free will and views behavior as determined by forces outside our control. The opposite may be closer to the truth.

Psychoanalytic therapists believe expanding our understanding of the meanings and causes of our behavior *creates* freedom, choice, and a freer will. People can change, people *do* change, and psychoanalytic therapy helps people change, sometimes in profound ways. Every psychotherapist, deep down, believes in the human capacity to grow, change, and experience a greater sense of freedom and equanimity in the face of life's inevitable hardships. If behavior were unavoidably determined, there would be no reason to practice psychoanalytic therapy or, for that matter, any form of therapy.[3]

_____

[3] A patient of mine was once deeply struck when I pointed out a repetitive pattern in his life. In a moment of soul-rattling insight, he realized he had repeated the same mistake in his life, time and again. He was highly intelligent but not terribly psychologically sophisticated. With the shock of recognition, he blurted out, "It's true, it's true! I do exactly what you say, I see it!" And then, with consternation: "Why do I

What's good for the goose

The reader may have noticed that I have written much of this chapter using the first-person pronoun "we." This is not an accident or literary convenience. It is meant to convey that the concepts and insights we apply to our patients apply equally to ourselves. The psychoanalytic sensibility draws no distinctions between the psychological principles that apply to patients and those that apply to therapists. As the psychoanalyst Harry Stack Sullivan (1954) observed, "We are all more simply human than otherwise." Patient and therapist alike view self and others through the lenses of past experience, have unconscious mental lives, disavow what is threatening, form transferences, and reenact past relationship roles.

Some of my students have held the unfortunate preconception that psychoanalysis is a hierarchical, "one up" relationship between an emotionally removed, authoritarian doctor and a disempowered patient. I cannot in good conscience say this never occurred; there was a time in the history of the profession when some psychoanalysts adopted a detached, distant stance toward patients.[4] The last half century has brought sea changes in psychoanalytic theory and practice and this phase in the development of the profession is, thankfully, behind us. Psychoanalytic therapy is not something done *to* or practiced *on* another person. It is something done *with* another person. Contemporary psychoanalytic practitioners strive to be warm, responsive, and engaged.

This does not mean that psychoanalytic therapy—or for that matter, any kind of therapy—is a symmetrical relationship. There is no point denying the fundamental reality that one person has come for help and the other to offer it, that one person is paying the other a fee, and these circumstances necessarily entail a power differential. The same holds true for any relationship in which one person is in need and another accepts the responsibility of trying to help. But it does mean that therapy is a

---

do this? Why do I keep doing it? Is this just the way I *am*?" I answered, "It's the way you've *been*." It was one of my favorite moments in therapy.

[4] I am inclined to think the best psychoanalysts never practiced this way, but certainly some mediocre ones did.

collaborative, shared effort between two humans who must struggle to make sense together.

The psychoanalytic therapists I know and respect consider it a deep privilege to share so intimately in the inner, private life of another person — and there is something in the work that breeds in them a deep humility regarding what we can and cannot know, and a deep humility regarding our capacity to help. I personally am not, by temperament, given to modesty or humility. I can nevertheless say sincerely that the longer I have practiced and the more I have learned, the more humble I have felt in my work with patients and the more deeply I have come to respect them. My patients and I share similar conflicts and struggles, and we know similar pain. I have never treated a person so disturbed that I could not see something of him or her in me. Truly, we *are* all more simply human than otherwise.

Psychoanalytic therapy requires of the therapist a degree of intelligence, a degree of professional knowledge and skill, a capacity for empathic attunement with another person, a willingness to immerse ourselves in another person's private, subjective world, an absolutely ruthless willingness to examine ourselves, and, for want of a better word, humanity. Of all the qualities that go into the making of a therapist, it is this last and most ineffable quality that may ultimately carry the day.

As for willingness to examine ourselves, it is difficult if not impossible to do meaningful psychoanalytic work without having a meaningful psychotherapy experience ourselves. Personal psychotherapy may be the single most important component of a psychotherapist's training. Also, there is something that strikes me as hypocritical in asking our patients to do something we have been unwilling to do ourselves, something improper and unbecoming in asking our patients to follow their thoughts without censorship wherever they lead, when we have been unwilling to do so ourselves.

There is nothing like the experience of being a patient to foster empathy for our patients and help us understand the powerful and often irrational feelings therapy can stir up. We cannot truly understand transference or resistance by reading about it in a book or observing it in someone else. We must experience it firsthand, as lived experience. Nor is it sufficient to enter psychotherapy for the sake of "professional development" alone. We must enter it, like our patients, as struggling human beings.

Beyond this, the more we understand of our own conflicts and relationship templates, the better we can resist reenacting them with our patients. Personal psychotherapy or psychoanalysis does not guarantee we will succeed in this, but it can at least give us a fighting chance. Too often, I have seen therapists recreate their personal psychopathology with their patients. Therapists with histories of sexual abuse, who have not worked through their experience in personal therapy, tend to be quick to pronounce their patients as victims, defining their experience for them instead allowing them to explore it for themselves.

It is my impression that the therapists (if they deserve to be called that) who have created furor over false memories fall into this category. Therapists who have unresolved issues with the other gender may be quick to join patients in bashing them, rather than helping their patients to better understand their own intimacy needs and the psychological obstacles to fulfilling them. Therapists who struggle with self-esteem difficulties may subtly demean their patients or offer them shallow validation and "affirmations" (like the kind caricatured by Stewart Smalley in old *Saturday Night Live* episodes), rather than offering an opportunity to explore and rework their sense of self in ways congruent with their personal histories and lived experience. These are relatively blatant examples. More often, therapists enact their conflicts and relationship templates in more subtle ways.

Finally, meaningful personal therapy engenders faith in the therapeutic process, and we require a great deal of faith when adrift in therapeutic seas. As Nancy McWilliams (2004, p. 67) eloquently observed, "The experience of an effective personal therapy or analysis leaves us with a deep respect for the power of the process and the efficacy of treatment. We know that psychotherapy works. Our silent appreciation of the discipline can convey that conviction to clients, for whom a sense of hope is a critical part of their recovery from emotional suffering." Without hope, there can be no therapy.

Bibliography

Ablon, J.S. & Jones, E.E. (1998). How expert clinicians' prototypes of an ideal treatment correlate with outcome in psychodynamic and cognitive-behavioral therapy. *Psychotherapy Research*, 8(1), 71-83.

Bettelheim, B. (1982). *Freud and Man's Soul: An Important Re-Interpretation of Freudian Theory*. NY: Random House.

Freud, S. (1904). *The Psychopathology of Everyday Life*. SE 6

Freud, S. (1912). *The Dynamics of Transference*. SE 12

Jones, E.E. & Pulos, S.M. (1993). Comparing the process in psychodynamic and cognitive-behavioral therapies. *Journal of Consulting and Clinical Psychology*, 61(2), 306 316.

Jong, E. (1977). *How to Save Your Own Life*. Holt, Rinehart & Winston.

McWilliams, N. (2004). *Psychoanalytic Psychotherapy: A Practitioner's Guide*. NY: Guilford.

Peebles-Kleiger, M.J. (2002). *Beginnings: The art and science of planning psychotherapy*. Hillsdale, NJ: The Analytic Press.

Schlesinger, H. (2003). *The Texture of Treatment: On the Matter of Psychoanalytic Technique*. The Analytic Press.

Shedler, J. (2022). That Was Then, This Is Now: Psychoanalytic Psychotherapy for The Rest of Us. *Contemporary Psychoanalysis*, 58:2-3, 405-437. https://doi.org/10.1080/00107530.2022.2149038

Sullivan, H.S. (1954). *The Psychiatric Interview*. New York: Norton.

Going Beyond the DSM with the Power Threat Meaning Framework, Open Dialogue Approach and Soteria

Radosław Stupak

Abstract: *This chapter provides a brief description of the Power Threat Meaning Framework (PTMF), which offers a way of framing human distress that may be a practical alternative to symptom-based categorical DSM diagnoses. PTMF, published by the British Psychological Society (BPS) in 2018, proposes replacing the stigmatizing labels that pathologize individuals (i.e., the "What's wrong with you?" approach) with a dialogical exploration and (re)construction of personal history, situations, events, and reactions shaped by culturally and socially influenced meanings (i.e., "What happened to you?"). This chapter also presents the main assumptions and practical solutions of the Open Dialogue Approach (ODA) and Soteria houses. ODA and Soteria, while studied and used mostly in the context of psychotic experiences, could prove to be successful in helping people in other kinds of difficult emotional situations and life experiences. They are compatible with the PTMF, reject the disease model of human distress, and allow going beyond the DSM while providing effective help.*

Introduction

Even if there seem to be emerging trends for the inclusion of a more nuanced perspective and a bigger emphasis on psychosocial interventions and human rights, as evidenced by recent World Health Organization and United Nations reports (UN Human Rights Commissioner, 2019; World Health Organization, 2021), the biomedical model of mental health is dominating (Stupak & Dobroczyński, 2021). Similarly, the biopsychosocial model favors interventions and conceptualizations operating within a biomedical perspective and could be seen as its mere extension, so that the "psychosocial" is colonized and subsumed by the "biomedical" (Read et al., 2013). According to the American Psychiatric Association (APA) former president, it actually seems to be a "bio-bio-bio model" (Sharfstein, 2005).

Psychiatric research and clinical practice focus on the biological level, but the progress in neuroscience does not lead to better treatments, and new drugs are no more effective or work on the same underlying principles as those discovered by accident in the middle of the 20th century (Deacon, 2013). Lack of progress in improving clinical outcomes, the iatrogenic harm of current model of care, and overprescription of psychiatric drugs is to a large extent connected with the nosological system current practice relies on — the *DSM* (as well as the ICD) (Fava & Rafanelli, 2019; Ghaemi, 2022; Van Os & Kohne, 2021).

The *DSM* and the categorical model of "mental disorders" has been criticized from many different perspectives, ranging from strictly scientific ones through sociological, philosophical, and political critiques (Karter, 2019). Some of the contemporary practical solutions to these problems are the Power Threat Meaning Framework (PTMF), Soteria, and Open Dialogue approaches. PTMF offers a non-pathologizing way of framing human distress and may be a practical alternative to *DSM*, while Soteria and Open Dialogue are clinical solutions, used mostly in the context of psychosis, that are compatible with the PTMF and allow going beyond the *DSM* while providing effective help. The goal of this chapter is to briefly present these approaches.

Power Threat Meaning Framework

The Power Threat Meaning Framework (PTMF) was developed by a collaborative team of mental health professionals and psychiatric survivors with Lucy Johnstone and Mary Boyle as leading authors. It received financial support from the Division of Clinical Psychology (DCP) within the British Psychological Society (BPS) and was published by the BPS in 2018, although it is not an official model used by the BPS.

In essence, PTMF aims to move beyond thinking in terms of diagnostic constructs as reified entities, which often occurs when research and clinical practice rely on categories from the *DSM*. Such reliance may lead to a number of negative cultural and social consequences for patients and the therapy process (Campolonghi & Orrù, 2023; Hayes & Hofmann, 2020). Furthermore, PTMF aims to creatively transcend the biopsychosocial model (Johnstone et al., 2018).

PTMF can be described as an effort to tackle the challenge of addressing "problems in living," a term used by Harry Stack Sullivan, without relying on psychiatric diagnostic systems (Harper, 2022). The fundamental premise is that what might be labeled as "psychiatric symptoms" are comprehensible reactions to frequently challenging circumstances. These responses, influenced by both evolutionary factors and socially conditioned, serve as protective mechanisms and are a sign of human agency and creativity. However, on occasion, they can contribute to the to the exacerbation and perpetuation of distress (Johnstone et al., 2018).

PTMF represents a stark departure from the *DSM* and, in doing so, blends a diverse array of theoretical and practical perspectives. These encompass radical behaviorism, cognitive, interpretive, and hermeneutic approaches as well as social constructionism, critical realism, systemic therapy, social justice, indigenous psychology, and narrative approaches (among others). Together, these perspectives offer a rich reservoir of ideas, theories, and methodologies that can be applied in practice that does not ignore the social, cultural, and even political dimensions underlying the problems people face (Harper, 2022).

Power

The fundamental aspect of the proposed approach is Power, understood broadly as various forms of biological/embodied power (related to the possession or lack of socially highly valued features), coercive or power by force, legal power (concerning specific legal solutions regulating various aspects of life and behavior), economic and material power (access to various types of services, goods, shelter, etc.), social and cultural capital, interpersonal power (the threat of withdrawal of emotional support in close relationships), and ideological power (Boyle, 2022).

These various manifestations of power are recognized in the PTMF as closely related and overlapping. Whether they have detrimental or beneficial effects, they function within the framework of social systems, institutions, and organizations, as well as within our physical surroundings. They are also at play in the realms of media, education, and social and familial interactions. Consequently, Power concerns, among others, control of meanings, language, stereotypes, policies, and specific practical solutions that influence our understanding of reality and shape individual subjectivity and behavior (Boyle, 2022) in alignment with the demands of economic ideologies such as neoliberalism (Teo, 2018).

In the context of mental suffering and disturbing behavior, Power also acts by creating cultural narratives about them (such as diagnostic systems), which become norms to which people submit themselves—or are forced to submit—and creates socially acceptable ways of responding to suffering. The discourse of psychiatry, psychology and psychotherapy, which can be also understood as a form of ideological power, can translate into very direct manifestations of violence and behavioral control (as, for example, in the case of the use of coercion and treatment without consent), which according to PTMF would belong to the area of power by force or power by coercion. Power may also contribute to distress, primarily by creating threats to the fulfillment of human needs (Boyle, 2022).

Threat and Meaning

Threat, as conceptualized in the PTMF, is closely related to the notion of needs. It is assumed that needs include but are not limited to (Johnstone et al., 2018, pp. 149-150): safety, close attachments to caregivers (as infants and children), positive relationships, control over our lives, basic physical needs, meaningful activity, and purpose.

Key areas where the operation of Power may create Threats to the fulfillment of needs could be framed as those relating to "childhood adversity, gender, 'race' and ethnicity" (Johnstone, 2022, p. 98). PTMF emphasizes that understanding the impact of these phenomena on individuals is impossible without placing them in a broader cultural context—that is, the context of individual and cultural meanings.

The very concept of "meaning" can be understood in many different ways, and there is a rich philosophical and linguistic tradition grappling with this problem. In the PTMF, Meaning is the third fundamental element and a thread that runs throughout all the other elements. Broadly, we can approach "meaning" as "meaning of life" as well as meanings that arise in the context of daily routines and social exchanges—even in commonplace, everyday situations. PTMF is interested in both of these dimensions (Cromby, 2022).

Meaning can extend beyond abstract sign systems, like language, and is embedded in tangible practices, actions, and the physical, institutional, and cultural environments. These elements serve as an enduring backdrop, collectively contributing to the interpretation of particular actions like speaking, listening, or other gestures and behaviors in material contexts influenced by the dynamics of Power (Cromby, 2022). Meaning can be conveyed in narratives that shape identities. The PTMF treats narratives as decentred and fluid while value judgments about them are avoided (e.g., pathological vs. non-pathological narratives).

Narratives can be expressed through a variety of mediums, extending beyond language, and can be non-chronological and non-linear (Vassilieva, 2016). "Therapeutic" narratives, in terms of their function, can emerge in a wide range of social, interpersonal, and relational contexts, encompassing creative forms like poetry, songs, music, art, and culturally-specific legends and beliefs. PTMF underscores individuals' agency in crafting their own narratives but concurrently seeks to avoid falling into the trap of "magical voluntarism" as described by Smail (Smail, 2016). This refers to the oversimplified notion that all that's required is a change in one's thinking or beliefs. Narratives, like meanings, are not isolated from the economic, material, and physical realities in which they are embedded.

In the PTMF, problematic behaviors and experiences—or as they are referred to in psychiatric terminology, "symptoms"—can serve multiple purposes. For example, they can help regulate overwhelming emotions, seek attachment, establish a sense of control, avoid perceived danger, maintain a sense of identity and self-esteem, or facilitate inclusion in a social or peer group. These behaviors can encompass both pre-reflective responses (unconscious, instinctual, or minimally influenced by language or culture but still shaped by learning) such as fight, flight, freeze, or heightened vigilance reactions, as well as behaviors subject to reflective influences (Boyle, 2022).

Threat responses shaped by Meaning

Specific Threat responses can have multiple functions. For instance, unusual beliefs can provide both a sense of purpose in life and a boost to self-esteem. Furthermore, various behaviors can serve the same purpose — for example, ritualistic actions, self-starvation, and resorting to violence may be all ways to establish a sense of control (Johnstone, 2022). In this context, the influence of Power is evident both in the creation of obstacles to meeting needs (for instance, due to working conditions or the actions of various institutions) and in shaping potential reactions to these challenges (such as advertising that may promote using substances as a way to manage distress or by highlighting different forms of expressing distress). This results in the development of a culturally influenced "pool of symptoms" that becomes cognitively accessible for people in order to communicate their problems.

Simply speaking, PTMF suggests replacing the key question for medicalization (e.g., "What's wrong with you?" or "What disorder do you have?") with "What happened to you?" Of course, this should not be understood literally, nor does it mean that such specific words should be used by a clinician — it illustrates a certain ontological and epistemological shift that is required (Harper & Cromby, 2022).

Instead of going over symptoms checklists to arrive at a diagnosis, the question "What happened to you?" emphasizes the importance of considering the dimension of Power. It encourages an exploration of the client's issues in terms of their personal history, potential significant or adverse life events that may have influenced them, and situating these problems within a broader social and cultural context. The next core question, "how did it affect you?", closely linked to the previous one, prompts an examination of Threats. "What sense did you make of it?" pertains to the analysis of Meaning. "What did you have to do to survive?" relates to Threat responses, specific behaviors, thoughts and feelings, coping strategies (Johnstone et al., 2018).

The questions "what are your strengths?" (referring to the identification of Power-related resources that a person can utilize to improve their situation and well-being, including skills, social support, and knowledge) and "what is your story?" (which focuses on the personal narrative) can be particularly helpful in a clinical setting. It's important to note, though, that these formulations apply to all people, not just those seeking professional support or described as "mentally ill" (Johnstone, 2022).

The PTMF proposes certain broad, evidence-based patterns of meaning-based threat responses to the negative operation of power, which provide a context for the co-construction of individual narratives in clinical context, as well as suggesting alternatives to diagnosis for purposes like clustering, administrative procedures, legal matters, service planning, and research (Johnstone et al., 2018). These regularities and responses are shaped by meanings, not biology, so they may change over time and across cultures (Johnstone, 2022). Therefore, it would advocate thinking in terms of "difficult situations" that people find themselves in rather than "disorders" that they supposedly "have" (Bergström, 2023).

The PTMF incorporates elements from various theoretical and therapeutic approaches and traditions. This versatility allows for a diverse range of therapeutic modalities, ranging from those grounded in radical behaviorism like Acceptance and Commitment Therapy to psychoanalytic, psychodynamic, existential, phenomenological, and humanistic therapies, to effectively utilize such a non-categorical diagnostic approach. The central aim of the PTMF includes shaping more beneficial narratives, which aligns well with the principles of the Open Dialogue Approach (ODA), initially developed in Western Lapland and increasingly adopted in various countries (Mosse et al., 2023).

Open Dialogue Approach

Open Dialogue Approach (ODA) is not just a therapeutic proposition but also a practical and pragmatic systemic approach to addressing the organizational aspects of mental health services. It may be as an important contribution to its success as the specific techniques and recommendations concerning therapy (Putman & Martindale, 2021). Even though ODA may be implemented differently in various healthcare settings, it's possible to describe its fundamental principles and values (Mosse et al., 2023).

ODA can be characterized as a crisis intervention, a distinctive narrative and systemic approach to family therapy delivered by mobile teams of professionals. Its core principles include (Seikkula et al., 2003; Seikkula & Olson, 2003):

1. provision of immediate help: an initial network meeting should be scheduled within 24 hours of first contact
2. a social network perspective: all significant members of the social network are invited to the first meeting, including those outside of the family
3. flexibility and mobility: methods are adapted to each case and change in response to current needs; no fixed treatment plans are made during the crisis
4. responsibility: the initially contacted staff member organizes the first meeting, and the team assumes responsibility for the process
5. psychological continuity: the same team oversees the whole process
6. tolerance of uncertainty: frequent (daily) meetings in the first two weeks to establish a sense of security and avoid premature decisions, particularly regarding medication use
7. dialogism: the goal is to facilitate a dialogue that enhances the patient's sense of agency and allows for the development of a new understanding of the situation

ODA underscores empathy, presence, attention and listening as core elements of practice. Much like the PTMF, it steers clear of interpreting others' experiences through symptom-oriented diagnoses. Instead, ODA is focused on meanings and narratives shared by individuals and their families (or other social networks) about challenging experiences and events.

Departing from a model where diagnostic labels designed and assigned by supposed experts guide the treatment, ODA places service users and their social network members at the core of a dialogical process. The dialogue becomes a pathway out of a crisis. One of the goals of this primarily psychotherapeutically oriented approach is to minimize or even abstain from the use of psychiatric drugs (Bergström et al., 2018).

In "network meetings," crucial care decisions are openly discussed. The diverse voices participating in Open Dialogue are given careful attention with an emphasis on sharing all relevant information and meanings. The objective is to ensure that every voice is heard, minimizing the impact of power imbalances in the support process. Thus, ODA is built on a mental healthcare epistemology that values everyday relationships and context-specific interpretations over symptom-focused nosological diagnoses (Mosse et al., 2023). There is also a trend to include psychiatric survivors as "peer" practitioners within the ODA teams (Lorenz-Artz et al., 2023).

Diagnostic labels become secondary or even irrelevant when problems are viewed as narratives constructed socially and interpersonally rather than as diseases. The core idea underpinning the principle of "dialogism" is the concept of a "polyphony of voices" that exists within individuals and between them. The emphasis lies not in categorizing and intervening but in nurturing a dialogue where all participants are regarded equally, aiming to harness the resources within the patient's family and other social networks.

Nevertheless, there is no predetermined blueprint for the team's efforts within the system and for the narratives to follow, or a pre-established objective guiding their form and construction. Instead, the clinicians, viewed as embodied emotional agents present in the moment, concentrate on empathetically responding to the clients. The primary focus is on ensuring that everyone is heard and does not experience feelings of abandonment, exclusion, or neglect—all with an aim to reestablish communication. Accordingly, the problems are understood primarily as survival strategies arising from blocked communication rather than as symptoms of an actual "disease" (Stupak & Dobroczyński, 2021).

While the principles of ODA might, at least on the surface, appear to be prevalent in mental health systems, especially in well-developed countries, a recent study detailing experiences with implementing an Open Dialogue-based approach in the United States revealed significant shifts in clinical practice. Staff reported notable changes, such as increased curiosity in listening, abandoning preconceived agendas, recognizing that solutions lie within the network, adopting a slower pace, and fostering more dialogue.

This unconventional approach was viewed as peculiar by other mental health professionals, and this, along with resistance to changing organizational culture, posed challenges to the implementation of Open Dialogue. Participants also noted reduced burnout and improved relationships among staff, clients, and their families (Florence et al., 2020). Overall, the ODA aligns well with the assumptions of the Power Threat Meaning Framework outlined earlier.

Soteria

The First Soteria home was established in 1971, offering an alternative to a simplistic biomedical model for explaining, understanding, and treating schizophrenia or psychotic states. Initially, there was only one house called Soteria located in San Jose, California; in 1974, another one followed, located near San Francisco and called Emanon ("No name" spelled backwards) (Stupak & Dobroczyński, 2019).

The Soteria model, though not necessarily remaining faithful to the original, has spread worldwide. Several Soteria homes have been established in the United States, Switzerland, the Netherlands, Sweden, Germany, Japan, the United Kingdom, France, and Hungary, although some have stopped functioning (Fabel et al., 2023). Originally, the goal of the Soteria Project, as a research programme, was to compare treatment in Soteria with minimal or no use of drugs to treatment-as-usual in hospitals. The outcomes showed comparable results after six weeks, with some aspects favoring Soteria long-term, and best results for those who did not use psychiatric drugs (Stupak & Dobroczyński, 2019).

Soteria homes offer care to people experiencing acute distress that may require round-the-clock treatment. Loren Mosher, the psychiatrist who established the original Soteria home, promoted a culture characterized by empathetic relationships and non-intrusive interventions for the person undergoing a psychotic episode (Friedlander et al., 2022). The Soteria approach resembles the ODA, both in theory and practice. It rejects the metaphor of illness—and views problems primarily as associated with interpersonal or systemic relationships, the meanings assigned to them, and as developmental crises (Mosher et al., 2004), which bears a resemblance to the PTMF perspective.

Essentially, Soteria is a home-like facility—originally with two members of the staff and up to eight patients, partly run by peers—with minimal hierarchy and where "being with" people in distress, instead of "doing to" (Mosher, 1999; Mosse et al., 2023), is crucial. The staff's primary responsibility could be described as facilitating a dialogue that leads to a new understanding of the situation. Originally, the staff consisted of people without formal psychological, therapeutic, or psychiatric training—chosen for their openness to unusual states of mind and given a brief training.

Patients are responsible for the day-to-day functioning of the home, which provides a safe space while also allowing residents to face the crisis and preserve personal autonomy without adopting the role or identity of a (chronic) patient. The approach to drug use in the original Soteria resembled that of the Western Lapland ODA; specifically, drugs are seen as substances that can provide temporary relief, are not seen as curative agents, and are not used without a patient's consent (Stupak & Dobroczyński, 2021).

In the words of Mosher (Mosher, 1999, p. 143):

> Basically, the Soteria method can be characterized as the 24 hour a day application of interpersonal phenomenologic interventions by a nonprofessional staff, usually without neuroleptic drug treatment, in the context of a small, homelike, quiet, supportive, protective, and tolerant social environment. The core practice of interpersonal phenomenology focuses on the development of a nonintrusive, noncontrolling but actively empathetic relationship with the psychotic person without having to do anything explicitly therapeutic or controlling. In shorthand, it can be characterized as "being with," "standing by attentively," "trying to put your feet into the other person's shoes," or "being an LSD trip guide" (remember,

this was the early 1970s in California). The aim is to develop, over time, a shared experience of the meaningfulness of the client's individual social context-current and historical. Note, there were no therapeutic "sessions" at Soteria. However, a great deal of "therapy" took place there as staff worked gently to build bridges, over time, between individuals' emotionally disorganized states to the life events that seemed to have precipitated their psychological disintegration. The context within the house was one of positive expectations that reorganization and reintegration would occur as a result of these seemingly minimalist interventions.

The house operated under certain "contextual constraints" (Read et al., 2013):

- do no harm
- treat everyone, and expect to be treated, with dignity and respect
- guarantee sanctuary, quiet, safety, support, protection and interpersonal validation
- ensure food and shelter
- the atmosphere must be imbued with hope—that recovery from psychosis is to be expected without antipsychotic drugs

In Soteria, in contrast to the ODA, the person most affected by the crisis was supposed to go through the process while largely *away* from their family of origin. The goal was to promote self-sufficiency and independence—and avoid further influencing the crisis by distressed family members who were also affected by it. Eventually, though, the family—together with the Soteria community—was supposed to become a part of a support network. The staff were encouraged to view the person in distress as a potential peer and maintain a shared equal relationship. Avoiding strict roles and hierarchy, encouraging friendly relationships, led to a development of an authentic bond, which continued after clients left the home (Stupak & Dobroczyński, 2019).

Recently, Soteria homes have been established in Israel, largely thanks to the initiative of Pesach Lichtenberg (Lichtenberg, 2017). Soteria Israel operates with eight basic principles (Friedlander et al., 2022; Lichtenberg, 2017):

1. care is given in a home, not an institution
2. groups are small, eight or less
3. communication is open
4. activities are client-centered
5. treatment is consensual
6. medication is de-emphasized
7. staff learns to "be with" the resident empathically and non-judgmentally
8. the group is the central therapeutic instrument

In Germany, some of the Soteria principles have been introduced in hospitals leading to less forced treatment (Fabel et al., 2023).

The concept of "being with" (as opposed to "doing to" and "coexisting" rather than "curing") a person had evolved from an idea to "keep vigil" with the client in acute distress within a dedicated room. This space, devoid of any rigid furniture except for a stereo set, was adorned with rugs and pillows, featuring a few small lamps for adjustable lighting based on the client's preferences. The room was positioned in the central part of the house as it was assumed that something hidden might seem more daunting—it was also supposed to encourage tenants to cooperate. Above all, the room was supposed to feel safe and provide minimal stimulation (Mosher et al., 2004).

It quickly became evident that the designated special room did not serve its purpose and ran counter to the structure-free essence of Soteria. It was found that the intended role for the isolated room could be effectively applied to the entire house, and any quiet room would suffice as long as the person in crisis had a trusted companion. These sessions of "being with" could extend for several hours or span two consecutive days. Shorter sessions occurred, for instance, twice a day, allowing patients to function more or less normally in between (Mosher et al., 2004).

Lichtenberg refers to the story of "Prince and the Turkey" told by the 18th century Rabbi Nahman of Breslov to explain the approach used in Soteria Israel:

> In this tale, a prince is convinced he is a turkey, and so he sits naked under a table and picks at crumbs on the floor. Nobody knows what to do, but finally a wise man comes. After a moment of contemplation, the wise man proceeds to take off his clothes and sit with the prince under the table. He is a turkey too! This goes on for a while, but then the wise man tells the prince he is cold; would it be okay if they got some clothes? He would of course still be a turkey! Then the wise man says turkeys can do better than eating crumbs from the floor; would it be okay if plates of food were served? Finally, the wise man says his back hurts from sitting under the table, and so would it be possible for them to sit at the table and eat? And with the prince clothed once more and sitting at the table, he was restored to his old self. (Whitaker, 2018, para. 40)

Of course, the question remains whether as a result the prince was convinced that he was not a turkey, or whether in the end he was or considered himself to be a turkey but behaved like a "normal" prince. Either way this may be enough, when assessed from the third-person perspective, to live a satisfying live in the community free of unnecessary medication and coercion.

Conclusion

Even though more research is needed, both Soteria and ODA, while minimizing iatrogenic effects of drugs, have encouraging treatment outcomes—comparable or even better than treatment-as-usual relying primarily on pharmacotherapy and symptom-based diagnoses. Together with the PTMF they provide a practical alternative that offers successful support for people in states of acute psychological distress (Stupak & Dobroczyński, 2021).

Going beyond *DSM* based diagnoses with PTMF, ODA and Soteria may prove useful not only in cases described as psychosis but also in other situations as the negative effects of trauma, difficult experiences and other adverse circumstances may present themselves in various ways that could be labeled with different diagnoses (Bergström, 2023). PMTF stresses the individual, social, and cultural aspects of distress—in addition to systemic and economic conditions—that shouldn't be overlooked and may provide a practical alternative to *DSM* diagnoses.

Both Soteria and ODA are interested in people's stories as shaped by events and circumstances via culturally influenced meanings attributed to them. In a similar way to the PTMF, they view psychological crises as understandable diverse human responses to adversities—survival strategies. Even though these strategies may sometimes prove ineffective and contribute to suffering, they are not inherently pathological as they stem from the mental processes and functions common to all people.

Fostering dialogue, accepting, empathetic, non-judgmental, and non-hierarchical communication in a safe space may create an opportunity for constructing a new narrative that allows to make sense of oneself and of the challenging experience without resorting to stigmatizing illness labels. This is particularly helpful if it allows transforming existing relationships or forming new ones while simultaneously changing the situation that could have contributed to the crisis. In this sense, Soteria and ODA are close to crisis interventions that concern people with problems rather than patients with diseases.

References

Bergström, T. (2023). From treatment of mental disorders to the treatment of difficult life situations: A hypothesis and rationale. *Medical Hypotheses, 176*, 111099. https://doi.org/10.1016/j.mehy.2023.111099

Bergström, T., Seikkula, J., Alakare, B., Mäki, P., Köngäs-Saviaro, P., Taskila, J. J., Tolvanen, A., & Aaltonen, J. (2018). The family-oriented open dialogue approach in the treatment of first-episode psychosis: Nineteen–year outcomes. *Psychiatry Research, 270*, 168–175. https://doi.org/10.1016/j.psychres.2018.09.039

Boyle, M. (2022). Power in the Power Threat Meaning Framework. *Journal of Constructivist Psychology, 35*(1), 27–40. https://doi.org/10.1080/10720537.2020.1773357

Campolonghi, S., & Orrù, L. (2023). Psychiatry as a medical discipline: Epistemological and theoretical issues. *Journal of Theoretical and Philosophical Psychology*, No Pagination Specified-No Pagination Specified. https://doi.org/10.1037/teo0000256

Cromby, J. (2022). Meaning in the Power Threat Meaning Framework. *Journal of Constructivist Psychology*, 35(1), 41–53. https://doi.org/10.1080/10720537.2020.1773355

Deacon, B. J. (2013). The biomedical model of mental disorder: A critical analysis of its validity, utility, and effects on psychotherapy research. *Clinical Psychology Review*, 33(7), 846–861. https://doi.org/10.1016/j.cpr.2012.09.007

Fabel, P., Wolf, T., Zyber, H., Rubel, J., & Jockers-Scherübl, M. C. (2023). Treatment with Soteria-elements in acute psychiatry—Effectiveness for acutely ill and voluntarily treated patients. *Frontiers in Public Health, 11*. https://www.frontiersin.org/articles/10.3389/fpubh.2023.1118522

Fava, G. A., & Rafanelli, C. (2019). Iatrogenic Factors in Psychopathology. *Psychotherapy and Psychosomatics*, 88(3), 129–140. https://doi.org/10.1159/000500151

Florence, A. C., Jordan, G., Yasui, S., & Davidson, L. (2020). Implanting Rhizomes in Vermont: A Qualitative Study of How the Open Dialogue Approach was Adapted and Implemented. *Psychiatric Quarterly*, 91(3), 681–693. https://doi.org/10.1007/s11126-020-09732-7

Friedlander, A., Tzur Bitan, D., & Lichtenberg, P. (2022). The Soteria model: Implementing an alternative to acute psychiatric hospitalization in Israel. *Psychosis*, 14(2), 99–108. https://doi.org/10.1080/17522439.2022.2057578

Ghaemi, S. N. (2022). Symptomatic versus disease-modifying effects of psychiatric drugs. *Acta Psychiatrica Scandinavica*, 146(3), 251–257. https://doi.org/10.1111/acps.13459

Harper, D. J. (2022). Framing, Filtering and Hermeneutical Injustice in the Public Conversation about Mental Health. *Journal of Constructivist Psychology*, 35(1), 68–82. https://doi.org/10.1080/10720537.2020.1773360

Harper, D. J., & Cromby, J. (2022). From 'What's Wrong with You?' to 'What's Happened to You?': An Introduction to the Special Issue on the Power Threat Meaning Framework. *Journal of Constructivist Psychology*, 35(1), 1–6. https://doi.org/10.1080/10720537.2020.1773362

Hayes, S. C., & Hofmann, S. G. (Eds.). (2020). *Beyond the DSM: Toward a Process-Based Alternative for Diagnosis and Mental Health Treatment* (1st edition). Context Press.

Johnstone, L. (2022). General Patterns in the Power Threat Meaning Framework – Principles and Practice. *Journal of Constructivist Psychology, 35*(1), 16–26. https://doi.org/10.1080/10720537.2020.1773358

Johnstone, L., Boyle, M., Cromby, J., Dillon, J., Harper, D., Kinderman, P., Longden, E., Pilgrim, D., & Read, J. (2018). *The Power Threat Meaning Framework: Towards the identification of patterns in emotional distress, unusual experiences and troubled or troubling behaviour, as an alternative to functional psychiatric diagnosis* (p. bpsrep.2018.inf299b). British Psychological Society. https://doi.org/10.53841/bpsrep.2018.inf299b

Karter, J. M. (2019). An Ecological Model for Conceptual Competence in Psychiatric Diagnosis. *Journal of Humanistic Psychology*, 0022167819852488. https://doi.org/10.1177/0022167819852488

Lichtenberg, P. (2017). From the closed ward to Soteria: A professional and personal journey. *Psychosis, 9*(4), 369–375. https://doi.org/10.1080/17522439.2017.1373842

Lorenz-Artz, K., Bierbooms, J., & Bongers, I. (2023). Introducing Peer-supported Open Dialogue in changing mental health care. *Frontiers in Psychology, 13*. https://www.frontiersin.org/articles/10.3389/fpsyg.2022.1056071

Mosher, L. R. (1999). Soteria and other alternatives to acute psychiatric hospitalization: A personal and professional review. *Journal of Nervous and Mental Disease, 187*(3), 142–149. https://doi.org/10.1097/00005053-199903000-00003

Mosher, L. R., Hendrix, V., & Fort, D. (2004). *Soteria: Through Madness to Deliverance.*

Mosse, D., Pocobello, R., Saunders, R., Seikkula, J., & von Peter, S. (2023). Introduction: Open Dialogue around the world – implementation, outcomes, experiences and perspectives. *Frontiers in Psychology, 13*. https://www.frontiersin.org/articles/10.3389/fpsyg.2022.1093351

Putman, N., & Martindale, B. (2021). *Open Dialogue for Psychosis: Organising Mental Health Services to Prioritise Dialogue, Relationship and Meaning* (1st ed.). Routledge. https://doi.org/10.4324/9781351199599

Read, D. J., Bentall, P. R., Mosher, L., Read, J., & Dillon, J. (2013). *Models of Madness: Psychological, Social and Biological Approaches to Psychosis.* Routledge.

Seikkula, J., Alakare, B., Aaltonen, J., Holma, J., Rasinkangas, A., & Lehtinen, V. (2003). Open Dialogue Approach: Treatment Principles and Preliminary Results of a Two-Year Follow-Up on First Episode Schizophrenia. *Ethical Human Sciences and Services, 5*(3), 163–182. https://doi.org/10.1891/1523-150X.5.3.163

Seikkula, J., & Olson, M. E. (2003). The Open Dialogue Approach to Acute Psychosis: Its Poetics and Micropolitics. *Family Process, 42*(3), 403–418. https://doi.org/10.1111/j.1545-5300.2003.00403.x

Sharfstein, S. S. (2005). Big Pharma and American Psychiatry: The Good, the Bad, and the Ugly. *Psychiatric News.* https://doi.org/10.1176/pn.40.16.00400003

Smail, D. J. (2016). *Power, interest and psychology: Elements of a social materialist understanding of distress.* PCCS Books.

Stupak, R., & Dobroczyński, B. (2019). The Soteria Project: A forerunner of "a third way" in psychiatry? *Psychiatria Polska, 53*(6), 1351–1364. https://doi.org/10.12740/PP/OnlineFirst/91731

Stupak, R., & Dobroczyński, B. (2021). From Mental Health Industry to Humane Care. Suggestions for an Alternative Systemic Approach to Distress. *International Journal of Environmental Research and Public Health, 18*(12), Article 12. https://doi.org/10.3390/ijerph18126625

Teo, T. (2018). *Homo neoliberalus*: From personality to forms of subjectivity. *Theory & Psychology, 28*(5), 581–599. https://doi.org/10.1177/0959354318794899

UN Human Rights Commissioner. (2019). *Right of everyone to the enjoyment of the highest attainable standard of physical and mental health: Report of the Special Rapporteur on the Right of Everyone to the Enjoyment of the Highest Attainable Standard of Physical and Mental Health.* https://digitallibrary.un.org/record/3803412

Van Os, J., & Kohne, A. C. J. (2021). It is not enough to sing its praises: The very foundations of precision psychiatry may be scientifically unsound and require examination. *Psychological Medicine, 51*(9), 1415–1417. https://doi.org/10.1017/S0033291721000167

Vassilieva, J. (2016). *Narrative Psychology*. Palgrave Macmillan UK.
   https://doi.org/10.1057/978-1-137-49195-4

Whitaker, R. (2018, February 11). *Soteria Israel: A Vision from the Past is a*
   Blueprint for the Future. Mad In America.
   https://www.madinamerica.com/2018/02/soteria-israel-a-vision-from-the-
   past-is-a-blueprint-for-the-future/

World Health Organization. (2021). *Guidance on community mental health*
   services: Promoting person-centred and rights-based approaches.
   https://www.who.int/publications-detail-redirect/9789240025707

Need-Based vs. Diagnostic-Driven Strategies for Helping People with Mental and Emotional Difficulties: A Systems Approach

Thomas E. Fink

Abstract: *The success of the medical model for diagnosing and treating physical illnesses has led to a mistaken attempt to apply the medical model to psychological problems. A medical-diagnostic model assumes that there are physical causes for psychological difficulties. This simplistic causal model ignores the dynamic, emergent nature of psychological disorders. Applying medical interventions to psychological difficulties may cause harm, both physically and psychologically, and often misses opportunities for more effective and humanistic interventions. Alternatively, it is argued that psychological problems emerge from a person's history of trauma and unmet psychological needs (e.g., for connection and belonging, predictability and control, self-esteem, safety, purpose and meaning). Problems occur in psychosocial contexts that necessitate interventions tailored to the level of arousal and dysfunction a person is experiencing. Effective treatment interventions involve different but interrelated strategies, varying from crisis and symptom reduction and interventions designed to interrupt dysfunctional patterns of thinking, feeling and behaving, to interventions designed to help people better meet their basic psychological needs.*

Diagnoses guide most forms of medical treatment. The medical model assumes that underlying biological pathology produces symptoms that present as aberrations of healthy functioning. Increasing scientific knowledge about the neurological and biochemical processes of the brain, along with the extraordinary success of the medical model in the area of physical disease, has led to an unfortunate and, in some ways, harmful attempt to apply these sciences and discoveries to mental and emotional problems.

This biological approach, while sometimes acknowledging psychosocial influences, focuses on genetics, neurotransmitters, and neuroanatomy as causal agents. What are considered symptoms of mental problems are assumed to be caused by underlying, errant neurological or biochemical processes. For example, hallucinations, extreme delusional ideas, personality decompensation and so on are considered symptoms of an underlying neurologically-based schizophrenia that causes these symptoms.

Sadness, an inability to sleep, social withdrawal, being stuck in despair and self-blame, and so on are considered symptoms of an underlying brain-based depressive disorder that generates these symptoms. This physicalist and reductionistic model dominates much of the mainstream mental health treatment community. The hope expressed in this approach is that increasing knowledge about what is going on in the brains of people with mental and emotional difficulties will yield information about the cause of these conditions and thus more effective intervention strategies.

The diagnosis of an assumed biological disorder accordingly will guide treatment choices, which will largely emphasize biological interventions such as drugs. In this model, psychosocial interventions are seen as supplements to the more basic biological treatment.

Empirically, however, the biological approach to the understanding and treatment of mental problems has not been particularly successful (see Whitaker, 2002, 2010, 2021). In fact, Robert Whitaker does an effective job in published work and lectures of dissuading us from the soundness of the medical/biochemical/genetic model of mental illness. It turns out there is limited empirical support for this approach in terms of long-term success and a good deal of evidence that drug-based treatment can cause harm.

Finally, philosophically, the bio-diagnostic approach embraces a mis-guided understanding of causality in the realm of the mental. It largely neglects the role of a person's developmental and psychosocial histories, assumes a simplistic and mistaken understanding of mind/body relationships, and ignores important and relatively recent advances in nonlinear dynamical thinking that provides an understanding about how order emerges in complex systems.

As an aside, while mental "disorders" are considered deviations from order, it will be argued that the disorders are actually overly organized, self-referential and self-maintaining patterns. In particular, it will be argued that if critical psychological needs are not met, coping patterns emerge as a way to adapt, albeit poorly, with the threats to a person's sense of safety and well-being.

Also, the classes or categories of mental illnesses that emerge are a set of patterns of behavior, thought, and feelings that have been given loose linguistic labels. The similarities within the various categories of problematic patterns (depression, anxiety disorders, psychoses, etc.), simply reflect similarities of emergent patterns. Within each category, there are family resemblances (Wittgenstein, 1966) as well as differences. The categories share overlapping similarities rather than a set of necessary and sufficient properties.

Because of this, the American Psychiatric Association's *Diagnostic and Statistical Manual of Mental Disorders (DSM)*, for example, uses checklists to help make diagnoses—with criteria that in order to apply a diagnosis, one doesn't need to display all of the symptoms, but only needs a key symptom or two and a few other possible symptoms. The lack of firm diagnostic criteria also explains why the *DSM* includes the "unspecified" designations for conditions that do not meet full diagnostic criteria within the checklist system.

In summary, similar patterns emerge from similar conditions and person-environmental interactions. The diagnostic labels do not designate underlying neurological conditions that produce symptoms but are emergent patterns that share similarities. What are considered symptoms are in essence part of a person's reactive, adaptive patterns. Treatment considerations informed by this understanding take into account critical psychological needs and the systemic nature of persons' behaviors and actions over time. The implications of this point of view will be elaborated below.

What are Mental Disorders? – Further Elaboration

What then are the variety of "disorders" that have been labeled as categories of mental illness—from the depressive (e.g., Major Depressive Disorders) and anxiety disorders (e.g., Obsessive Compulsive Disorder, Panic Disorder, Generalized Anxiety Disorder), psychoses, (e.g., Schizophrenia, Delusional Disorder), and attention difficulties (Attention-Deficit/Hyperactivity Disorder)? First, with regard to causality, a critical distinction needs to be made between true neurological and biological diseases such as Alzheimer's and Huntington's, and the maladaptive patterns that emerge in persons with adequately functioning brains but problematic behavioral patterns.

Neurological disorders do, indeed, produce brain anomalies and associated behavioral and emotional symptoms. But what are considered mental disorders are actually labels for emergent patterns of maladaptive responses, rather than casual conditions. The responses arise or emerge from the interaction of variables in a complex web of psychological and environmental variables. They are linguistic classifications within a psychiatric language game (Fink, 2022).

The problematic patterns that emerge do share similar characteristics within each category—family resemblances à la Wittgenstein (1966). And the labels do have some communicative as well as predictive value because the terms reflect similarities in pattern. If one uses the rules of diagnosis assignment to label a person as having schizophrenia, for example, one can assume, tautologically, the person will have a cluster of behaviors associated with the label—hallucinations, delusions, social deficiencies, et cetera.

But clusters of behaviors do not connote causality. In order to assert causality, underlying conditions must be found that could be a cause (biochemical imbalances, neurological lesions, etc.) And, as noted, attempts to identify such causal agents, even in the more severe mental conditions such as schizophrenia, have not borne fruit (see Joseph, 2017, Valenstein, 2002).

In summary, what are mental disorders? They are emergent ways of thinking, feeling, and behaving that have been given linguistic labels and are used in a mental health language game to refer to classes of similar patterns of dysfunction.

A second point needs to be made with regard to the relationship between physical variables and mental conditions. There is no argument that the brain (its physiology, neurotransmitters, genetic sensitivities, etc.) is involved in the unfolding manifestations (feelings, overt behavior, thoughts, etc.) associated with what we consider mental illness. But as already noted, except in the case of true neurological diseases, the notion that what we classify as psychological pathology is related to neurological pathology is unsupported.

We now know, for example, that serotonin deficiencies do not appear to be the cause of the attribution of depression (Moncrieff, 2022). The search for biological or genetic causality in schizophrenia has not yielded reliable data (Joseph, 2017). In addition, the relationship of psychological processes to biochemical or neurological processes is quite complex, if not impossible to ascertain (Khalidi, 2023). From this context, discussions of higher order relational concepts, such psychological needs, is both appropriate and useful.

Third, the concept of causality itself turns out to be complex and, with regard to mental phenomenon, debate continues in the philosophical community about bottom-up vs. top-down causality (Ellis, 2008; George et al., 2012). For example, if someone believes their life is in imminent danger when entering a particular building or room, the person will be aroused, alert and anxious—all emotional states that will change brain chemistry. The notion of brain-behavior relationships is also complicated by issues raised many years ago about what comes first—avoidant behavior in the face of a threat or the emotional responses of arousal and fear (Lang, 1994).

Finally, on a practical level, the relationship between biological/neurological processes and psychological problems appears to be so complex it can reasonably be argued that practitioners in the mental health field are left with the option of embracing philosophical pragmatism (see

Fink, 2022; Margolis, 1978; Moron, 2008). The language of psychology cannot be substituted for descriptions of underlying neurological or biological processes.

Descriptions of neurological/biological processes do not allow for discussion about important psychological issues critical to the work of psychotherapy—concerns about a person's belief systems, motivations, memories, needs, goals, desires, skill levels, and so on. From this context, it will be argued that discussions of higher order concepts that have no simple physical mapping are a necessary part of identifying effective intervention strategies. In particular, the concept of psychological needs and ways in which they may be or historically have been frustrated and unmet, is explanatory and both appropriate and necessary (see Flanagan, 2010).

In summary, it will be argued that the classes of dysfunctional conditions that are categorized as disorders in the psychiatric classification systems are emergent, self-referential, and self-maintaining adaptations to real or perceived threats, unmet critical psychological needs, and personal emotional distress. They arise out of a person's attempts to understand and deal with real or perceived stresses, and threats to important relationships a person has with self, others, and their environment.

The patterns are driven by arousal and anxiety and, on examination, often are closed systems that consist of repetitive thoughts, associated feelings, and behaviors. Without effective intervention, these patterns often are impervious to change. Clues to treatment will be found in understanding how key psychological needs could be better met for identified persons, as well as understanding that these "disorders" are unfolding, self-reinforcing and repetitive patterns that need to be interrupted.

Psychological Needs

Don't think, but look.
   – Wittgenstein, 1966, p. 66

You can observe a lot just by watching.
   – Yogi Berra

If the language of neuroanatomy, neurochemicals, and genetics doesn't provide an adequate understanding about what psychological problems are, how they develop, and what can be done practically to help people with those difficulties, what is an alternative approach—particularly if we resist the illusion that getting to the bottom of things comes from physical reductionism? Instead of looking to reductionistic biological models for explanations, let's act like ethologists.

Let's look and observe human behavior. Let's examine the psychosocial histories, belief systems, and relationship patterns of people who psychologically appear to be functioning well versus persons not functioning well psychologically and notice what is different between these two groups.

There is a long history in psychology of identifying psychological needs—characteristics of a person's relationship with self and others as well as their broader psychosocial environments—that if not met, or are thwarted, contribute to mental and emotional issues. The most well-known theoretician in this area is Abraham Maslow (1946), who suggested that there is a hierarchy of needs, that met or unmet, affect a person's psychological functioning and well-being.

Maslow suggested that these needs vary from basic safety and survival needs to higher order psychological needs such as social acceptance and belonging, a sense of self-worth, and ultimately self-actualization. Others espousing the concept of needs include Viktor Frankl (1959) who stressed the importance of meaning and purpose in surviving in an abusive and hostile environment. Bandura stressed the importance of self-efficacy (1982). Gliner (1972) demonstrated predictability in the administration of aversive stimuli helps mitigate its negative psychological effects.

More recently, Ryan and Deci (2017) suggested that there are three classes of essential psychological needs—autonomy, competence, and relatedness. Marker (2003) suggested a large collection of needs that include both individual and cultural factors. Her list of needs consisted of safety and security, belongingness and love, self-esteem, personal fulfillment, identity, cultural security, freedom, distributive justice, and participation.

The need for connection, attachment, and belonging has been well documented by many (Baumeister & Leary,1995; Cacioppo & Patrick, 2009; Hari, 2018; Lynch, 2000).

The need for perceived control was well demonstrated in the early animal research of Seligman (1975) and further elaborated in the learned helplessness model of depression (Langer, 1983; Miller & Seligman, 1975; Seligman & Beagley,1975). Others have demonstrated the need for perceived control for both healthy physical and mental health (Pagnini et al., 2016). (See Skinner, 1995 for further discussion of the behavioral impacts of perceived control.)

In summary, there is no periodic table of psychological needs because the complexity of human behavior and the variety of uses of language creates many ways of talking about people and their behavior. However, the broad concept of critical psychological needs provides a pragmatic and nonreductive way of talking about and understanding human actions as well as developing ways to intervene. Incorporating psychological needs into our understanding of human behavior provides a language game that allows us to talk about concepts such as intentions and reasons rather than physical causality (see Ossorio, 2006; Schwartz, 2019).

Threats to or conditions that interfere with important psychological needs being met, especially during the developmental period, produce a cacophony of problematic emotional, behavioral, and cognitive responses. Unmet psychological needs produce a variety of unpleasant and problematic emotional reactions including anxiety, despair, hopelessness, sadness, panic, fear of death, and anger. Reactions to these emotions and the adaptive responses that follow create categories of psychological dysfunction.

System Concepts: Chaos Theory, Order/Disorder and Emergence

A final and critical point needs to be made with regard to intervention strategies for people experiencing challenges due to unmet psychological needs, and the reactive and coping strategies that emerge. These reactions unfold over time and lead to ordered, albeit dysfunctional, patterns. Order emerges in complex systems in a manner that produces repetitive, self-reinforcing patterns in many physical (see Gleick, 1987; Newman, 1996) as well as psychological systems (Wagman, 2010).

These psychological patterns are self-reinforcing and lack openness and flexibility. For example, depressive reactions often are characterized by repetitive, ruminative behaviors (Papageorgiou & Wells, 2003). Anxiety disorders and, in particular, Obsessive Compulsive Disorder, are self-evidently characterized by repetitive behavior and thought. The mental disorders appear overly organized and often closed to outside input.

Treatment Implications

Treatment options from the perspective elaborated above thus involve therapeutically engaging with withdrawn, disturbed, agitated, and anxious individuals who are locked into recurring patterns of repetitive, dysfunctional behaviors. Access to these persons appears to typically require steps to:

1. induce calm
2. interrupt the dysfunctional behavioral and thought patterns
3. find ways to support these persons in getting their basic needs better met

These are not necessarily distinct or mutually exclusive steps. Obtaining psychotherapeutic access to an agitated person can be difficult. Fortunately, from a systems perspective there are a variety of ways to help someone achieve calmer states, to interrupt pathological and recurrent behavioral and emotional patterns, and to support a person in finding ways to have important psychological needs met.

Because intervention strategies need to be sensitive to the level of arousal and severity of the behavioral patterns exhibited, initial interventions during a severe psychological crisis, for example, will often involve actions such as removal from a perturbing environment, and then steps to reduce anxiety and arousal. Interestingly, the so-called antipsychotic medications, previously labelled, "major tranquilizers," do appear to reduce many of the active signs of psychosis by simply suppressing the central nervous system. Their long-term negative effects are well-known, but the administration of these drugs does produce a quieting, if not deadening, effect because they suppress all thoughts, feelings, and behavior (including those considered problematic).

The argument that these drugs treat mental illness by correcting chemical imbalances or faulty circuits as suggested by, for example, Insel (2010) is demonstrably incorrect (Deacon, 2013; Valenstein, 2002). The willingness to use these drugs can be understood because they do quiet and suppress undesirable behaviors. There was a brief history, at least in Pennsylvania's state hospital system, when the overuse of antipsychotics was considered a chemical restraint and thus highly discouraged. I was a psychological consultant at a local state hospital in those days who was occasionally called on to provide behavioral recommendations for disturbed individuals, including those with active psychotic symptoms.

However, psychotherapeutic and behavioral interventions were not usually effective when the patient was in an acute psychotic state. A nurse with a long history of working in the intake ward of this hospital commented to me that she missed the "old days" when a patient with psychosis would be admitted in an agitated state and then immediately placed on heavy doses of a neuroleptic medication such as chlorpromazine (Thorazine). Patients, then highly tranquilized, would be allowed to sleep, sometimes for days. The nurse reported that these newly admitted patients would eventually awaken and often be essentially free from active psychotic symptoms.

Sleep therapy was frequently espoused as a treatment for schizophrenia in Europe and Russia (Windholz & Witherspoon, 1993). Similarly, insulin coma therapy, which induces a lengthy coma, was even used in the United States up to the early 1960s to treat schizophrenia. Insulin coma therapy was based on the notion that hypoglycemia-induced coma could basically "jolt" patients out of their psychoses. The approach was eventually discredited and is no longer used, for good reason. Among other problems, there was an unacceptable death rate with this procedure.

In any event, sleep, which profoundly quiets the mind, was seen as a way to quiet agitated patients prior to the advent of the "major tranquillizers" (now labeled antipsychotic medication). Quieting the system appears to be an essential part of even a humane psychiatric intervention for highly disturbed individuals. As a student intern in the late 1960s, I remember watching training films developed in the early 1960s (prior to the extensive use of drugs like chlorpromazine) that illustrated the use of warm whirlpool baths to induce calming effects. For less disturbed individuals, a therapeutic relationship itself can provide a calming effect. And, perhaps, a calming or anti-anxiety effect is one of the seemingly beneficial consequences from the use of various "antidepressant" and "anti-anxiety" medications.

Negative effects aside, the antidepressant or anti-anxiety drugs appear to quiet the emotional reactivity of its users, often to the point that users simply don't care as much about what had previously been upsetting (Levy et al., 2014; Perkins et al., 2013). This apathy may explain why one of the seldom discussed negative effects of antidepressant medication can be an alteration in users' moral judgment. Overall, people who are prescribed these medications simply do not care as much about other people's discomfort or the circumstances in which they find themselves. Users may be more willing to stay in dysfunctional relationships, for example.

Concurrent with calming, changing dysfunctional behaviors, by definition, involves interrupting in some way the problematic patterns of thinking, feeling, and behaving. Even though it is not typically conceived of in this way, some form of interruption of problematic states appears to be involved in all therapeutic interventions whether, for example, it involves behavioral techniques such as thought stopping, the variety of the cognitive behavioral techniques, or simply suggestions made in psychotherapy to consider other ways of thinking and behaving.

The most extreme form of interruption still in use is electroconvulsive therapy (ECT). ECT does appear to have at least a short-term impact on persons' problematic patterns of feeling, thinking, and behavior for crude and obvious reasons. After ECT, a patient has difficulties with thinking and memory. However, the positive changes are usually transient and often dissipate (Read et al., 2021). Accordingly, current strategies in ECT often involve repeated administration of ECT, sometimes on a monthly basis for years.

Finally, with regard to psychological needs and interventions to aid people's ability to have key psychological needs better met, there are a host of individual and psychosocial interventions that address these needs. The therapeutic relationship itself begins to address issues related to social isolation and lack of interpersonal connection. Therapeutic relationships are affirming and supportive.

Having someone listen to one's complaints on issues can itself be affirming and calming. The relationship itself can be calming if patients are entrained to the therapist's calm demeanor. Skill-building done in the context of individual or group therapies addresses the need for effective interpersonal relationships. Individual therapy may address issues about meaning, purpose and, if the client is so inclined, existential concerns. With increases in understanding gained from considering another perspective, people in therapy may develop a better understanding of their own behaviors and that of others. More in-depth psychotherapy helps in advancing self-awareness, altering negative introjects, and, as possible, supporting positive personality restructuring. Psychotherapeutic engagement thus directly or indirectly addresses a range of key psychological needs.

With regard to the need for control and positive interactions with one's environment, I am reminded of my experience in the 1970s and 1980s when I was providing behavioral consultation to staff in institutional and community group home and apartment settings who were working with challenging populations. At the height of enthusiasm for behavior modification techniques, I was hired to develop behavioral programs. I was young and needed the work.

What I usually did in the context of behavioral programing was restructure staff interactions and, in ways I came to realize, that stopped many negative behaviors of staff which gave clients clear goals they were able to achieve. These interventions gave clients an ability to exercise control of their environment, receive positive feedback, and increase their sense of self-efficacy. Sometimes very simple goal setting and feedback systems produced surprisingly positive results. These behavioral plans were more about controlling staff behavior than directly controlling client behavior. These interventions helped clients better meet a number of important psychological needs.

One additional note about systemic interventions: Recognizing that there is a need for pattern interruption and calming effects, which is often necessary before serious therapeutic work can begin, can help explain why a number of non-traditional techniques being used to aid the treatment of psychological difficulties have some support. These techniques include a range of procedures that don't appear directly related to psychological problems. These techniques include procedures such as EEG biofeedback, vagus nerve stimulation, brain spotting, eye movement desensitization (EMDR), transcranial alternating current stimulation (tACS), Stanford neuromodulation therapy (SNT), transcranial magnetic stimulation (TMS), and even the use of ketamine and psychedelics.

The notion that these techniques treat mental disorders is a curious assertion, in my opinion. But these interventions do interrupt behaviors, including brain-related processes in the case of EEG biofeedback, and they often promote relaxation and calming effects. All these interventions can have therapeutic impact and aid the ultimate goals of psychological treatment.

Summary

The mental disorders that are categorized and described in the two dominant psychiatric diagnostic systems, the *International Classification of Diseases* (*ICD*) (World Health Organization, 2019) and the *Diagnostic and Statistical Manual of Mental Disorders* (*DSM*) (American Psychiatric Association, 2013), are labels applied in a psychiatric language community to the variety of emergent and largely dysfunctional patterns of human actions, feelings, and thoughts that present to psychiatric and psychological communities for treatment. These reactive patterns occur in response to trauma, threats to a person's well-being and survival, and deficits in the ability to have critical psychological needs met.

Of course, there are brain processes occurring while dysfunctional behaviors are occurring, but the relationship between brain processes and the psychological and behavioral patterns is complex, if not theoretically impossible to track. Not only does a strictly biological approach to psychological problems dehumanize humans and our approach to them (Eccles, 1994), it also undermines the belief in self-efficacy and control that is central to good mental health.

The idea that a biological understanding of psychiatric disorders is humanistic because it removes a sense of personal blame for disturbed persons is ultimately countertherapeutic. Persons suffering from psychological distress are often seized by these conditions for which they have little control. One of the goals of therapy is to empower individuals and help them gain improved control of their lives. In addition, the notion of biological causality is a flawed concept that has little, if any, support in the area of problematic mental conditions.

The language of psychology, which embraces common sense notions of psychological needs, offers us a pragmatic way to understand and then support people suffering from dysfunctional and distressing psychological conditions. A systems approach also provides an orientation that is useful to understand and for applying a variety of available techniques to reduce anxiety and agitation that can stand in the way of change as well as ways to interrupt stuck problematic patterns.

References

American Psychiatric Association. (2013). *Diagnostic and statistical manual of mental disorders* (5th ed.). https://doi.org/10.1176/appi.books.9780890425596.

Bandura, A. (1982). Self-efficacy mechanism in human agency. *American Psychologist, 37,* 122–147.

Baumeister, R. F. & Leary, M. (1995). The need to belong: desire for interpersonal attachment as a fundamental human motivation. *Psychological Bulletin, 117,* 497-529.

Cacioppo, J.T., & Patrick, W. (2008). *Loneliness: Human nature and the need for social connection.* New York: W.W. Norton & Company.

Deacon, B. J. (2013). The biomedical model of mental disorder: A critical analysis of its validity, utility, and effects on psychotherapy research. *Clinical Psychology Review, 33,* 846-861.

Eccles, J. (1994). *How the self controls its brain.* Springer.

Ellis, G. F. R. (2008). On the nature of causation in complex systems. *Trans. R. Soc. South Africa* 63, 69–84. http://www.mth.uct.ac.za/~ellis/Top-down%20Ellis.pdf

Fink, T. (2022). Language Games in Contemporary American Psychiatry and Psychology: A critical look at how language shapes our understanding and approach to mental and emotional difficulties. In E. Maisel & C. Ruby (Eds.), *Critiquing the psychiatric model* (pp. 50-61). The Ethics International Press.

Flanagan, C.M. (2010). The case for needs in psychotherapy, *Journal of Psychotherapy Integration, (20, 1),* 1-36.

Flanagan, C. M. (2014). Unmet needs and maladaptive modes: A new way to approach longer-term problems. *Journal of Psychotherapy Integration,* 24 (3), 208-222.

Frankl, V.E. (1959). *Man's search for meaning.* New York: A Touchstone Book.

George, F. R. Ellis, D. N., & O'Connor, T. (2012). Top-down causation: an integrating theme within and across sciences? *Interface Focus.* Feb 6; 2(1): 1–3. Published online 2011 Nov 23. doi: 10.1098/rsfs.2011.0110

Gleick, J. (1987). *Chaos: Making a new science.* New York: Penguin Books.

Gliner, J. A. (1972). Predictable vs. unpredictable shock: Preference behavior and stomach ulceration. *Physiology and Behavior.* 9 (5), 693-698. https://doi.org/10.1016/0031-9384(72)90036-4

Hari, J. (2018). *Lost connections: Uncovering the real causes of depression and the unexpected solutions.* New York: Bloomsbury.

Insel, T. R. (2010). Faulty circuits. *Scientific American, 302,* 44-51.

Joseph, J. (2017). *Schizophrenia and genetics: The end of an illusion.* Routledge.

Khalidi, M.A. (2023). *Cognitive ontology: Taxonomic practices in the mind-brain sciences.* Cambridge University Press.

Lang, P. J. (1994). "The Varieties of Emotional Experience: A Meditation on James–Lange Theory". *Psychological Review*. 101 (2): 211–221. doi:10.1037/0033-295x.101.2.211.PMID8022956.

Langer, E.J. (1983). *Psychology of control*. Beverly Hills, CA: Sage.

Levy, N., Douglas, T., Kahane, G., Terbeck, S., Cowen, P., Hewstone, M., & Savulescu, J. (2014). "Are You Morally Modified?: The Moral Effects of Widely Used Pharmaceuticals, *Philosophy, Psychiatry, & Psychology*, 21(2), 111- 125. https://doi.org/10.1353/ppp.2014.0023.

Lynch, J. J. (2000). *A cry unheard: New Insights into the Medical Consequences of Loneliness*. Baltimore, MD: Bancroft Press.

Margolis, J. (1978). *Persons and minds: The prospects of nonreductive materialism*, Boston: D. Reidel Publishing Company.

Marker, S. (2003). Unmet Human Needs. In G. Burgess & H. Burgess (Eds.) *Beyond Intractability*. Conflict Information Consortium, University of Colorado, Boulder. Posted: August 2003. http://www.beyondintractability.org/essay/human-needs.

Maslow, A. H. (1943). A theory of human motivation. *Psychological Review*, 50(4), 370-396.

Miller, W. R., & Seligman M. E. (1975). Depression and learned helplessness in man. *Journal of Abnormal Psychology, 84*, 228-238. http://dx.doi.org/10.1037/h0076720

Moncrieff, J., Cooper, R.E., Stockmann, T., Amendola, S., Hengartner, M. P., & Horowitz, M. A. (2022). The serotonin theory of depression: a systematic umbrella review of the evidence. *Molecular Psychiatry*. https://doi.org/10.1038/s41380-022-01661-0

Morin, E. (2008). *On complexity*, Denver, CO: Hampton Press.

Newman, D. V. (1996). Emergence and Strange Attractors. *Philosophy of Science, 63*(2), 245–261. http://www.jstor.org/stable/188472.

Nolen-Hoeksema, S. (2000). The role of rumination in depressive disorders and mixed anxiety/depressive symptoms. *Journal of Abnormal Psychology, 109*(3), 504–511. https://doi.org/10.1037/0021-843X.109.3.504

Ossorio, P. G. (2006). *The behavior of persons. The collected works of Peter G. Ossorio*, Vol. V. Ann Arbor, MI: Descriptive Psychology Press.

Perkins, A. M., Leonard, A. M., Weaver, K., Dalton, J. A., Mehta, M. A., Kumari, V., Williams, S. C. R., & Ettinger, U. (2013). A dose of ruthlessness: Interpersonal moral judgment is hardened by the anti-anxiety drug lorazepam. *Journal of Experimental Psychology: General, 142*(3), 612–620. https://doi.org/10.1037/a0030256

Papageorgiou, C & Wells, A. (2003). *Depressive rumination.* Wiley & Sons.

Pagnini, F., Bercovitz, K, & Langer, E. (2016). Perceived control and mindfulness: Implications for clinical practice. *Journal of Psychotherapy Integration, 26* (2), 91 - 102.

Read, J., Kirsch, I., & McGrath, L. (2021). Electroconvulsive therapy for depression: a review of the quality of ECT versus sham ECT trials and meta-analyses. *BJPsych Advances, 27*(5), 284. https://doi.org/10.1192/bja.2021.25

Ryan, R. M. & Deci, E. L. (2017). *Self-determination theory: Basic psychological needs in motivation, development, and wellness.* New York: Guilford Publishing.

Seligman, M. E. (1975). *Helplessness: On Depression, Development and Death.* W.H. Freeman.

Seligman, M. E & Beagley, G. (1975). Learned helplessness in the rat. *Journal of Comparative and Physiological Psychology, 88,* 534-541.

Schwartz, W. (2019). *Descriptive psychology and the person concept: Essential attributes of persons and behavior.* Elsevier Academic Press.

Skinner, E. A. (1995). *Perceived control, motivation, & coping.* Sage Publications.

Thomasson, N., Pezard, L., Allilaire, J. F. Renault, B., & Martinerie, J. (2000). Nonlinear EEG Changes Associated with Clinical Improvement in Depressed Patients. *Nonlinear Dynamics Psychol Life Sci 4,* 203–218. https://doi.org/10.1023/A:1009580427443.

Valenstein, E.S. (2002). *Blaming the brain.* Free Press.

Wallston, K.A., Wallston, B.S., Smith, S. & Dobbins, C. J. (1987). Perceived control and health. *Current Psychology 6,* 5–25 (1987). https://doi.org/10.1007/BF02686633.

Wagman, J.B. (2010). What is responsible for the emergence of order and patterns in psychological systems? *Journal of Theoretical and Philosophical Psychology.* 30 (1), 32-50.

Whitaker, R. (2002). *Mad in America: Bad Science, Bad Medicine, and the Enduring Mistreatment of the Mentally Ill.* Cambridge, MA Perseus Pub.

Whitaker, R. (2010). *Anatomy of an Epidemic: Magic Bullets, Psychiatric Drugs, and the Astonishing Rise of Mental Illness in America,* New York: Crown Publishers.

Whitaker, R. (2021). The scientific collapse of the DSM model of care. https://www.youtube.com/watch?v=29WKzcRaUGM

Windholz G. & Witherspoon L. H. (1993). Sleep as a cure for schizophrenia: a historical episode. *History of Psychiatry.* 4(13):83-93. doi:10.1177/0957154X9300401304

Wittgenstein, L. (1966). *Philosophical Investigations.* (G.E.M Anscombe, Trans), New York: The Macmillan Company. (Original work published 1953).

World Health Organization. (2019). *International statistical classification of diseases and related health problems* (11th ed.). https://icd.who.int/

Stalked by Stress, Abandoned to Predation: The Appeal of Suicide in a Modern World

Sarah Knutson

Abstract: *This chapter challenges the mainstream conception of suicide as sick, crazy, or irrational. The author argues that suicidal thoughts, impulses, and acts are in fact a logical outgrowth of troubling developments affecting the larger cultural context. In the author's view, modern life has become increasingly stressful and challenging while mainstream culture has become increasingly predatory and abandoning. The author provides numerous examples of how predatory and abandoning dynamics have inserted themselves into everyday experiences and relationships. The author illustrates from personal experience how these factors operate to deprive natural and clinical relationships of their protective value and instead operate to increase the sense of isolation, despair and loss of social value that make suicide appealing. The author further argues that, far from signifying weakness or illness, rising suicidality is a beacon and a warning about relational trends in the culture at large that are dangerous to everyone's health. The role of stress as a contributing factor in leading causes of illness and death - whether accidental, organic or psychological - is pointed out, raising the question of whether the stress of modern living is killing us all - just in different ways.*

Acknowledgement: A version of this chapter was first published by Mad in America on January 16, 2020.

Suicide, for me, is about overwhelming, inescapable stress. The conditions of life are stalking me in a way that feels insurmountably scary and bad. At first blush that may seem strange to you. After all, it's not like I live in a particularly rough neighborhood. Nor do I have to forage for my dinner or fight off predators who want to eat my young.

Even so, my life has some disadvantages compared to my mammalian forebears. It's not like I'm that lucky rabbit in the wild who can sniff the air, slip out of my hole for a few nibbles, and then burrow back into safety for the rest of the day—rinse and repeat tomorrow, and the day after that, and the next and next, ad infinitum.

Modern problems aren't like that. They're more like a shadow that goes wherever I do:

> *Where to live? How to afford it? Who do I have to keep happy to keep it? How big of an ask will they make of me? Will I ever escape if I piss them off?*

Add to all this: databases, identity tracking, employment records, rap sheets, taxes, standardized tests, et cetera. My failings are never forgotten. The same basic requirements, standards and regulations are everywhere— all requiring me to recall, disclose and defend the density I reported for lint particles in my navel at age six. Even with family or long-term friends, there is always a new obligation to be met or graciously evaded. Social media virtually assures it.

Modern society would have me believe that I'm crazy if this stuff kills my desire to live. In mainstream fairyland, no stress is happening:

> *Nothing is wrong, damaging, or intentional. Hardship is avoidable, temporary, and my fault. I need to be patient, persistent, and responsible. The people in charge will make it all better. My attitude is the problem. If I weren't so bad or my genes were good, I would be coping like everyone else.*

Frankly, those messages don't make me feel better—they put another nail in my coffin.

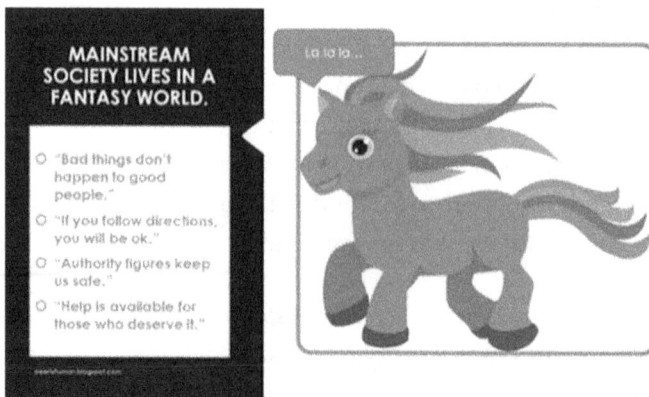

But here's a message that perked up my ears. It didn't come from the culture—it came from my own body. At the height of suicidal stress—feeling demoralized, paralyzed, utterly despairing—the following questions floated into my dazed awareness:

- *What if some conditions are beneath the dignity of the Life Spirit?*
- *What if the effects of chronic stress are killing me not because I'm "mentally ill," but because the human race needs to find a better way to live?*

For me, those simple questions lit the Life in me on fire. I began to look for evidence. Here is what I found.

Head Start on Stress

The stressors cited above are First World problems. They are issues that anyone who can access the resources needed to read this chapter is up against—and has to reckon with on some level. Due to various kinds of social inequality, however, many of us also experience Second, Third and Fourth World problems, even in relatively prosperous nations (Deaton, 2018). This includes poverty, violence, abuse, neglect, labor exploitation, homelessness, environmental hazards, intentional exclusion, substandard education, barbaric healthcare, predatory targeting, police brutality, unresponsive government, callous indifference…the list goes on.

Statistically speaking, these kinds of stressors have a huge impact on health and life expectancy. That's what the emerging field of study on the "social determinants of health" is all about. Here's the concept, pioneered by international social epidemiologist Richard Wilkinson (2003) in a nutshell:

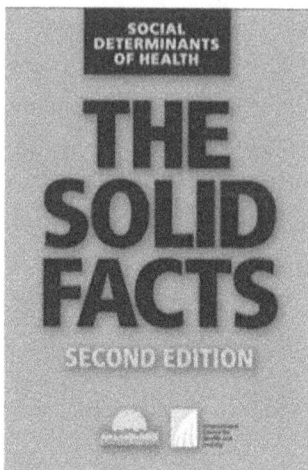

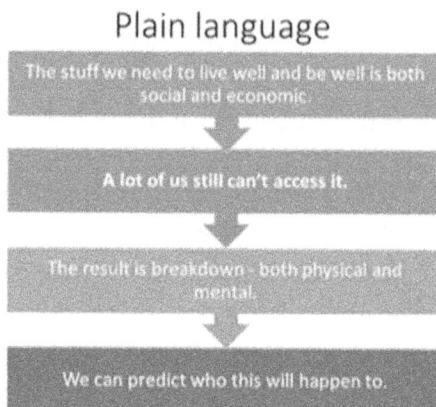

The potential impact of stressors like these on mental well-being is shocking. In 2011, the National Council for Community Behavioral Healthcare reported that an estimated 90% of us in the public mental health system are survivors of pre-existing childhood adversities, including abuse, neglect, violence, poverty, discrimination, et cetera (National Council for Community Behavioral Healthcare, 2011).

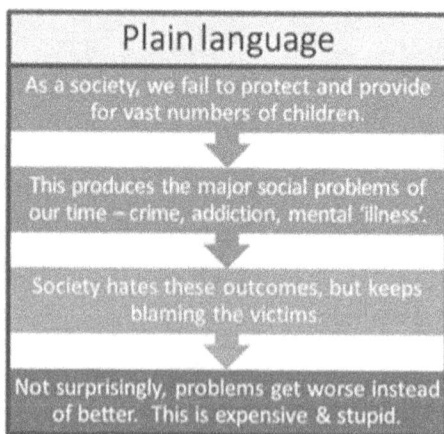

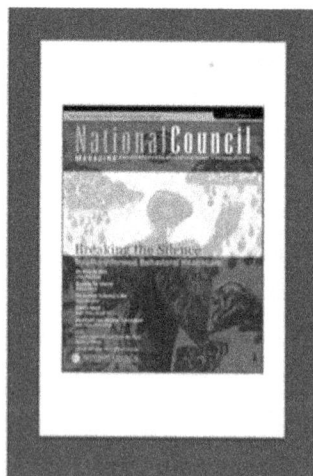

Thus, if I have a mental health diagnosis and I'm contemplating suicide, in all probability I have a lifetime of disadvantage, adversity and resultant stress preceding that. This isn't mere statistical correlation—it is easy to see the reasons this happens once I understand how the stress response works.

As a child, my rapidly developing body makes me vulnerable to whatever is happening around me. If I'm growing up in a war zone, physically or metaphorically, my body is going to accommodate that (Sapolsky, 2017).

High idle mode

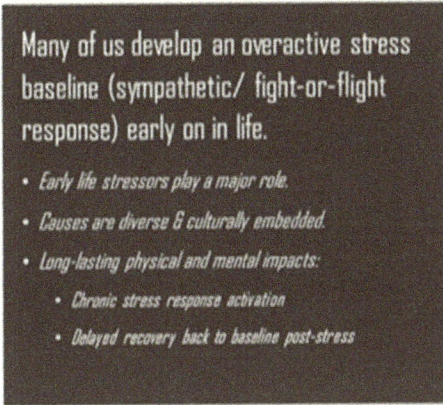

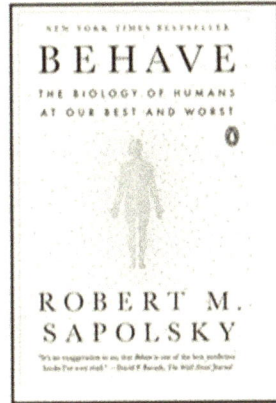

Many of us develop an overactive stress baseline (sympathetic/ fight-or-flight response) early on in life.

- Early life stressors play a major role.
- Causes are diverse & culturally embedded.
- Long-lasting physical and mental impacts:
  - Chronic stress response activation
  - Delayed recovery back to baseline post-stress

BEHAVE

THE BIOLOGY OF HUMANS AT OUR BEST AND WORST

ROBERT M. SAPOLSKY

(Sapolsky, 2017, p. 194)

As a result, a lot of us develop an overactive stress baseline as children. "High idle" becomes our natural normal. This can lead to enduring, devastating effects on both physical and mental health.

The way this played out for me was that I almost never felt comfortable in my own skin. It was hard to rest, relax, or let down my guard. The continual discomfort took a toll and wore me down, both physically and mentally.

Also, the elevated level of baseline pain made other life setbacks and frustrations feel more intense. That, in turn, affected my judgment and my relationships with others. All of this contributed to the progressing trainwreck of demoralizing circumstances and experiences that, ultimately, made me vulnerable to giving up on life.

The Social Inequality Game

When you look at the data on stress-related disease, it's not just that modern life is stressful. It's not just that some of us take harder knocks than others. No—a huge source of stress for humans is...each other. (Sapolsky, 2004).

More specifically, it's how I've been socialized to view and treat you—and vice versa. We don't talk about it much where I live because, you know, we're Americans and we're all supposed to be equal. But underneath, practically everyone knows how to play the game:

> Rule 1. Pick a measure of social worth (wealth, appearance, education, sports, culturally relevant access, or knowledge).
> Rule 2. Compare myself with you.
> Rule 3: Whoever has more of what the culture values wins.

This is the Social Inequality Game. It's habitual, ingrained and played every day by practically everyone everywhere. I might not even know I'm doing it—unless I'm the loser. Then, I notice it. Ouch. That hurts. I don't measure up. According to Wilkinson (Social Science Bites, 2018, para. 6), this kind of "status anxiety—and its ill effects such as worsening health—affects everyone, the super-rich and the dirt-poor."

The more inequality, the more status anxiety. Tortuously, privilege still has to beat out privilege. So even if I'm filthy rich and have the biggest yacht or boobs, the next Kardashian private jet or nose job can still put mine to shame. Also, there are endless categories to compete in. Literally, I could feel bad about my lesser knowledge of bacterial life in Antarctica or Spencer Tracy movies in 1949.

Far more insidious is the way that status competition permeates the entire fabric of conscious existence:

> [T]hanks to urbanization, mobility, and the media that makes for a global village, something absolutely unprecedented can now occur— we can now be made to feel poor, or poorly about ourselves, by people we don't even know. You can feel impoverished by the clothes of someone you pass in a midtown crowd, by the unseen driver of a new car on the freeway, by Bill Gates on the evening news, even by a fictional character in a movie. Our...modern world makes

it possible to have our noses rubbed in it by a local community that stretches around the globe. (Sapolsky, 2004, pp. 191-92)

While probably no one is "up there" orchestrating it, status competition is demoralizing and destructive in a socially deadly kind of way. In the view of Robert Sapolsky (2004), professor of biology and neurology at Stanford University and world-renowned stress researcher, "when humans invented poverty, they came up with a way of subjugating the low-ranking like nothing ever before seen in the primate world" (p. 192). In other words, making each other feel poor has turned into an art.

If played to its logical conclusion, the outcome (literal and metaphoric) is mutually assured destruction:

1. We've created a highly status-conscious society.
2. Everyone is taught not only to seek high status for themselves, but also to police social status rules as a condition of being a good citizen.
3. It's a zero-sum game that I can only win by beating you out and keeping you down.

What is worse, to play at all I have to buy into the idea that human beings have relative worth. Otherwise, I don't create worth for myself by trouncing friends and neighbors. No less disturbing, to stay on top, I must repeatedly make a loser of you to maintain my illusion of superiority.

The end result is that I end up competing with you for virtually everything all the time. Also, the stakes are really high. For most of us, the Social Inequality Game is not played for luxury vacations. We're competing for life and death necessities—safe neighborhoods and housing, nutritious food, adequate healthcare, the means to make a living and support a family.

This is not only frightening and traumatizing for the losers—it's even bad for the winners:

Basically, more unequal societies have worse quality of life. Across countries and among U.S. states, more inequality, independent of absolute levels of income, predicts higher rates of crime, including homicide, and higher incarceration rates. Add in higher rates of kids being bullied at schools, more teen pregnancies and lower literacy. There are more psychiatric problems, alcoholism and drug abuse, lower levels of happiness and less social mobility. And there is less social support—a steep hierarchy is the antithesis of the equality and symmetry that nourish friendship. This grim collective picture helps to explain the immensely important fact that when inequality increases, everyone's health suffers. (Sapolsky, 2018, para. 5)

What is worse, it's not just material needs that we're denying each other. It's basic social courtesies like respect, dignity, regard, time, attention, patience, fairness, an invitation to belong, the opportunity to take part, and a meaningful audience. Can any of us grow up feeling okay—or stay feeling okay—without this?

Sadly, this is all stuff that we could freely offer each other—without any grants, public funding or costing the taxpayer a dime. Quite possibly, we would be offering it—if our culture encouraged us to invest half as much in each other as we are encouraged to invest in "getting ahead."

But that's not all.

Little Fish, Big Pond

A close cousin of status inequality is living at the mercy of concentrated wealth and power. Did you know that, since the 1920s, all it takes is a few media giants and a single concerted effort to straitjacket the collective cultural conscience (Radcliff, 2004)? Within a few hours, days, months or years, there's a routinely recited "same page" I need to be on with the rest of my relevant social world (Chomsky, 2017).

If I dare to think, believe, or voice out loud anything at odds with this—no matter how personally authentic or seemingly important—I risk widespread re-education from upstanding citizens who "got the message." Given what I hear from others, I also risk unemployment, community suspicion, monitoring for danger to self or others, and possibly end up in the psychiatric system, corrections, or homeless on the streets.

Next, there's the marketers, corporations, and political machines (Kruse, 2015). How they maintain even the pretense of fairness is a mystery to me. Day in and day out, they devote unfathomable economic, intellectual, and technical resources to studying and manipulating the rest of us and the rules of a game we are bound by.

The rules are so complex most of us don't even know they exist. Yet, every minute of every day, behind impenetrable firewalls, the world's top minds are getting six or seven figure salaries to crunch the numbers of my existence—and to ensure that the thumb on the scale pushes the odds to favor their investors and special interests.

Consider the likelihood that all of these players cross-pollinate (Hanretty, 2014). Then factor in their likely strongholds in education, curricula, and research. Add to that their likely influence on the experts and outcomes selected for public news reporting (Levy, 2019).

My first serious awakening to this clandestine advantage was in law school. We were studying a famous tort case involving Ford motors. Landmark punitive damages were awarded after it was shown that Ford executives knowingly refused to recall exploding vehicles due to an internal "cost-benefit analysis."

They intentionally decided it was cheaper to let an estimated 500-900 innocent unsuspecting consumers burn up inside their cars than change the design (American Museum of Tort Law, n.d.). That's how much, and how callously, corporations are studying us—and selling us out, even unto death—to keep shareholders happy.

It's not like this was an isolated incident. It's big business as usual. Tobacco, Enron, the Gulf of Mexico oil spill, the mortgage crisis—not to mention the iatrogenic Psychiatry-Pharma alliance that Mad in America[1] is exposing.

And it's not just the big life and death stuff that kills me. There is also the excruciating long, slow death that comes in nickels and dimes. Does anyone remember the annoyingly long and hard-to-skip Verizon voicemail

---

[1] https://www.madinamerica.com/

greetings? Not an accident. The extra time such greetings ran aggregated into billions of extra billable minutes for phone carriers over millions of voicemails daily, monthly, and yearly (Pogue, 2009, 2010; see also Mai, 2016; Reardon, 2012).

And that's just the tip of the iceberg. I haven't even scratched the surface of cable TV, cars, computers, electric and fuel companies, internet service providers, healthcare and pharmaceutical marketing and zillions of other products that modern consumers interact with daily.

I'm not saying the big fish are lying and cheating on everything—I'm just too limited to know when they are or aren't. What I do know is that all of this scares me and stresses me out. I don't trust—or feel particularly safe with—what appears to be standard operating procedure for the lion's share of high-level business and political players these days.

Big Brother is Watching

Now factor in the impact of technological surveillance. Not only in the interests of "national security," as Edward Snowden finally proved, but also the major industrial players. My habits, location, purchases, opinions, and associations are either known or knowable by powerful others with a proven track record of throwing the little guy under the bus. And the government that's supposed to protect me from that? Given wealth disparities in who gets elected, it's pretty clear that it's mostly the foxes guarding us chickens (Thompson, 2011).

Just as important from a stress standpoint, how much weight do you think my opinion is going to carry if push ever comes to shove? I'm a lone citizen with a documented "serious mental illness." They are experts with fancy degrees and corporations with big lawyers and friends in high places. Even if I'm right, almost no one in their right mind is going to bother pressing my case. The potential downside for everyone who can safely stay under the wire is simply too great.

Modern Predators, Modern Jungle

I used to think I was making a mountain out of a mole hill. Obviously, this stuff was just all in my head. Certainly, my brain knows the difference between a lion and intentionally bad customer service or an obviously self-dealing politician. And it has to be smart enough to know that it shouldn't go into blowout stress mode just because my health insurance "lost" my claim again.

Actually, no — it's not just weapons and fangs that kill me. Being stalked by industry, bureaucracy, and social sentiment is deadly, too. Mammalian bodies are not wired to endure chronic, pervasive threat and vulnerability (Sapolsky, 2004). Yet this stuff is ubiquitous and embedded into mainstream culture.

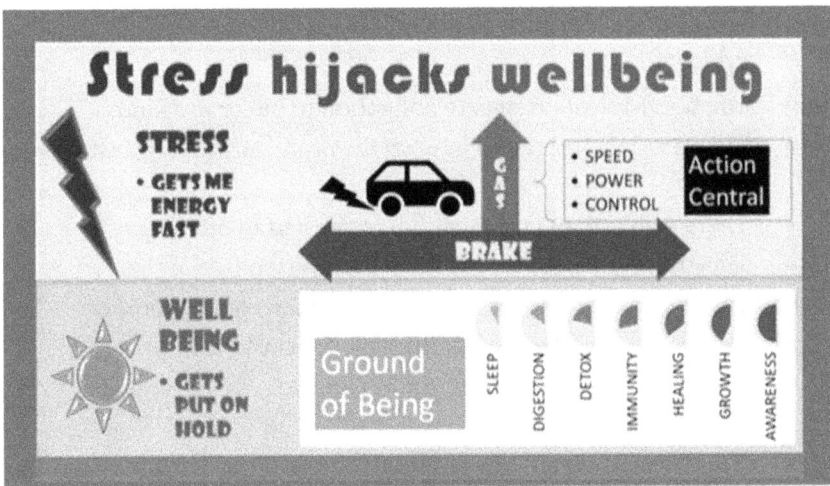

Thus, I don't need a lion or natural disaster to experience the ill-effects of stress. Anything that matters to me, including my future, will capture the attention of this system and erode my long-term health (Sapolsky, 2004, pp. 7-8).

All of that used to make me feel a lot of shame. At the outer extremes, succumbing to the grip of stress can feel a bit like being possessed. I must be weak or crazy to let this stuff get to me. I'm wasting my life. It's so unproductive.

More recently, however, I've come to see stress activation as resulting far more from my gifts than my failings. It is the logical outcome of a brain that allows me to self-reflect, know my limits, and appreciate the vastness that is out there. It's kind of amazing when I think about it:

I have hard-wired mental capacities that let me travel through time such that I can actually project my past experiences into the future and, based on that, make educated guesses about how to live today. On the downside, this same capacity allows me to be aware (24-7-365) of the millions of things about life (past, present, future) that are beyond my ability to manage or control. If the world I live in is generally benevolent and protective, then all good—having control isn't such a big deal then because my relevant universe has my back.

On the other hand, suppose:

- I'm a tiny fish in a big pond.
- The big fish feel no sincere obligation to me or my kind.
- They are only interested in what they can get and how fast they can get it.
- There's little they want that I'm interested in offering.
- They have the potential to track my every move.
- There's little protection or recourse if they come after me.
- They have friends in every high place I could turn to.
- There are many ways they could make my life miserable or get rid of me if they wanted to.
- The rest of my kind is as vulnerable and scared as I am, so we don't stick up for each other.

Clearly this does not bode well for letting the "soft animal of your body love what it loves" (Oliver, 1992, p. 110). To the contrary, given my capacity to appreciate vulnerabilities, project into the future, and hold my awareness of likely outcomes 24-7-365, it is pretty clear that stress is going to create problems for me.

Please pause here, and allow just a moment to take this in, because this is an important distinction to get:

The problem of the modern world for me is not so much the stress of having a present threat to survival. It is a continual uncertainty about future survival given the conditions of life as I have come to know and experience them.

The Perfect Storm for Suicide

This is how I think mainstream culture has become deadly for me, and possibly for a lot of other people. It sets up a perfect storm of predation and abandonment, wrapped together in a never-ending, ever-escalating cycle.

The pervasive predation virtually assures that many of us will, at some point, find ourselves hopelessly in over our heads. The pervasive abandonment separates us from each other—and, therefore, cuts us off from naturally-occurring human support that is arguably our most powerful evolutionary resource in these circumstances.

The predictable outcome is the "Sisyphus Cycle" depicted below:

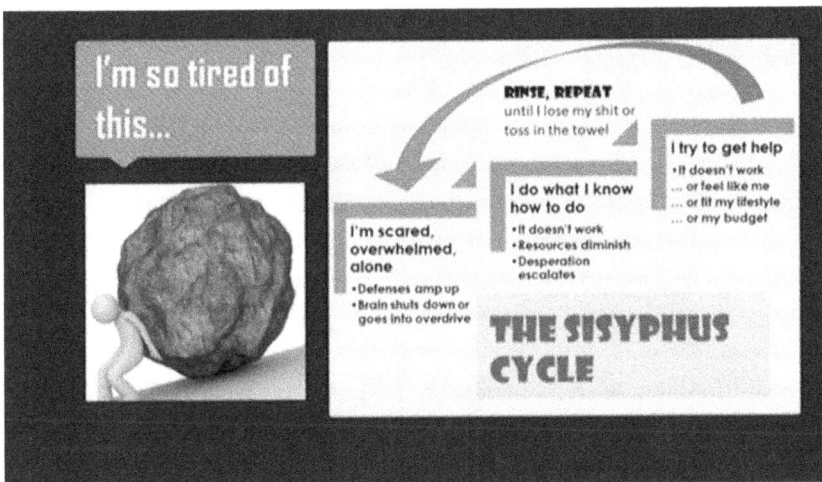

(Knutson, 2019)

The Sisyphus Cycle basically works like this:

1. The stress of trying to survive a predatory, abandoning culture leads to physical and mental breakdown.

2. The breakdown itself makes me even more vulnerable to predation and abandonment, leading to progressive loss of material, social and emotional resources.
3. Once I'm in it, the continual drain on my energy and resources, combined with progressive loss and depletion, makes it incredibly hard to get out.

A good example is what happens in mainstream mental health. Economic predation has led the mental health professions to market the message that "mental illness" is dangerous, complicated and beyond the capacity of untrained citizens. The pharmaceutical industry has teamed up with them to market their predatory message that these are brain issues—not stress or life issues—requiring professional services, preferably drugs.

Both of these so-called "helpers" have used their considerable social and economic power to up their relative status and limit the array of options available. This is done both at the expense of society (much of healthcare is funded by tax dollars) as well as at the expense of the vulnerable people they claim to serve.

These industries also create a subsidiary class of predators. This includes ordinary citizens who are eager to take advantage of the status differentials that make them socially "better than." The fact of my psychiatric label not only makes me fair game for this group, but it also creates a natural tension with family and friends who now fear the downward status consequences of guilt by association.

The real-life impacts are painful and cruel. When I try to talk about what I see happening—how devastating and frightening this is, how much it is killing my motivation to live—responsible citizens mostly follow the directions they are given by professionals and experts through mass media. Time again, respected others politely decline to offer basic human courtesies like attention and interest, and, instead, suggest I see a professional.

The repeated effect of such socially diminishing responses in a status-conscious world is devastating. The relative status of the disengaged and dismissive advice-giving person goes up. They have done their duty, followed directions, and proven themselves a good citizen. So now, they get to feel better about themselves.

The effect on me is the opposite. The person has literally added insult to my injury. Consequently, my status goes down, basic human needs go unmet, and I feel even worse. Yet, this happens over and over, even with family and close friends.

The next stop on the train is the therapist's office. Here I try to express my pain as I honestly see it:

- Widespread mainstream denial
- Rampant status competition
- The professional guild privilege that siloed me into treatment and away from authentic human conversation
- Social outsider status resulting from the psychiatric diagnosis, the history of which will follow me and make me vulnerable to social and professional exclusion for the rest of my life—even if I beat the odds and "get better"

If I honestly say, as I often have, that this makes me feel like my life is over, and that everyone, including me, would be better off if I were dead, then out comes the suicide assessment. The repeated effect of this socially diminishing response in a status-conscious world is also devastating. The relative status of the diminishing, rejecting, assessment-giving professional goes up. They have done their duty, followed directions, proven themselves a good clinician.

Now they are in full compliance with the ethical advice of their profession, their legal obligation to society, and the organization they work for. Society even tells them they have "no choice" because the legal profession predators and the surviving relative predators will team up and get them if they don't.

Not surprisingly, in this social world, I get worse instead of better. My basic human needs for honest conversation and meaningful connection about my painful state in a painful world are still going unmet. Plus, my status is continually decreasing relative to others—simply as a result of voicing my sincere, honest, and seemingly reasonable concerns.

Again, power is used by important others in predatory or abandoning ways, and I am paying good money for this. All of this increases my stress and discomfort, decreases my connection with others, and destroys my hope of things ever changing while putting me at a loss for reasons to stay alive.

But do you know what's just as deadly?

Everyday Responses

Practically everyone knows that the kind of stuff I'm bringing up here is happening. There are new abuses every minute, much of this documented. But if I call it as I see it, in most people's eyes, I'm paranoid, obsessed, overreacting, negative, dysfunctional, toxic, and/or diagnosable.

I think that's really interesting. In fact, it kind of proves my point about how stressful it is to be alive these days:

- Most people know that power is being abused at very high levels.
- Most people know that higher-ups can take advantage of us and actively are.
- Yet, we're all being told by the experts that healthy people cope with this.

And thanks to mass media and mass marketing, I'm bombarded with tips for coping. The social message is that if I get distressed by the moral outrages of social, economic and political power brokers, it means something is wrong with *me*. It's like: *Well, boys will be boys. The mature citizen recognizes that and lets it go.* In the end, every citizen is an "expert" and happy to share or enforce the coping message on us reluctant lag-behinds.

And just to prove that the social predators truly have no shame, they have turned coping into an industry as well. As a result, there are now countless services and products I can buy to feel better while I am being ripped off (e.g., Google "Stress Relief Products" to see my point).

If I put all this together, I get a clear and concise recipe for wanting to die:

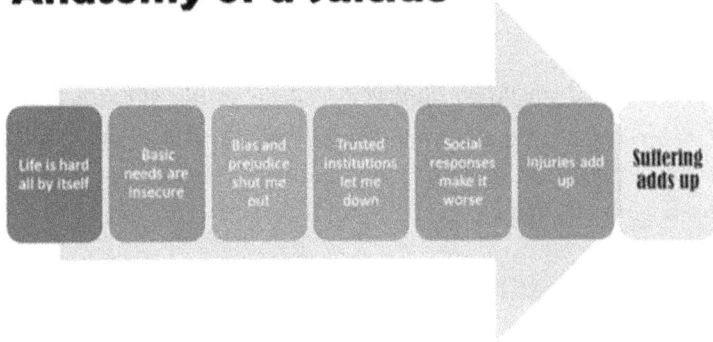

Anatomy of a Suicide

Life is hard all by itself | Basic needs are insecure | Bias and prejudice shut me out | Trusted institutions let me down | Social responses make it worse | Injuries add up | **Suffering adds up**

No bad genes or broken biology required. It's simply a matter of stress and chronicity. Challenges and injuries accumulate. Suffering compounds. At some point, there are too many injuries, in too many ways, that have happened too often and been too painful for far too long. It becomes too much.

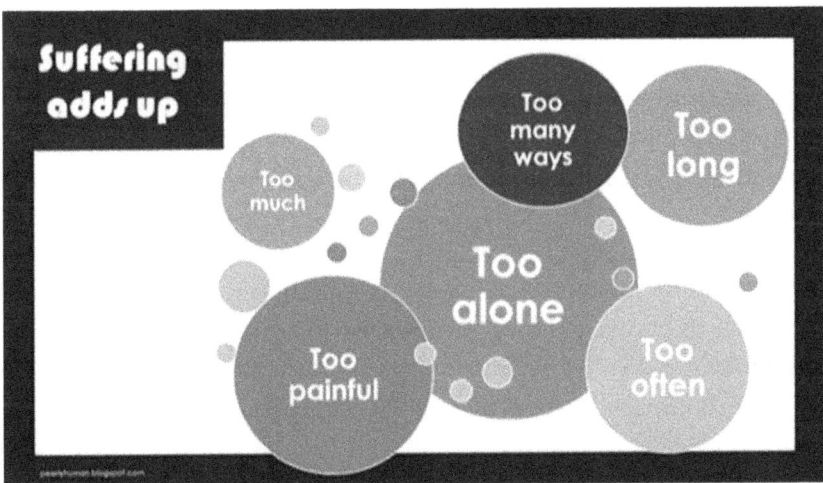

Suffering adds up

Too much

Too many ways

Too long

Too alone

Too painful

Too often

Ultimately, I reach a point where life feels disconnected, pointless and unbearable. I, then, decide I have had enough. I am going to get out of the Sisyphus Cycle.

The next time I get energy, I take my opportunity. Some might call this a coward's escape, but it can also be seen as a Hero's Journey. The only weapon I have left is my life. Now, I'm using it to send you one last message:

> *Whatever the hell you people think you are doing on planet Earth, it is not okay with me. As much as I value my life, I'll take my chances with death. Given what you are offering, I'm betting my eternity that death is not the worst thing that can happen to me.*

If Stress is So Deadly and Pervasive, Why Isn't Everyone Breaking Down?

It's a legitimate question. After all, statistics suggest that suicide and "mental illness" are related. Roughly 50% of suicide completers in the past two decades had "known mental health conditions" (Stone, 2018). A seemingly logical conclusion is that stress only gets to emotionally vulnerable people who are on their way to "crazy" already.

The problem with that kind of logic is that it assumes there is only one kind of breakdown from stress (i.e., psychological). Clearly, that is not the case. Stress affects all sorts of functions in my body—digestion, heart rate, blood pressure, respiration, circulation, immune function, liver, kidneys, detoxification, sleep, healing, and growth and development (Sapolsky, 2004).

It also makes for poorer judgment and reasoning since it diverts resources from brain to brawn, priming my muscles to act and makes me want to jump out of my skin. If I put all that together, I get a more complete picture of the actual impacts of stress and who it is impacting. It goes like this:

1. Wear and tear, plus lousy choices, increases vulnerability to breakdown.

2. Only a fraction of the breakdown we are seeing is actually psychological.

3. A more complete model of stress impacts includes a myriad of common maladies: high blood pressure, high cholesterol, heart disease, diabetes, fibromyalgia, ulcers, acid reflux, allergies, colds, flu, pneumonia, asthma, emphysema, bronchitis, cancer, kidney and liver disease, anxiety, depression, addiction, et cetera (Agnvall, 2014; Blake, 2017).

4. Under the influence of chronic stress, such problems compound, potentially leading to system failure and death.

This becomes even clearer when you take a look at the leading causes of death in modern times: diabetes, cancer, stroke, flu/pneumonia, Alzheimer's, accidents, and suicide (Heron, 2019). They are all potentially mediated by stress, including effects like those mentioned above (e.g., Bisht et al., 2018; Bruce et al., 2015; Everson-Rose et al., 2014; Glaser et al., 2000; Justice, 2018; Kiecolt-Glaser et al., 1996; Lehrer, 2006; Moreno-Smith et al., 2010; Rosiek et al., 2016; Turgeman-Lupo & Biron, 2017; U.S. Department of Labor, n.d.).

In other words, stress is getting to all of us, not just some of us. Quite possibly, as a species, we are dishing out to each other more than any of us can safely take. In a very real way, we are all breaking down. We are all dying—it's just that we're all dying differently.

That only makes sense. Diversity is a strength of our species. Our bodies have different gifts as well as different challenges. Stress feels out frailties and makes the kill from there. Whether mental or physical, however, stress gets most of us in the end.

Now I am at the interface between the gift of stress and the gift of wanting to die. Stress is my body's gift to me. It tries to wake me up to the fact that I'm in over my head and something needs to change. I ignore or kill the messenger at my peril.

Wanting to die is my gift to you. It's my attempt to share with you my sincere and desperate conclusion:

Some conditions and terms of life may not be worthy of the human body, mind, or spirit. I think the culture we live in is deadly.

I have been dying inside from this. Unless something changes, you could be too.

References

Agnvall, E. (2014, November). Stress! Don't Let It Make You Sick. *AARP Bulletin.* Retrieved from https://www.aarp.org/health/healthy-living/info-2014/stress-and-disease.html.

American Museum of Tort Law. (n.d.). The Ford Pinto: Grimshaw v. Ford Motor Company 1981. In American Museum of Tort Law. Retrieved from https://www.tortmuseum.org/ford-pinto/.

Blake, H. (2017, August 9). How Your Body Reacts to Stress. *Smithsonian Magazine.* Retrieved from https://www.smithsonianmag.com/science-nature/what-happens-your-body-when-youre-stressed-180964357/.

Bisht, K., Sharma, K., & Tremblay, M. È. (2018). Chronic stress as a risk factor for Alzheimer's disease: Roles of microglia-mediated synaptic remodeling, inflammation, and oxidative stress. *Neurobiology of stress, 9,* 9-21.

Bruce, M. A., Griffith, D. M., & Thorpe, R. J. (2015). Stress and the kidney. *Advances in Chronic Kidney Disease, 22*(1), 46–53. https://doi.org/10.1053/j.ackd.2014.06.008

Chomsky, N. (2017). The five filters of the mass media. In *Public Reading Rooms: The art of politics and vice versa.* Retrieved from https://prruk.org/noam-chomsky-the-five-filters-of-the-mass-media-machine/.

Deaton, A. (2018, January 24). The U.S. Can No Longer Hide from Its Deep Poverty Problem (Op-Ed.) *New York Times.* Retrieved from https://www.nytimes.com/2018/01/24/opinion/poverty-united-states.html.

Everson-Rose, S. A., Roetker, N. S., Lutsey, P. L., Kershaw, K. N., Longstreth, W. T., Sacco, R. L., Roux, A. V. D., & Alonso, Á. (2014). Chronic stress, depressive symptoms, anger, hostility, and risk of stroke and transient ischemic attack in the Multi-Ethnic Study of Atherosclerosis. *Stroke, 45*(8), 2318–2323. https://doi.org/10.1161/strokeaha.114.004815

Glaser, R., Sheridan, J., Malarkey, W. B., MacCallum, R. C., & Kiecolt-Glaser, J. K. (2000). Chronic stress modulates the immune response to a pneumococcal pneumonia vaccine. *Psychosomatic medicine*, 62(6), 804-807.

Hanretty, C. (2014). Media outlets and their moguls: Why concentrated individual or family ownership is bad for editorial independence. *European Journal of Communication*, 29(3), 335-350.

Heron, M. (2019, June 24). Deaths: Leading Causes for 2017. National Vital Statistic Reports, 68(6). Retrieved from https://www.cdc.gov/nchs/data/nvsr/nvsr68/nvsr68_06-508.pdf.

Justice, N. J. (2018). The relationship between stress and Alzheimer's disease. *Neurobiology of Stress*, 8, 127–133.

Kiecolt-Glaser, J. K., Glaser, R., Gravenstein, S., Malarkey, W. B., & Sheridan, J. (1996). Chronic stress alters the immune response to influenza virus vaccine in older adults. *Proceedings of the National Academy of Sciences of the United States of America*, 93(7), 3043–3047. Retrieved from https://www.ncbi.nlm.nih.gov/pmc/articles/PMC39758/.

Knutson, S. K. (2019). Anatomy of a Suicide: Stress and the Human Condition. *Mad in America*. Retrieved from https://www.madinamerica.com/ 2019/12/anatomy-of-a-suicide-stress-and-the-human-condition/

Kruse, K. M. (2015). *One nation under God: How corporate America invented Christian America*. Basic Books.

Lehrer, P. (2006). Anger, stress, dysregulation produces wear and tear on the lung. *Thorax*, 61(10), 833–834. Retrieved from https://www.ncbi.nlm.nih.gov/pmc/articles/PMC2104758/.

Levy, A. R. (2019, September 16). The Incredible Belief That Corporate Ownership Does Not Influence Media Content. In *Fairness & Accuracy in Reporting (FAIR)*. Retrieved from https://www.commondreams.org/ views/2019/09/17/incredible-belief-corporate-ownership-does-not-influence-media-content.

Mai, J. (2016, February 25). 9 sneaky ways cell phone companies get you to pay more. *Business Insider*. Retrieved from https://www.businessinsider.com/sneaky-ways-cell-phone-companies-get-you-to-pay-more-2016-2.

Moreno-Smith, M., Lutgendorf, S. K., & Sood, A. K. (2010). Impact of stress on cancer metastasis. *Future oncology*, 6(12), 1863–1881. Retrieved from https://www.ncbi.nlm.nih.gov/pmc/articles/PMC3037818/.

National Council for Community Behavioral Healthcare (2011). Breaking the Silence: Trauma-informed Behavioral Healthcare. *National Council Magazine*. Retrieved from https://www.thenationalcouncil.org/wp-content/uploads/2012/11/NC-Mag-Trauma-Web-Email.pdf.

Oliver, M. (1992). *"Wild Geese" in New and selected poems, volume one*. Beacon Press.

Pogue, D. (2010, October 4). Verizon Comes Clean. New York Times. Retrieved from https://pogue.blogs.nytimes.com/2010/10/04/verizon-comes-clean/.

Pogue, D. (2009, July 30). 'Take Back the Beep' Campaign. *New York Times*. Retrieved from https://pogue.blogs.nytimes.com/2009/07/30/the-mandatory-15-second-voicemail-instructions/.

Rosiek, A., Rosiek-Kryszewska, A., Leksowski, Ł., & Leksowski, K. (2016). Chronic Stress and Suicidal Thinking Among Medical Students. *International journal of environmental research and public health*, 13(2), 212. Retrieved from https://www.ncbi.nlm.nih.gov/pmc/articles/PMC4772232/.

Radcliff, P. (2004). Lecture Seven: The Origins of "Mass Society". *Interpreting the 20th Century: The Struggle Over Democracy (Course Guidebook)*. Chantilly, VA: The Teaching Company. Retrieved from http://download.audible.com/product_related_docs/BK_TCCO_000156.pdf.

Reardon, M. (2012, March 27). Why you can't sue your wireless carrier in a class action. In C|Net. Retrieved from https://www.cnet.com/news/why-you-cant-sue-your-wireless-carrier-in-a-class-action/.

Sapolsky, R. M. (2017). *Behave: The biology of humans at our best and worst*. Penguin.

Sapolsky, R. M. (2004). *Why Zebras Don't Get Ulcers, 3rd Edition* (New York: Holt Paperbacks).

Sapolsky, R. M. (2018, November 1). How economic inequality inflicts real biological harm: The growing gulf between rich and poor inflicts biological damage on bodies and brains. *Scientific American*. Retrieved from https://www.scientificamerican.com/article/how-economic-inequality-inflicts-real-biological-harm/.

Social Science Bites. (2018, July 3). Richard Wilkinson on how inequality is bad. In *Social Science Space*. Retrieved from https://www.socialscience space.com/2018/07/richard-wilkinson-on-how-inequality-is-bad/.

Stone, D. M., Simon, T. R., Fowler, K. A., Kegler, S. R., Yuan, K., Holland, K. M., ... & Crosby, A. E. (2018). Vital signs: trends in state suicide rates—United States, 1999–2016 and circumstances contributing to suicide—27 states, 2015. *Morbidity and Mortality Weekly Report*, 67(22), 617. Retrieved from https://www.ncbi.nlm.nih.gov/pmc/articles/PMC5991813/.

Thompson, D. (2011, December 27). Why Does the Wealth Gap Between Congress and Voters Matter?. In *The Atlantic*. Retrieved from https://www.theatlantic.com/business/archive/2011/12/why-does-the-wealth-gap-between-congress-and-voters-matter/250546/.

Turgeman-Lupo, K., & Biron, M. (2017). Make it to work (and back home) safely: The effect of psychological work stressors on employee behaviour while commuting by car. *European Journal of Work and Organizational Psychology*, 26(2), 161-170.

U.S. Department of Labor. (n.d.). Safety and Health Topics / Long Work Hours, Extended or Irregular Shifts, and Worker Fatigue. In *Occupational Health and Safety Administration (OSHA)*. Retrieved from https://www.osha.gov/SLTC/workerfatigue/hazards.html.

Wilkinson, R., & Marmot, M. (2003). *Social determinants of health: The solid facts (2nd ed.)*. Copenhagen: World Health Organization. Retrieved from http://www.euro.who.int/__data/assets/pdf_file/0005/98438/e81384.pdf.

Referring Clients to Stoic Writing Practices: Exploring Principles, Techniques, and Challenges

Kate Hammer and William Van Gordon

Abstract: *Social prescription or community referral is a means for clinicians to refer people to non-clinical local services for meeting a range of social, emotional, and/or practical needs. A novel domain of activities that could be socially prescribed derives from Stoicism, a practical life philosophy from the ancient world that has informed culture and psychotherapy. Research indicates that approaches based on Stoicism can improve emotional clarity, psychological flexibility, and personal death awareness, as well as reduce worry, rumination, and death taboos. Using the example of an open, affordable program called 28 Days Joyful Death Writing with the Stoics, we consider what practical role contemporary Stoicism might contribute to community-oriented mental health and wellbeing provision. More specifically, this chapter discusses the key principles, techniques, and challenges associated with socially prescribing Stoic practices, and proposes future directions for the evaluation of Stoic writing communities for mental health.*

Including community referral in a therapeutic model

The present chapter critically evaluates the rationale for including Stoic writing activities in a clinical practice that is shifting from the medical model of diagnosis towards a more holistic conception of the individual client/patient. We begin with the terminology and therapeutic model.

Social prescribing is a recognized means for referring an individual to "a local voluntary, community and[/or] social enterprise organization" (Polley et al., 2017, p. 14) so that "social, emotional or practical needs" can be addressed by "a variety of holistic, local non-clinical services" (Kimberlee, 2015, p. 105). Such community referrals "view a person not as a 'condition' or disability, but quite simply as a person" (Polley et al., 2017, p. 11).

Viewing clients as persons coheres with critical psychiatry and critical psychology movements to which this volume contributes. Here we apply the synonymic term "community referral" to avoid any authoritative overtones carried by the term "prescribe." The purpose of choosing this term over "signposting" is to engender an integrative approach whereby clinicians and clients form a mutual understanding of a given activity's relevance to therapy.

Underpinning our perspective on community referral is a model for therapy that diverges from the medical model. The contrasting model assumes the client is an active agent of their personal change and the expertise of the therapist is a process expertise, related to the therapist's capacity to be with their client in the here-and-now, come what may. Supported by research findings, Bohart and Tallman (2022) formalize this therapeutic orientation as the meeting of the minds model, characterized in terms of:

- Collaboration between client and therapist, who "cothink, coexperience, and coconstruct strategies and solutions" (p. 35) in a "workplace" the therapist creates where the client has "permission to feel, think, imagine, and solve problems" (p. 36).
- Change results from "creative problem-solving by the client" where ideas and interventions from the therapist are taken as "offerings" each client "sculpts [...] to suit [their] own life context" (p. 35) or "cocreated by client and therapist" (p. 36).

The meeting of the minds model diverges from a model of therapy in which a therapist assigns clients "homework" and gauges client "compliance" with the aim of "treating" resistance.

Benefits are known to arise for both clients and clinicians when activities in the community are integrated into therapy (Chatterjee et al., 2017; Tomlinson et al., 2020). For clients, the community-based activity has the potential to draw the individual's energy and attention both beyond the consulting room and beyond their focus on their problem or suffering.

Furthermore, activities can engage individuals in proto-social or social interchange who might otherwise be isolated (Hughes et al., 2019). Finally, well-chosen activities can elicit the individual's capacities or interests that may have been dormant (Stickley & Hui, 2012).

For clinicians, the community referral process can leverage the benefit of therapeutic activities that the clinician is not themselves initiating or orchestrating. Such benefits are threefold. Firstly, leaving the design and running of the activity to the community provider saves the clinician time and energy. Second, when referring, the clinician avoids the client perceiving them as a stakeholder in the activity, leaving the client more latitude to determine for themselves whether the activity is worthwhile or beneficial. This marks a very different position to the therapist setting "homework" for their client, whereby compliance is implicitly sought (Kazantzis, 2021). Rather, come what may from the client's undertaking, the clinician can stay in a relational space with them, expressing as much empathic concern and interest in a client's reasons for not yet starting or not continuing the activity as required. Third, this neutrality removes the cloud of failure which, in turn, promotes a distance a therapist can use not only for dialogue and rapport, but also to model a healthy self-distance (Kross & Ayduk, 2011).

Stoicism for therapy

A fertile ground for community referral is modern Stoicism. Stoicism, an ancient philosophy of everyday life developed in classical Greece before spreading to the Roman Empire, has endured over centuries as well as influencing major Western philosophers from St Augustine to Adam Smith and Immanuel Kant (Pigliucci, n.d.). Stoicism's key themes include (Farnsworth, 2018):

1. the inevitability of death
2. the limits of personal control
3. the value of developing habits of retrospection, mental rehearsal, and emotional equanimity to become better prepared for life's vicissitudes

Ancient Stoicism was concerned with *eudaimonia*, meaning flourishing. Stoics maintained a worthwhile life could be fashioned by following a middle way between the aristocratic virtue ethics Aristotle taught, and the ascetic minimalism promoted by a rival school called the Cynics (Pigliucci, 2017). Thus, Stoicism, like Buddhism, offers practical wisdom people can apply to their attitudes and daily life practices (Sellars, 2019). Teaching focuses on four core Stoic virtues: wisdom, justice, courage, and temperance (Polat, 2022).

The Modern Stoicism movement takes up Stoic ideals and teachings by applying them in a contemporary context. According to philosopher Massimo Pigliucci (n.d.), Viktor Frankl's logotherapy, Aaron Beck's Cognitive Behavioral Therapy (CBT), and Albert Ellis's Rational Emotive Behavioral Therapy (REBT) provide the roots of Modern Stoicism (see Menzies & Whittle, 2022 for a brief historical summary from a psychotherapeutic perspective; and Robertson, 2018 for a more detailed account).

People encounter Modern Stoicism through online conferences, blogs, books and in-person conferences. Academics in disparate fields—from classics, philosophy, history, to social theory and sustainability studies—contribute to or comment appreciatively on the Modern Stoicism movement (Love, 2021). As a collaboration beginning in 2012 between psychotherapists and academics, *modernstoicism.com* hosts a blog and holds public events, including Stoic Week where participants practice "living as a Stoic." Stoic Week has in turn prompted the development of a Stoic psychometric called Stoic Attitudes and Behaviours Scale, now in its fifth iteration (LeBon, 2020).

For the wider public, Stoic philosophy's revival follows the 1998 publication of Tom Wolfe's novel *A Man in Full* (Rainey, 1999; Wolfe, 1998). In April 2020, Penguin Random House shared annual sales figures for Stoic philosopher Marcus Aurelius' *Meditations*, which steadily increased from 16,000 in 2012 to over 100,000 in 2019 before a rapid upturn during the first coronavirus lockdown (Flood, 2020).

Preparing the ground for this upswelling attention, blockbuster movies have brought Stoic themes to audiences for generations. For example, Frank Capra's classic Christmas film, *It's a Wonderful Life* (1946) strikes a Stoic chord, with its message that a good life is what an individual does, not what happens to them. This theme is more expansively explored in the 1995 film, *The Shawshank Redemption*.

Even more centrally than in *A Man in Full*, *The Shawshank Redemption* is about prison life and the tagline on its movie poster was: "fear can hold you prisoner; hope can set you free." The narrator, the world-weary Red (played by Morgan Freeman) was serving a life sentence, when he takes on the sage role to a younger man Andy Dufresne who was wrongfully imprisoned for a double murder. Red's edict was: "Get busy living or get busy dying." Dufresne incorporates this advice by adopting a dignified and proactive stance to his circumstances while safely navigating his escape from prison.

More explicitly, the *Star Wars* character Yoda resembles a Stoic sage, both in his mentoring of his protégé Luke Skywalker and in his declarations. In *The Empire Strikes Back* (1980), the Jedi Master Yoda explained to an angry Luke, "Fear is the path to the Dark Side. Fear leads to anger. Anger leads to hate. Hate leads to suffering" (quoted Stephens, 2005, p. 19). Later in the film, Yoda coins the aphorism: "Anger… fear… aggression. The Dark Side of the Force are they" (ibid).

For philosopher William O. Stephens, these are vices. Under Yoda's tutelage, wisdom to distinguish the Light Side and Dark Side of the Force will come to young Skywalker when he is "calm, at peace, passive." By passive, we understand Yoda to mean composed and receptive as contrasted with reactive and agitated. Taking up Jedi practices, Luke will cultivate the Jedi virtues. Stephens draws out the philosophical resemblance:

> [T]he virtues the Jedi shares with the Stoic sage are patience, timeliness, deep commitment, seriousness (as opposed to frivolity), calmness (as opposed to anger or euphoria), peacefulness (as opposed to aggression), caution (as opposed to recklessness),

benevolence (as opposed to hatred), joy (as opposed to sullenness), passivity (as opposed to agitation), and wisdom. (2005, p. 22)

These mainstream movies suggest that Stoicism may already be familiar and perhaps even interesting to clients. (See Schulenberg, 2003 about incorporating movie recommendations to clients; and Norcross, 2006 on self-help more broadly).

Stoic writing activities

Stoic philosophy lends itself to writing activities for several reasons. First, Stoicism is a practical philosophy oriented to everyday matters: saving time, friendship, crowds, aging, self-control, riches, fame, travel, grief, ill health, death. The themes are accessible to people from all walks of life and often resonate with people's worries, anxieties, and suffering. Second, the ancient Stoics wrote prolifically. The Roman Seneca, also a playwright, encapsulated his Stoic philosophy in a series of 124 letters addressed to Lucilius Junior, a state official but apparently intended for wider publication. While the *Discourses* of Epictetus were lecture transcripts by his pupil Arrian, the emperor Marcus Aurelius cited Epictetus in the meditations he wrote for himself.

Their legacy is a body of work that has been re-translated through the centuries, that is freely available online. This makes ancient Stoicism readily accessible for personal study and creative transformation.

Using Stoic writings in therapy provides scaffolding for interpretation and introspection. Wright and Chung (2001) define writing therapy as "client expressive and reflective writing, whether self-generated or suggested by a therapist/researcher" (p. 279), and Ruini and Mortara (2022) adopt this definition in their subsequent literature review. Therapeutic writing differs from journaling because it incorporates contents and methodologies whereas for Ruini and Mortara, journaling is freeform.

An example of therapeutic writing is the thought record recommended in standard Cognitive Behavioral Therapy (National Health Service [NHS], n.d.). Thought records are notational and analytic rather than expressive.

As envisaged by Aaron Beck (see Beck et al., 1979), these self-observations contribute to cognitive restructuring.

A contrasting approach is expressive writing. Since the 1980s, social psychologist James W. Pennebaker has studied the influence of expressive writing on traumatic processing and overall health (cf. Pennebaker, 1997). An early champion of clients writing more expressively was poet/ practitioner/researcher Gillie Bolton, who highlighted that writing is "for" and "by" clients, not something done "to" them (qtd. Wright & Chung, 2001, p. 280). Bolton's attitude accords with the therapeutic meeting of the minds model described above. In Bolton's experience:

> People are composed of a stewpot of beliefs, understandings, memories, terrors and hopes. Different elements bubble up at different times, wanting and needing to be attended to. Dealing with these in an appropriate way then and there will lead to a more balanced and happy individual. (1999, p. 200)

Using Stoic passages as a resource in writing therapy can combine the cognitive restructuring and expressive aspects highlighted above. Next, we outline two approaches to Stoic writing: stimulus and copywork.

Stoic stimulus for therapeutic writing

Brittany Polat's book *Journal Like a Stoic: A 90-day Stoicism program* was recently published by Quercus, a division of the major multinational publisher, Hachette Group. The subtitle of Polat's book states its purpose: "to live with greater acceptance, less judgment, and deeper intentionality."

The 90-day writing challenge is organized in three sections, called "courses" entitled:

1. "Examining the Inner Critic"
2. "The Road to Acceptance"
3. "Living with Virtue"

They are intended to be engaged in order. Each section has prompts for 30 days. Polat invites the journaling reader to spend 10-15 minutes each day, choosing either one of the day's prompts with encouragement to "tackle them all if you feel inspired" (2022, p. 29). Each day's journal entry consists of five elements:

1. Prompt title.
2. Ancient Stoic excerpt.
3. 1-2 paragraphs explaining the excerpt for contemporary readers.
4. 2 prompts for introspection and writing.
5. Lined space to write by hand in the book.

For example, the prompt on Day 12 of the "Examining the Inner Critic Course" is titled "Calming Your Nervous System," supported by a 25-word quote from Seneca in a letter to Lucilius about the capacity of someone with a "well-ordered mind" to "linger in their own company" (Polat, 2022, p. 54). One prompt invites the writer to switch off their digital devices and notice how they feel. The other prompt invites the writer to cast themselves into a future where they spend 15 minutes each day in their own company and imagine what they learn about themselves.

In summary, using *Journal Like a Stoic*, an individual can expect to learn something about Ancient Stoicism, become familiar with its most celebrated exponents, and receive focused prompts for introspection. The promise of the subtitle is that, by way of cognitive restructuring and increased self-awareness, shifts are experienced in acceptance, judgement, and intentionality.

To assess the value in therapy of Stoic writing as a response to informative stimuli oriented towards self-awareness and self-conduct, it is worth taking a moment to consider how a practical philosophy such as Stoicism is learned. According to Owen (2020), the model of information processing is complex because it involves declarative knowledge, procedural knowledge, and reflective knowledge. "Knowing that" is the basic form where familiarity can stimulate recognition. "Knowing how" is more demanding because familiar principles need to be applied in action, and the experience reflected upon for integration to occur.

To take the Day 12 prompt above, I can only know I can satisfactorily "linger in" my "own company" if I try in practice, repeatedly. *How it is for me to attempt this self-presence -- if I am recovering from heartbreak or loss, lonely in an unfamiliar place, socially isolated by dint of deprivation, disability, or exhaustion -- is a theme I could bring to my therapy session. Maybe self-companionship evades me, but the passage sparks in me an aspiration about developing or regaining a "well-ordered mind" possessed of this capacity to be in good company alone? Or perhaps in contemplating the excerpt, I recollect the peace and connection I've previously felt in the company of an animal I can stroke and tend? And in so recollecting, I resolve to include in my "own company" a pet I adopt or borrow? Or I realize I can linger alone best in nature.*

Stoic copywork

Stoic copywork as defined by Kathryn Koromilas offers another way to access Stoic wisdom. Copywork is the term for copying word for word a passage by hand. In more archaic schooling, it was one means by which children learned handwriting, spelling, grammar, and rhetoric. The value now of copywork is that it engages the hand as the first step towards the writer taking ownership for and eventually restating ancient wisdom in their own words. The reformulation of standard passages can be profoundly creative (see Hammer & Gordon, 2023).

Koromilas includes copywork in the Stoic training program offered online she created called *28 Days of Joyful Death Writing with the Stoics. 28 Days* uses email and a web app called Slack to create a temporary community of Stoic contemplators. An identical daily email prompt is sent to each a participant (see Figure 1).

The prompt contains a passage by the Roman emperor Marcus Aurelius, the facilitator's reformulation of it, and recommendations for activities involving contemplation and copywork (see Figure 1). All participants encounter the same passages from Marcus Aurelius' *Meditations* each day. Everyone decides whether to participate in a wholly solitary way or to also enter the community. This dual character adds a level of complexity and richness to the solo Stoic journaling discussed above.

Each day, a participant faces the decisions: Do I open the email? Do I engage the activity? Do I reflect on the passage I've copied, or do I also reformulate it? On Slack, people can share their daily reflections and respond to one another using text, emojis, images and web links. Sharing reformulations and reflections online draws the solitary introspection into a community setting where people can spark off one another. When I enter the Slack channel, do I share my reformulation of the day's passage? Or have I come only to read the reformulations or commentaries on others' posts? Do I comment on what others have posted, or do I read only? If someone reacts or responds to what I post, do I engage them?

Some participants will move easily between solitary and sharing modes, others will weigh up how they engage and how openly they disclose their own contemplations (Hammer & Gordon, 2023). Moreover, meditations and activities vary day by day. Therefore, each day a participant may find themselves answering these participation questions in different ways.

Time's passage becomes a factor in the group experience because the prompts will arrive daily, and the Slack community will eventually close. As the program progresses, email subject lines count down from 28, which serves as a memento mori (a reminder that the end is coming).

The benefits of "a dose of Stoicism"

A study conducted by the present authors into daily Stoic writing highlights writers' experiences undertaking copywork using meditations from Marcus Aurelius in *28 Days* (Hammer & Van Gordon, 2023). Participants were adults over aged 18, fluent in English and who were not currently experiencing mental distress or at risk of self-harming. Data was not collected relating to whether participants were currently or had ever been in therapy. Overall, participants reported three types of gain:

1. Beneficial behaviors and activities: daily exercise, focused attention (contrasted with distraction), friendship, and engaging in a collegial way with other people.
2. Positive experiences and emotions: calm, equanimity, at-homeness, joy, delight, freedom, sense of reinforcement, and intimate connection with others.
3. Purpose: life priorities, sense of calling, life meaning, resolve, and commitment.

28 Days of Joyful Death Writing with the Stoics

5 Days Left . . .

Today's meditation is from Marcus Aurelius's Meditations, Book 7.6, about our legacy.

> All those once remembered are now forgotten
> and those who remembered them are gone too.

Legacy

When my time is up, who will remember me? How will I be remembered? What will I be remembered for? However much I try, I cannot control whether others will remember me or think about me when I'm not around. I can't even control that while I'm alive.

So, I need to rethink what legacy means to me and how important being remembered is. As soon as I make it important, I can feel the tension arise inside me. As soon as I make it unimportant, desirable sure, maybe, but not something my well-being depends on, then I feel relief. Then I can stop worrying and start living.

We say we'd like to live on beyond the grave. But what if we change that to living before the grave? In this case, if we live good lives now, if we focus on what is right, if we care for our community, if we excel in our own personal way, we will live lives worthy of being remembered. If we happen to be remembered, we will be remembered for being excellent humans. If we are forgotten, we will still have been excellent humans.

Today's Writing Exercise

If you have 5 minutes

- Read the above meditation (here or in the translation of your choice) out loud.
- Write down a single keyword or phrase to capture this meditation.
- Two or three times during the day, repeat this keyword or phrase.

If you have 10 minutes

- The above, plus copywork. Copy out the meditation word for word; slowly, attentively, meditatively.
- Try to memorise a portion of it.
- Try recalling this meditation throughout the day.

If you have 20-60 minutes

- The above, plus reformulation. Summarise and/or reformulate (reexpress/rewrite) the meditation using your own words and voice. Try to memorise.
- Personal, expressive writing. Set the timer for 5-10 minutes.
  - Respond to Marcus Aurelius's meditation.
  - Write about being forgotten.
  - How does this feel?
  - Reframe this as Marcus Aurelius might, come up with a helpful thesis.
  - Reflect on this. How does this death contemplation help?

Don't forget your daily 5-second practice

Two or three times during the day, just as you are about to enjoy something or someone you love, say this to yourself: '*Tomorrow, you will die.*' We will repeat this little mental exercise for 5 seconds once or twice a day for the entire 28 days.

28DaysOfJoyfulDeathWriting.com

Figure 1: *Sample Prompt by Kathryn Koromilas for 28 Days*

The Stoic "dichotomy of control" expresses the idea that individuals are not responsible for their circumstances but are responsible for the attitudes they adopt and the actions they take (however circumscribed the options). One study participant eschewed copywork because of physical discomfort when writing and, instead, reflected daily on the prompts:

> I've found that process of: "OK, what are we going to do today? How much of this do I control? How much of it is outside my control? What my *will* towards this will be. What my attitude to all this will be." That's sort of becoming a practice and I think receiving this message every day kept that in the forefront. (Hammer & Gordon, 2023, p. 20)

Another participant wrote daily, posted in the Slack channel, and discussed her *28 Days* experience with a friend outside the group. She subsequently reported that her "daily dose of Stoicism" changed the attitude she brought to interactions with her mother which had previously been stressful. These are examples of psychological flexibility. Additionally, participants spontaneously spoke about life, relationships, and self-worth. In doing so, they identified and described distinct emotions.

Furthermore, *28 Days* confronted participants with the finite nature of life and the inevitability of death. A participant confronted evanescence: "The breath that you've had is the breath that you'll never get back, and that probably was the biggest revelation coming out of that 28 Days" (Hammer & Gordon, 2023, p. 15). Faced with finitude, the question of values became paramount to this participant: "Right, Harry, what are you doing and why are you doing it?" he asked himself and repeated in the interview (p. 18). Other participants found the taboo about death they carried "dissolved," or how the infirmities they experienced due to aging or disease could be reframed in Stoic terms about the inevitability of decay (ibid, pp. 17-18). A further participant followed Marcus Aurelius in her resolve to exit life gracefully and subsequently wrote a death plan she shared with her adult children.

In terms of psychological processes underpinning these benefits, Terror Management Theory posits that morality salience inductions impact us, even below our conscious awareness (Solomon et al., 2015). The kind of mortality salience induction Stoic writing activities provide is one that "encourage[s] participants to think about death with acceptance or curiosity" (Pyszczynski et al., 2015, p. 56). Stoicism teaches that all things die, including people, and none of us are exempt. This makes the death contemplation personal and concrete, not general and abstract.

For this reason, it can be likened to the death reflection concept advanced by Cozzolino which promotes "open and authentic considerations of death" (Cozzolino et al., 2014, p. 419). Cozzolino's model posits that when fear of death and denial of death are low, self-esteem, self-concept clarity, locus of control, self-realization, and existential well-being are high. Cozzolino et al. (2014) also assert that self-actualization predicts death acceptance, although of course in the present chapter we are regarding the correlation from the other direction: does cultivating death acceptance through Stoic contemplation contribute to self-actualization?

More modestly, we could assess Stoic writing's impact on the development of emotional clarity (Gohm & Clore, 2000), emotional freedom from the persistence of negative emotions (Park & Naragon-Gainey, 2020), and psychological flexibility while bearing in mind that the Acceptance and Commitment Therapy (ACT) paradigm regards psychological inflexibility as a major contributor to psychopathology (Hayes et al., 2006).

Cautions and contraindications

Stoic writing activities will obviously not suit all clients or contexts and key considerations in this regard include the following:

- Suicidality. Safety plans and authentic co-presence take precedence. The client should feel unconditional positive regard for them in their suffering without feeling this is in any way dependent on their engaging in semi-structured activities or introspective writing.
- Cognitive capacity. If an individual's capacity is diminished by disability, exhaustion, or illness, the demands of learning and introspection may be too burdensome. Use a lighter touch in introducing Stoic themes.

- Self-image. If an individual's self-image is organized around perceived low status or victimhood, focus first on fostering their capacity and agency. When they are more empowered, titrate Stoic ideas as prompts for discussion. If they like the material, invite them to journal or do copywork/reformulation.
- Repetition can lead to rumination. Lyubomirsky et al. (2006) found reduced well-being in individuals after they wrote about their happiest moments. Similarly, Pennebaker and Evans (2014) found the act of writing can increase cognitive rumination by emphasizing negative thoughts and feelings.

Limitations and barriers

People who have internet access, a willingness to write, and a curiosity about the paradox of "joyful death writing" may be surprised at what participation in a program like *28 Days* brings. Even less coordination is required to undertake Stoic journaling following the program Brittany Polat outlines as it is self-guided (Polat, 2022).

Both designs make scaling relatively easy. However, it is important to be realistic about the limitations and barriers of community-based Stoic writing and solitary Stoic journaling. Consequently, the following outlines six limitations and barriers to Stoic writing activities, which are divided in terms of writing communities and writing activities:

1. Community writing presupposes linguistic homogeneity. In settings where a single language is not shared to a proficient or fluent level by all participants, a solitary writing therapy approach may be more suitable.
2. Not everyone feels entitled to write expressively. Pennebaker and Evans (2014) make the link between interpersonal exposure through expressive writing and feelings of shame and embarrassment. Susceptibility may be tied to individual differences but, equally, there may be a cultural dimension at play. Ruini and Mortara's (2022) narrative review of the research highlights that individualistic and collectivist cultures differently value self-expression even of gratitude towards others. Bungay et al. (2023)

summarizes group dynamics in Arts on Prescription programs while Wakefield et al. (2019) highlights the harmful impact of in-group divisions.

The next set of concerns pertain both to community and solitary writing:

3. Reading, reflecting, and responding to Stoic prompts takes time and quiet surroundings. Not everyone can regularly accommodate this in their daily lives, particularly if their living situation is crowded or unstable or if their domestic workload is high.

4. Sharing writing can be stressful. The academic associations with writing being "graded" can make it hard for people to willingly share what they write due to lack of confidence, feeling fragile or nervous. One way to address this is to turn the dialogue towards the individual's experience of reflecting and reformulating rather than their estimation of what they ultimately wrote. The focus needs to be on the experience the individual has of writing, not its perceived merits in the eyes of individuals with power in the system. Bungay et al. (2023) emphasize the importance of withholding stigma and judgement to enable play and exploration.

5. It follows that neither the writing facilitator nor therapist should assume a role of literary critic.

The final barrier may impede both clinicians and clients taking up Stoic writing activities. This is the stereotype of a Stoic as being emotionally repressed. For example, in the psychology of interpersonal relationships, small-s stoicism has been defined as triple lack of emotional involvement, emotional expression, and emotional spontaneity (Wagstaff & Rowledge, 1995). The same deficit model was used in a recent study by Johnson and Samp (2021) into overt aggression and partner-directed violence occurrences when pent-up emotion is released.

A negative view of stoicism also appears in health psychology and sociology studies. For example, Moore et al. (2013) catalogued studies where patient stoicism was labelled as a maladaptive coping strategy— while for others, such as Pathak et al. (2017), it was a belief system. Overall, psychologists' negative evaluation of "being stoic" combined with the vagueness of the term has contributed to a gap in knowledge about the potentially beneficial application of explicit Stoic philosophic principles and practices to well-being.

An example of how stereotypes about Stoicism are widespread can even be seen in the way Thomas Newman, the highly successful composer of *The Shawshank Redemption,* named the song accompanying the prison scenes "Stoic theme." Music critic Jonathan Broxton (2004) describes the "downbeat" tune as "a grinding bass passacaglia to underline the drudgery of life in the slammer." If drudgery and downbeat are the connotations people bring to Stoic writing, whether clinicians or clients, they may be disinclined to spend their time trying it.

Future directions

We'll learn more about possibilities and pitfalls of introducing Stoic writing activities into the lives of people undergoing therapy as it becomes more commonplace. Research into therapeutic writing/expressive writing research can provide one set of benchmarks and contemplative psychological research can provide another. For example, Lyubomirsky and others (2006) developed experimental writing, thinking, and replaying study designs and applied them with university students. Their studies found that positive life events and negative life events evoke different responses depending on how they are engaged by the study design.

The analytic activities evinced in the writing activity reduced the beneficial impact of wonderful life moments, which were savored when replayed but not written; whereas analysis and sense-making were beneficial when applied to negative life events, although replaying those negative events led to rumination. Consequently, the authors concluded as follows:

> Our research suggests that systematic step-by-step analysis (which presumably tends to occur while writing or speaking) is worthwhile and beneficial when directed at unhappy, stressful, or traumatic life events, but may be harmful when applied to happy times. In contrast, repetitive, circular replaying (which presumably is inclined to occur during private thought) is somewhat advantageous when

the target is one's highest moment, but may be damaging when the target is one's lowest ebb. (Lyubomirsky et al., 2006, p. 706)

In other words, there is no one-size-fits-all when it comes to the benefits of rendering life experiences in speech, writing, or mental recollection. Similarly, in the subfield of emotional studies, emotional clarity and attention to emotions may coordinate differently for positive and negative emotions (Boden & Thompson, 2017).

Given that Stoic writing activities engage analysis, thinking and replaying, using writing prompts that also confront people with a mix of emotions (e.g., joy, delight, grief, and loss), the expressive writing and positive psychology study paradigms may not be suitable. Appropriately designed future studies are therefore needed to shed light on the inner processes involved in Stoic reflection.

Mindfulness and self-compassion training efficacy study designs (Kotera & Van Gordon, 2021) provide useful examples. Mixed methods study design is recommended by Chatterjee et al.'s (2017) systematized review of non-clinical community interventions studies. To evaluate the impact of Stoic writing activities on clients, a pre-post within-subject study could use a range of instruments, including those useful in assessing within-subject impact such as:

1. The 9-item Acceptance and Action Questionnaire which uses a 7-point Likert scale (Hayes et al., 2004).
2. The 36-item Difficulties in Emotional Regulation Scale which uses a 5-point Likert scale (Gratz & Roemer, 2004).
3. The 46-item Existence Scale assessing personal fulfilment which uses a 6-point Likert Scale (Längle et al., 2003).
4. The 14-item Warwick-Edinburgh Well-being Scale which uses a 5-point Likert Scale (Tennant et al., 2007).

Since the cohorts in experimental studies of Stoic writing activities are likely to be small, robustness of findings will be limited (Cooper et al., 2022). Nonetheless, as in all innovative undertakings, starting small and soon is probably advisable. As Epictetus wrote in his Discourses 1.2.37b: "We don't abandon our pursuits because we despair of ever perfecting them." Instead of perfection, strive for progress instead. Progress, as Marcus Aurelius reminds us, is a daily matter.

References

Beck, A., Rush, J., Shaw, B. F. & Emery, G. (1979). *Cognitive Theory of Depression*. Guilford Press.

Boden, M. T., & Thompson, R. J. (2017). Meta-Analysis of the Association Between Emotional Clarity and Attention to Emotions. *Emotion Review, 9*(1), 79–85. https://doi.org/10.1177/1754073915610640

Bohart, A. C. & Tallman, K. (2022). Client expertise: The active client in psychotherapy. In J. N. Fuertes (Ed.) *The other side of psychotherapy: Understanding clients' experiences and contributions in treatment* (pp. 13-43). American Psychological Association. https://psycnet.apa.org/doi/10.1037/0000303-000

Bolton, G. (1999). *The Therapeutic Potential of Creative Writing: Writing Myself.* London: Jessica Kingsley.

Broxton, J. (2004). The Shawshank Redemption -Thomas Newman. Movie Music UK. https://moviemusicuk.us/2004/09/23/the-shawshank-redemption-thomas-newman/

Bungay, H., Jensen, A., & Holt, N. (2023). Critical perspectives on Arts on Prescription. *Perspectives in Public Health*, 175791392311707. https://doi.org/10.1177/17579139231170776

Chatterjee, H. J., Camic, P. M., Lockyer, B., & Thomson, L. J. M. (2017). Non-clinical community interventions: A systematised review of social prescribing schemes. *Arts & Health, 10*(2), 97–123. https://doi.org/10.1080/17533015.2017.1334002

Cooper, M., Avery, L., Scott, J., Ashley, K., Jordan, C., Errington, L., & Flynn, D. (2022). Effectiveness and active ingredients of social prescribing interventions targeting mental health: A systematic review. *BMJ Open, 12*(7), e060214. https://doi.org/10.1136/bmjopen-2021-060214

Cozzolino, P. J., Blackie, L. E., & Meyers, L. S. (2014). Self-related consequences of death fear and death denial. *Death Studies, 38*(6), 418-422.

Farnsworth, W. (2018). *The Practicing Stoic: A philosophical user's manual*. David R. Godine Publishers.

Flood, A. (2020, April 16). "Dress rehearsal for catastrophe": How Stoics are speaking to locked-down readers. *Guardian*. https://www.theguardian.com/books/booksblog/2020/apr/16/how-stoics-are-speaking- to-locked-down-readers

Gohm, C. L., & Clore, G. L. (2000). Individual differences in emotional experience: Mapping available scales to processes. *Personality and Social Psychology Bulletin, 26*(6), 679– 697. https://doi.org/10.1177/0146167200268004

Gratz, K. L., & Roemer, L. (2004). Multidimensional assessment of emotion regulation and dysregulation: Development, factor structure, and initial validation of the difficulties in emotion regulation scale. *Journal of Psychopathology and Behavioral Assessment, 26*(1), 41–54. https://doi.org/10.1023/B:JOBA.0000007455.08539.94

Hammer, K., & Van Gordon, W. (2023). Joyful Stoic Death Writing: An Interpretative Phenomenological Analysis of Newcomers Contemplating Death in an Online Group. *Journal of Humanistic Psychology*, 00221678231178051. https://doi.org/10.1177/00221678231178051

Hayes, S., Strosahl, K., Wilson, K. G., Bissett, R. T., Pistorello, J., Toarmino, D., Polusny, M. A., Dykstra, T. A., Batten, S. V., Stewart, S. H., Zvolensky, M. J., Eifert, G. H., Bond, F. W., Forsyth, J. P., Karekla, M., & McCurry, S. M. (2004). Measuring experiential avoidance: A preliminary test of a working model. *The Psychological Record, 54*(4), 553-578. http://dx.doi.org/10.1007/BF03395492

Hayes, S. C., Luoma, J. B., Bond, F. W., Masuda, A., & Lillis, J. (2006). Acceptance and Commitment Therapy: Model, processes and outcomes. *Behaviour Research and Therapy, 44*(1), 1–25. https://doi.org/10.1016/j.brat.2005.06.006

Hughes, S., Crone, D. M., & Sumner, R. C. (2019). Understanding well-being outcomes in primary care arts on referral interventions.pdf. *European Journal for Person Centered Healthcare, 7*(3). http://www.ejpch.org/ejpch/article/view/1768

Johnson, E. P., & Samp, J. A. (2021). Stoicism and Verbal Aggression in Serial Arguments: The Roles of Perceived Power, Perceived Resolvability, and

Frequency of Arguments. *Journal of Interpersonal Violence.*
https://doi.org/10.1177/0886260521994583

Kazantzis, N. (2021). Introduction to the Special Issue on Homework in
Cognitive Behavioral Therapy: New Clinical Psychological Science.
Cognitive Therapy and Research, 45(2), 205–208.
https://doi.org/10.1007/s10608-021-10213-9

Kimberlee, R. (2015). What is social prescribing? *Advances in Social Sciences
Research Journal, 2*(1). https://doi.org/10.14738/assrj.21.808

Koromilas, K. (n.d.). *28 Days of Joyful Death Writing with the Stoics.*
http://28daysofjoyfuldeathwriting.com/

Kotera, Y., & Van Gordon, W. (2021). Effects of Self-Compassion Training on
Work-Related Well-Being: A Systematic Review. *Frontiers in Psychology, 12,*
630798. https://doi.org/10.3389/fpsyg.2021.630798

Kross, E., & Ayduk, O. (2011). Making Meaning out of Negative Experiences
by Self-Distancing. *Current Directions in Psychological Science, 20*(3), 187–
191. https://doi.org/10.1177/0963721411408883

Längle, A., Orgler, C., & Kundi, M. (2003). The Existence Scale. *European
Psychotherapy, 4*(1), 135–151.

LeBon, T. (2020). *Report on SMRT 2020: Stoicism is not all about the stiff upper lip.*
Retrieved from:
https://www.researchgate.net/publication/344284690_Report_on_SMRT_2
020_Stoicism_is_not_all_about_the_stiff_upper_lip

Love, S. (2021, June 29). The revival of Stoicism. *Vice.*
https://www.vice.com/en/article/xgxvmw/the-revival-of-stoicism

Lyubomirsky, S., Sousa, L., & Dickerhoof, R. (2006). The costs and benefits of
writing, talking, and thinking about life's triumphs and defeats. *Journal of
Personality and Social Psychology, 90*(4), 692–708.
Pennehttps://doi.org/10.1037/0022-3514.90.4.692

Menzies, R. E., & Whittle, L. F. (2022). Stoicism and death acceptance:
Integrating Stoic philosophy in cognitive behaviour therapy for death
anxiety. *Discover Psychology, 2*(1), 11. https://doi.org/10.1007/s44202-022-
00023-9

Moore, A., Grime, J., Campbell, P., & Richardson, J. (2013). Troubling
stoicism: Sociocultural influences and applications to health and illness

behaviour. *Health: An Interdisciplinary Journal for the Social Study of Health, Illness and Medicine, 17*(2), 159–173. https://doi.org/10.1177/1363459312451179

National Health Service (n.d.). Better Health. Thought Record. https://www.nhs.uk/every-mind-matters/mental-wellbeing-tips/self-help-cbt-techniques/thought-record/

Norcross, J. C. (2006). Integrating self-help into psychotherapy: 16 practical suggestions. *Professional Psychology: Research and Practice, 37*(6), 683–693. https://doi.org/10.1037/0735-7028.37.6.683

Owen, J. (2020). Understanding Stoic and Epicurean ethical 'training' in light of the DPR model. *Ancient Philosophy Today, 2*(2), 145–170. https://doi.org/10.3366/anph.2020.0033

Park, J., & Naragon-Gainey, K. (2020). Is more emotional clarity always better? An examination of curvilinear and moderated associations between emotional clarity and internalising symptoms. *Cognition and Emotion, 34*(2), 273–287. https://doi.org/10.1080/02699931.2019.1621803

Pathak, E. B., Wieten, S. E., & Wheldon, C. W. (2017). Stoic beliefs and health: Development and preliminary validation of the Pathak-Wieten Stoicism Ideology Scale. *BMJ Open, 7*(11), e015137. https://doi.org/10.1136/bmjopen-2016-015137

Pennebaker, J. W. (1997). Writing about emotional experiences as a therapeutic process. *Psychological Science, 8*(3), 162-166. http://www.jstor.org/stable/40063169?origin=JSTOR-pdf

Pennebaker, J. W. & Evans, J. F. (2014). *Expressive writing: Words that heal.* Idyll Arbor.

Pigliucci, M. (n.d.) Stoicism. In *Internet Encyclopedia of Philosophy.* Retrieved 20 May 2022, from https://iep.utm.edu/stoicism/

Pigliucci, M. (2017). *How to be a Stoic: Ancient wisdom for modern living.* Rider/Penguin Random House Group.

Polat, B. (2022). *Journal Like a Stoic: A 90-day Stoicism program to live with greater acceptance, less judgment, and deeper intentionality.* Quercus.

Polley, M. J., Fleming, J., Anfilogoff, T. & Carpenter, A. (2017). *Making sense of social prescribing.* London University of Westminster. Retrieved from:

https://westminsterresearch.westminster.ac.uk/item/q1v77/making-sense-of-social- prescribing

Pyszczynski, T., Solomon, S., & Greenberg, J. (2015). Thirty years of terror management theory. In *Advances in Experimental Social Psychology* (Vol. 52, pp. 1–70). Elsevier. https://doi.org/10.1016/bs.aesp.2015.03.001

Rainey, J. (1999, March 11). A new season of Reason. *Los Angeles Times*.

Robertson, D. (2018). *The Philosophy of Cognitive-Behavioural Therapy (CBT): Stoic Philosophy as Rational and Cognitive Psychotherapy*. Routledge.

Ruini, C. & Mortara, C. C. (2022). Writing techniques across psychotherapies – From traditional expressive writing to new positive psychology interventions: A narrative review. *Journal of Contemporary Psychotherapy*, 52, 23-34.

Sellars, J. (2019). *Lessons in Stoicism: What Ancient Philosophers Teach Us About How to Live*. Penguin.

Schulenberg, S. E. (2003). Psychotherapy and Movies: On Using Films in Clinical Practice. *Journal of Contemporary Psychotherapy, 33*(1), 35-48.

Solomon, S., Greenberg, J., & Pyszczynski, T. (2015). *The worm at the core: On the role of death in life*. Penguin Random House.

Stephens, W. O. (2005). Stoicism in the stars: Yoda, the Emperor, and the Force. In K. Decker & J. Eberl (Eds.), Star Wars and philosophy (pp. 16-28). Open Court Publishing. Retrieved from: https://philarchive.org/rec/STESWA

Stickley, T., & Hui, A. (2012). Social prescribing through arts on prescription in a UK city: Participants' perspectives (Part 1). *Public Health, 126*(7), 574–579. https://doi.org/10.1016/j.puhe.2012.04.002

Tennant, R., Hiller, L., Fishwick, R., Platt, S., Joseph, S., Weich, S., Parkinson, J., Secker, J., & Stewart-Brown, S. (2007). The Warwick-Edinburgh Mental Well-being Scale (WEMWBS): development and UK validation. *Health and Quality of Life Outcomes, 5*(1). https://doi.org/10.1186/1477-7525-5-63

Tomlinson, A., Lane, J., Julier, G., Grigsby-Duffy, L., Payne, A., Mansfield, L., Kay, T., John, A., Meads, C., Daykin, N., Golding, A., & Victor, C. (2020). Qualitative findings from a systematic review: Visual arts engagement for adults with mental health conditions1. *Journal of Applied Arts & Health, 11*(3), 281–297. https://doi.org/10.1386/jaah_00042_1

Wagstaff, G., & Rowledge, A. (1995). Stoicism: Its Relation to Gender, Attitudes Toward Poverty, and Reactions to Emotive Material. *Journal of Social Psychology, 135*(2), 181–184.

Wakefield, J. R. H., Bowe, M., Kellezi, B., McNamara, N., & Stevenson, C. (2019). When groups help and when groups harm: Origins, developments, and future directions of the "Social Cure" perspective of group dynamics. *Social and Personality Psychology Compass, 13*(3), e12440. https://doi.org/10.1111/spc3.12440

Wolfe, T. (1998). *A Man in Full.* Farrar, Straus & Giroux.

Wright, J. & Chung, M. C. (2001). Mastery or mystery? Therapeutic writing: A review of the literature. *British Journal of Guidance and Counselling, 29*(3), 277-291. http://dx.doi.org/10.1080/03069880120073003

Sense and Nonsense in Psychotherapy — and Some Possible Solutions

Louis Wynne

Abstract: *The creation of practical alternatives to the current treatment of the so-called mentally ill must begin with changing the way we talk about it. This chapter argues that the language we presently use is ill-conceived and based on long-standing cultural misconceptions regarding the brain, thinking, dreaming, deviance, and the place of the profession of medicine in dealing with distressing conduct. The reader is introduced to the definition of illness in general; the metaphorical nature of mental illness; the representational and the pragmatic approaches to language; and the First Person and Third Person universes of discourse. Within this framework, the brain is shown to be irrelevant; the use of medications dangerous and ineffective; the existence of the Diagnostic and Statistical Manual of Mental Disorders useless; why some techniques within the armamentarium of the psychologist are also ineffective; and which others deserve more emphasis. The key concept from which all distressing conduct derives is trauma — in all its variegated versions — and it is this concept on which clinical psychologists should place their entire therapeutic emphasis.*

Throughout the western world, mad people have for centuries been seen as sick — as having a special kind of illness called *mental* illness. Claudius, Hamlet's uncle, says of his nephew, "Madness in great ones must not unwatched go." More to the point to be made in this chapter, the author of the Shakespearian Canon noted that madness is beyond the scope of a physician's practice (Macbeth, Act V, Scene 1). And, when the Inquisition commanded Saint Teresa of Avila to turn over her charges to them for "treatment," she refused, saying that they acted "*as if* they were sick."

The situation today, several hundred years later, is little different. The subtitle of Szasz' *The Manufacture of Madness* (1970) says it well: *A Comparative Study of the Inquisition and the Mental Health Movement.* My direction in this chapter will be to insist that we must change the way we talk about the so-called mentally ill. That is, we will start by making a study of the language we use when we talk about human behavior, generally, and deviant behavior, specifically.

I begin with the wry assertion, in agreement with Lewis Carroll's Cheshire Cat, that *we are all mad here*. I, the author of this piece, am mad; you, dear reader, are also mad; and so is everyone else. What differentiates us from each other, and whether or not we are invidiously labelled "mentally ill," is how well each of us deals with the mad-making environments that we are all living in.

Just because a person is brought, usually forcibly, to a mental health facility does not automatically mean that the person is mad and in need of a mental health professional. Quite frequently, in my evaluation of applicants for services, I find that the person might be better off retaining a lawyer.

We must stop using the term "mental illness." To medicalize deviancy is to encourage the use of the physician's armamentarium: drugs, psychiatric commitment, electroconvulsive stimulation, et cetera, and to overlook the psychological impacts on the individual of violence, alcohol, loss in the family, and excessive demands for compliance with usually unspoken family rules as well as general societal factors such as unemployment, homelessness, and discrimination.

In dealing with conduct distressing to others, *we are not confronting any sort of illness*. Szasz (2001) noted the schema laid out by Rudolph Virchow in 1847 that in order for an ailment to be considered an illness, it must meet four criteria:

  (a) consistent symptoms between patients presumed to have the illness
  (b) a predictable course
  (c) tissue pathology
  (d) etiology

No so-called mental illness meets more than the first of these criteria—and even that one is open to question. Indeed, many *medical* illnesses don't meet all of them either. Many diseases are merely agglomerations of symptoms. I discussed the term "mental" itself in my review of Szasz' *The Meaning of*

Mind (Wynne, 2005) and I will not repeat that discussion here but will simply assert that *there is nothing happening inside the head of a healthy, uninjured, functioning human being that is of any interest to a behaviorist.*

One might ask—is the mind not inside the head? No, it is not. The mind occupies neither time nor space, and the word "mind" is a *linguistic contrivance born of the human need for a sense of agency*—that each of us is in control of our existence. A few examples: "I've made up my mind;" "I changed my mind;" "Pay it no mind;" "You've been on my mind;" "I'll keep it in mind;" "I lost my mind;" and, "I have half a mind to…"

This contrivance is related to our notion of free-will, a religiously-inspired concept: without it, how can we be held accountable in our final judgement? Both the Jewish and Christian traditions, as well as recent Western philosophers (chiefly, German and French) have taught us to believe that there is within each of us an entity that motivates and energizes our otherwise inert bodies. Where this entity is located was originally thought to be in the heart, but for the past two millennia it is generally acknowledged, *on the basis of the flimsiest of data,* to be located in the brain. We call this "thing" the mind and, for some, it seems in a vague way to be related to something called the soul.

These issues were lurking long before they were brought to prominence by Gilbert Ryle in his *The Concept of Mind* (1949); by Thomas Szasz, MD in his *The Myth of Mental Illness* (1960); and by Iris Murdoch in her dissertation on Sartre (1953) in which she quotes Dostoyevsky's atheist character Kirillov as saying, "I would like to believe in free will. I just haven't been able to find even a single example of it!" I raise these issues here to point out that, until some resolution of them is reached, they will continue to roil and confuse our attempts to bring order out of the chaos that is our mental health system.

Mental illness, then, is a metaphor—a *dead* metaphor. That is to say, a metaphor that has been in common use for so long that it is no longer recognized as such—even by behavioral scientists. This oversight has for at least a century led us down many blind alleys in our efforts to deal with madness.

There are two conceptualizations of language. The more popular by far is *representational*; that is, words *mean* something. They refer to, or designate, things in the real world. The study of these meanings is called semantics. The second conceptualization is *non-representational*. It sees words as tools by which we deal, more or less effectively, with the world and the people in it. This view of language was incorporated into the only philosophy originating in the New World: the pragmatism of William James, America's first psychologist. Conceiving of language in this way makes it easy to make the following distinction.

Every language is comprised of two vast universes of discourse: the Third-Person and the First-Person. Understanding this distinction is vital to any rethinking of so-called mental illness. We employ Third-Person discourse when each of us talks about the world outside our skins: the world of people, animals, and their activities—and objects, large and small, as well as their behaviors. It is the language of sports and of the sciences such as physics, chemistry, biology, botany, geology, zoology, and that part of psychology known as behaviorism. (I believe that "cognitive science," behaviorism's chief competitor as psychology's philosophy of science, is a contradiction in terms.)

The second universe is First-Person discourse, the language each of uses when we are talking about our own experiences: our thoughts, dreams, feelings, emotions, needs, fears, urges, memories, impressions, and preferences. It is the language of drama, tragedy, comedy, music, theater, poetry, literature, theology, and broadcast journalism (with its emphasis on, "How did you feel when . . .?"). It also includes all of our statements about the future: our plans, objectives, wants, goals, wishes, and desires.

This means that, as the title of Chapter 5 in *Warm Logic* (Wynne and Klintworth, 1990) points out, the future is fictitious. But it is not that statements about the future have no *referents*; it is the more pragmatic view that statements purporting to be about the future cannot be used to help us deal reliably with the present. This is why we treat the predictions of stock market analysts with suspicion!

First-Person discourse is also, significantly, the discourse that our clients are employing when they tell us why they are coming to us for help. However, as we therapists respond to what our clients say, *we must not be seduced into using First-Person discourse with them.* To fall into that trap (no doubt to convince them that we are empathizing with them) is to threaten our attempts to help them.

Our task is ultimately to shape their discourse to match our own—to focus their attention where it can do the most good. This can best be done with the simple admonition: "Don't look inward—look outward!" That is: what is happening in your world; what has been happening to you that you have been unable to change; indeed, that people close to you have prevented you from changing—often by confusing you regarding what you *should* want or how you *should* feel. *Time spent talking to clients about their feelings of anger, depression, anxiety, et cetera is time wasted.*

The most serious confusion occurs when we go from one universe to the other without realizing it. In such a way, one might say, "Such a horrendous act can only be the product of a diseased or sick mind." This sounds reasonably intelligent apropos to the situation it presumably describes, and it would probably be accepted with little question by a court as expert testimony.

It is, however, intellectual drivel because it conflates terms from the two universes of discourse. The term "disease" or "sickness" belongs in the Third-Person universe. Its symptoms are observable by anyone—often including the person who has the disease. The term "mind," on the other hand, belongs in the First-Person universe because it is "observable" only by the person whose mind we are talking about. It is even a stretch to say that one sees or knows his/her *own* mind. Knowing one's own mind is nothing more than one more figure of speech of dubious value.

Readers familiar with the writings of Wittgenstein and, especially, of his student, Drury (1996), will remember Drury's distinction between Psychology A: the writings of such people as Tolstoy, Simone Weil, and Simone de Beauvoir; and Psychology B: the work of, say, Uttal (2001) and

Sarbin and Mancuso (1980) — a distinction much in agreement with the one I am proposing here.

Within the field of psychology there are two major groups of techniques that have been developed to remediate the unwanted behaviors of madness. The first enjoyed enthusiastic support in the 1960s and 70s although there were earlier attempts in this direction by such psychologists as Knight Dunlap, author of *Habits: Their Making and Unmaking* (1932). I refer here to applied behavior analysis, also called behavior modification. My paper, "The Missing Theory" (Wynne, 2004), emphasized the chief weakness of this approach: unwanted behaviors are frequently not operants; that is behaviors that are reinforced or punished by the history of their consequences.

One clue why this is so, is that symptoms of intra-familial stress usually appear full-blown, usually in mid- to late-adolescence, rather than being shaped over a long period of time through successive approximations. Hence, the futility of using operant techniques with autism, with the gluttony of Prader-Willi syndrome, or with the conduct labelled schizophrenia. Of equal importance is that, while some aspects of the client's distressing conduct might be operant, these are usually *avoidant* and highly resistant to extinction — and they give rise to a variety of symptoms along the continuum of "anxiety": thumb-sucking in children, panic, phobias, trichotillomania, obsessive and compulsive conduct, hoarding, and visceral and other somatic complaints.

To illustrate, I ask the reader to consider the conversation that took place recently between two experimental subjects in an operant conditioning chamber, also known as a Skinner box, after its inventor. Scene One of this scenario begins with a white rat alone in the chamber. There is a bar set into one of the walls of the box that, if pressed, operates according to two random parameters. The first is the Shock-Shock Interval: the amount of time programmed to elapse between electric shocks delivered to the rat through a grid on the floor of the box *if the bar in the wall is not pressed.* The second parameter is the Response-Shock Interval: the amount of time programmed to postpone the next shock *following the rat's pressing the bar.*

Scene Two begins after several months with the introduction into the box of a second rat. The rats sniff each other, and then Rat 1 goes over and presses the bar.

> Rat 2: "What are you doing?"
> Rat 1: "I'm pressing the bar. What does it look like I'm doing?"
> Rat 2: "Yes, I can see that, but why?"
> Rat 1: "'Cos if I don't, we're both gonna get shocked, and I assure you, you won't like that one bit!"
> *And Rat 1 presses the bar again.*
> Rat 2: (After a short pause during which Rat 1 presses the bar two or three more times) "There's something you ought to know. Please stop pressing the bar while I tell you this!"
> Rat 1: "No, I can't!"
> Rat 2: "Look! Just before the psychologist put me in here with you, I saw her pull the plug out of the wall. So you don't have to press the bar any longer. The circuit is broken!"
> Rat 1: "I don't believe you!"
> Rat 2: "Why should I lie to you? If I'm lying, I'll get shocked, too!"

The question is: How long will it take Rat 1 to realize that Rat 2 is telling the truth, and that the shocks will no longer occur? The answer: a very long time. And, in the meantime, Rat 1 will suffer much anxiety and other symptoms, and might even fight with his partner to press the bar. This is the challenge the psychotherapist has in trying to help the client who has been for many years on a schedule to avoid pain—from an abusive parent or an alcoholic partner—who now might even be deceased.

The second group of techniques in the repertoire of the psychologist is the myriad of verbal methods called psychotherapy, and much of the remainder of this chapter deals with these. But first, I note in a brief aside that *language*, the vehicle by which psychotherapy is carried on, is a field to which academic psychology has paid scant attention: there is no division within the American Psychological Association called the Division of Language. How ironic that humanity's one idiosyncratic attribute—its most obvious defining characteristic—continues to be explicitly abjured by that august body!

One consideration that we must pay attention to in our search for practical alternatives is what happened in the 1980s in addition to the advent of DSM-III. This includes the sweeping changes toward the "medical model" that included a wild expansion of the number of psychiatric diagnoses health insurance companies would support, and the parallel expansion that continues to this day of the number of psychiatric drugs made available to "treat" these diagnoses.

In this regard, therapists are enjoined to use only "evidence-based treatments"—a self-serving slogan used by the constituencies benefitting from the current arrangements. If the professional community did indeed consider the all the evidence accompanying the use of neurotoxic drugs in the treatment of the so-called "mentally ill" (especially the pernicious side-effects), we would stop using them immediately! More generally, one may surmise that the astronomical increase in obesity in the US is not due to Americans' lack of exercise or poor diet so much as it is our profligate use of prescription drugs, one of whose side effects is weight gain.

The 1980s also saw the disappearance in America—in all but the large coastal cities—of Sigmund Freud's psychoanalytic approach to human behavior. This did not occur because of its perceived patriarchal emphasis, although feminism certainly played a part in its demise. More importantly were that Freud's views of the unconscious, et cetera, went very much against the American grain, and his views would have eventually disappeared, social revolution or not.

We Americans are, after all, Children of the Enlightenment—that French world-view standing firmly on the Primacy of Nature (think of the current prevalence of the climate-change movement, and the almost universal presence in TV commercials of greenery having nothing to do with what is being sold); the Inevitability of Progress (our preoccupation with national decline); and most of all that human beings are "Rational." It is this last point that I think is wrong (and that Freud was right).

I believe we are *not* governed chiefly by Reason. Our Enlightenment culture has taught us that thought precedes—is indeed *necessary*—to action. René Descartes even went so far as to assert that thinking was the only thing he could be sure of: "I think, therefore I am," a statement *par excellence* within the First- Person universe of discourse. But "thinking" is demonstrably separate from, although it frequently accompanies—and even follows, action. As I noted in my review of Szasz' *The Meaning of Mind* (2005), thinking while playing the piano or baseball is a guarantee you'll do neither very well.

To make the most consequential choices in our lives, we might make up lists of pros and cons, but in the end we will "go with our guts": whether or not to marry someone; whether to have a baby now (or ever); whether to move to Florida; et cetera. Yes, we would like to see ourselves as rational but, to borrow a current quandary from the AI world, we have already designed computers "smarter,"—that is, more rational—than we are! This is because intuition, which is seen as non-rational, cannot be, at least now, coded into them.

It might be more fruitful to adopt the approach of the Indian mystics who say that we do not have either dreams or thoughts—they have us. And, whether behaviorists realize it or not, this is a view close to their own perspective. Further, while thoughts and dreams can be conceptualized alongside the five senses (touch, taste, hearing, vision, and smell), there is one very important difference. We know the locations in the brain where vision and hearing are located, but where are thoughts located? There are neuroscientists who believe that "executive function" is located in the frontal cortex—and in the past, there were those who believed that the disordered thinking of people labelled "schizophrenic" could be ameliorated by a lobotomy in that area. Indeed Egas Moniz, MD, the chief promoter of that barbaric procedure, was awarded the Nobel Prize for his efforts!

I suggest, on the contrary, that we have not been able to locate thoughts, disordered or normal, in the brain because we are looking in the wrong place. *How* we have looked—that is, by damaging the brain—deserves a chapter all its own but consider the ridicule we would suffer if we were to experimentally damage the liver or the thyroid in attempts to discover their contribution to intellectual activity. We do not do such experiments because we have already decided *in advance* that the brain is where purposive actions are initiated.

Our belief that thoughts are a product of brain activity is, then, ultimately an act of faith dating back to Homer (but not before, when the heart was seen as the locus of cognition), and well-established in our language and our gestures. For example, we scratch or tap our heads when trying to remember something. One may say that the English language is woefully inadequate when it comes to dealing with what B. F. Skinner (1953) called "private events." Indeed, Wittgenstein noted that there is no such thing as a private language. My own linguistic preference is to say paradoxically that *our bodies have minds of their own!* I also like Woody Allen's remark in his film, *Manhattan:* "The brain is the most overrated organ."

More important than Freud's anti-Enlightenment views, though, has been the vacuum their disappearance left behind: psychological approaches to so-called mental illness are no longer informed by any theory of deviancy. This leaves the field in the hands of psychiatry whose theory of deviance is "chemical imbalance"—an idea as old, outdated, and ill-conceived as Hippocrates.

Perhaps the most eloquent statement of the current state of affairs regarding deviancy was the late Senator Daniel Patrick Moynihan's article, "Defining Deviancy Down" (1993), in which he noted just how much conduct, unconventional and societally disapproved of just a few decades ago, is now accepted as conventional if not entirely approved of. Consider tattoos, from the simple and amateurish to the elaborate and artistic (and expensive), covering much of the bodies of women.

One might have anticipated that the acceptance of bizarre and distressing behavior would lessen the prevalence of mental illness, but the opposite seems to be true. There seems to be no limit to the number of dubious illnesses with which pharmaceutical companies seek to frighten the gullible: "You might have ABC disease!" and to encourage them to, "Ask your doctor if Chemical X may be right for you!"

We should initiate change in the mental illness racket by examining just what brings the client to the psychologist in the first place, and the following approach is based on my own experiences over a fifty-year period beginning in 1973 as a statistician in a large multifaceted mental health center; then as Clinical Director of a 626-bed inpatient psychiatric hospital; as a surveyor of mental health and substance abuse clinics and hospitals for the Joint Commission on Accreditation of Healthcare Organizations (JCAHO); as Co-Editor-in-Chief of a professional journal; as an examiner of applicants for social security disability benefits; and, for the past 35 years, as a solo practitioner in an outpatient psychotherapy clinic serving adults.

I usually ask a new client: Why do you need someone like me to solve your problem? Why can't you solve it yourself? The question is rhetorical; the reason the client can't solve the problem is that his/her initial statement of it is not the actual problem. He/she has already been taught to verbalize his/her difficulties in terms of diagnoses, (e.g., "I'm bipolar.")

No. It is far more likely that there have been for years, operating within the family of origin, values and rules that unobtrusively and subtly function to prevent the client from acting in his/ her own best interest. This is the thrust of my *Healing the Hurting Soul: A Survival Manual for the Black Sheep in Every Family* (Wynne, 2008). Over the next few sessions with the client, I point out, for example, that episodes of panic very likely result from the client's unwitting moves that contravene these family rules. It is important to realize that labelling such a client with anxiety, psychosis, or bipolar disorder adds nothing to our knowledge of either how he/she developed these troublesome behaviors, or what sort of intervention would likely be effective with them.

A large group of clients present as depressed—a condition best seen within the context of the client's history. Many of these clients were unwanted children, but it is not a good move to ask that question straight out. Instead, the client should, in what one of my colleagues calls my Socratic technique, be asked questions such as, if s/he were the firstborn of the sibship:

- "How soon after your parents married were you born?" "Were they married then?"

- "As far as you know, did your mother's pregnancy with you alter any career plans she had?"
- "Were they happily married, or did the pregnancy glue together a relationship that your mother was not sure of?"
- "Did your grandparents welcome your parents' marriage and your mother's pregnancy with you?"

Or, if s/he was the last-born of the sibship:

- "Was your mother's pregnancy with you planned, or had she decided she didn't want any more children, and you were an accident?"
- "Did your mother ever have a miscarriage or an abortion? When?"

Note how this approach—of asking questions that search for details in the history of the client's family—is different from the conventional approach of many clinical psychologists and psychiatrists. Their approach has been to make a frontal assault on the anxiety, depression, intrusive thoughts and urges, et cetera of the new client. Behavior modification, cognitive behavior modification, systematic desensitization (now called "exposure therapy"), and biofeedback have been four such techniques employed by psychologists, while the wholesale use of neurotoxic drugs has long been the stock-in-trade of American psychiatry.

To what end? As I pointed out in *Healing the Hurting Soul*, psychiatric outcomes in third-world countries, where psychiatric medications are used as a last resort, are better than in advanced countries where drugs are the first response and are consumed almost by the bushel. Indeed, as I have already intimated, one of America's best-kept secrets is that our epidemic of obesity is largely the result of widespread drug use.

As this chapter was in preparation, the latest drug "breakthrough" was one for postpartum depression. I am sure there are many reasons why this tragic condition occurs, but one I have seen that will *not* be resolved by any drug is the mother's deep ambivalence over having the baby. However, in our drug-besotted culture, I'm betting that the new drug will be the *first*, possibly the only, mode of intervention.

Symptoms leading to society's labelling people as mentally ill do not just *happen*. They are *caused*, sometimes in the short-term, but more often over a long period of time beginning in early childhood and, whenever possible, the intervention should attack those presumed causes. For example: when a veteran of convoy duty in Iraq was unable to drive between towns in the southwestern US because of strong visceral responses and stomachaches, I suggested he post a sign on his vehicle's dashboard: "This is NOT Iraq!" The technique, by helping him to discriminate his situation, ameliorated the symptoms.

When a client is clearly, often by his/her own admission, the family black sheep, I suggest posting a sign on the refrigerator or the bathroom mirror such as, "Nancy's feelings don't count for anything in this family." Such a sign would likely infuriate members of her family, but this fury is a validation of the sign's truth, and it is part of the price that must be paid by the client as she regains her sense of autonomy and dignity. I call this note-posting technique "directed discrimination"—statements of reality that have brought about the client's confusion, anxiety, gastric disturbances, depression, or even violence and psychosis. These realities have been vehemently denied or even hidden by the family, so that they are not discriminated by the client and have, therefore, remained "unconscious."

There are some symptoms that are particularly resistant to all treatment regimens. Most obdurate is dissociation—the report by both the client and his/her family that there are periods of time during which s/he seems to the family to be functioning normally but of which s/he has no memory. This seems to occur most frequently in women who were repeatedly molested over several years from early childhood until puberty by one or more family members but, when these women appealed to their mothers for help, they were called liars, sluts, or whores. Frequently, they were put in foster care. Do I need to add that the probability of molestation in foster care is not insignificant? I have also seen dissociation in men but, again, there was sexual abuse in their histories.

Why dissociation is very difficult to treat directly is that the therapist does not know that an episode is occurring, and the client only knows when his/her close associates tell him/her following an episode that, "We just talked about that!" My solution has been to listen sympathetically and assure the client that I believe every word of his/her account of the trauma. And I encourage him/her to cry and say, "You have not cried enough."

Probably the most important obstacle the effective therapist has to overcome is the client's own beliefs regarding not only the problem but also what therapeutic procedures are likely to be effective. The more the client has investigated—in popular books and magazine articles or on the Internet—what s/he believes his/her problem to be, the more difficult is the therapist's task. The therapist should remember that *psychotherapy is not an intellectual exercise, a debate, or a lecture.* It is not, as Sigmund Freud's patient, Anna O., said, "The Talking Cure." Its goal is to help the client to *feel* again, to shed the suit of armor s/he put on as a defense against further hurt.

Indeed, I characterize psychotherapy as "emotional reconditioning" that *can* be achieved by talking but better by exposing the client to certain films. My favorite for men is Jack Lemmon's Oscar-winning performance in *Save The Tiger.* For women, I recommend Mary Tyler Moore's equally heart-rending performance in *Ordinary People.* Katharine Hepburn in *The African Queen* shows how a meek and submissive spinster can be transformed into a confident, assertive, and unafraid modern woman. Another film, one that portrays what I call Sigmund Freud's Oedipus Complex in reverse, is the adaptation of D. H. Lawrence's *Sons and Lovers* with Trevor Howard and Wendy Hiller.

The Oedipus Complex was Freud's use of Sophocles' play, *Oedipus Rex,* to demonstrate his belief that little boys—unconsciously, of course—want to kill their fathers and marry their mothers. My experience with hundreds of cases suggests the reverse: a mother wants (unconsciously) to sideline her son's father and forge a tight bond with her son, usually the first-born. This frequently results in the son's stunted emotional and sexual development. Pointing this out to a mother will, of course, be hotly denied, and could cost the therapist his/her client. Pointing it out to the father will likely be received with a wry smile and a nod.

Almost all behavioral deviance emerges from family issues—which are currently being dealt with through the forced drugging of the "identified patient" under the euphemism of Assertive Community Treatment (ACT) or drugged incarceration in an inpatient psychiatric facility. Unfortunately, for the family's black sheep, the clinical intervention in such facilities is meager and formulaic with every inpatient receiving the same one-size-fits-all round of daily medication and group therapy. It should not be surprising, then, that little if any improvement in the client's functioning is accomplished there—beyond what might have been achieved from a stay of equal length at a local 3- or 4-star hotel. Despite the prevailing belief that an inpatient stay is psychiatry's most intensive level of care, a once- or twice- weekly outpatient session with a psychologist is actually much more intensive.

Much of the improvement I have seen in clients in any venue, including psychiatric long-term care units, has been due to what I call non-specific effects. This is very much in line with the observations of Hubble, Duncan, and Miller (1999) who wrote that as much as 40% of the success of psychotherapy is due to events happening during the episode of care over which neither the therapist nor the client had any control or could have predicted. This observation has led me to discourage clients from setting goals. Objectives can destroy spontaneity and the opportunity to take advantage of unforeseen developments.

Clients do get better in therapy, but they do so in ways neither they nor their therapists could have predicted. In addition, roughly 30% of client improvement is, according to Hubble and colleagues (1999), due to the quality of the relationship between the therapist and client—another non-specific effect. In other words, we should deal with clients, especially those in long-term care units, as we would deal with anyone else. One of my greatest successes was with a long-term, very disturbed inpatient—psychotic and enuretic—whose only characteristic we shared was a love of cigars!

As we have already seen, clients usually express their difficulties in terms of a diagnosis, but they also use the vaguely defined terms of First-Person discourse: depressed, anxious, phobic, obsessed, irritable, guilty, frustrated, angry, et cetera. In either case, the psychologist's primary task is *not to give advice,* but to re-focus the client *outward* to the environments presumed to have elicited these uncomfortable feelings.

The client should be encouraged to look, first, to the current situation at home, at work, and in the world at large—and then to the salient historical events of her/his life (particularly the traumatic events), some of which might well have occurred before the client was born (e.g., the mother's earlier miscarriage, the death of a child by accident or unrecognized illness, or the death of the client's father during the mother's pregnancy). The list of possibilities is endless, and the therapist must be relentless in hunting them down.

Some of these might not even be known to the client, their having been kept secret from him or her—but they are often suspected, and the client will be guarded about revealing what are seen as family secrets. In this regard we must acknowledge that it is the *family reactions to trauma* that are significant, and that the most important communications within a family are frequently non-verbal: giggles, glances, frowns, smiles, shrugs, ignoring, gifts, not caring for others' things that have sentimental value, etc.

Many family secrets, often revealed in these gestures, emerge in response to the therapist's question: Why were you treated differently from your siblings? It might turn out, for example, that the person the client was raised to think was his/her mother was actually not. This was revealed to one of my clients first by my asking such questions as: which parent do you look like? ("neither"); do you look like any of your siblings? ("no").

Summarizing, then, much can be done to help the so-called "mentally ill" by:

1. Ending the use of the term "mental illness." Why not just call them "emotionally damaged"?
2. Abolishing the *Diagnostic and Statistical Manual of Mental Disorders.* We should return to something like the *DSM-II* classificatory scheme, but explicitly based on trauma.
3. Providing (ideally by the state) residential facilities, meals, transportation, and a telephone so that applications for

psychological intervention can be accomplished independently of their families' coaching from the sidelines.

4. Closing all inpatient psychiatric hospitals.
5. Funding, preferably by the state, psychological interventions to permit:
   a. more than 60 minutes per session
   b. more than one session per week
   c. day treatment for severe cases
6. Permitting prospective clients to seek help without a referral from a physician.
7. Recognizing that "going off medications" is an action beneficial to the client and not something to be vilified.
8. Training psychologists to:
   a. illuminate the part played in the lives of their clients by early childhood trauma
   b. train their clients to focus outward rather than inward
9. Separating the evaluation function from the psychotherapy role.
10. Separating interventions with the so-called mentally ill from substance, including alcohol, abusers.
11. Re-establishing orphanages to replace the foster care cottage industry.
12. Funding the services of lawyers to advocate on behalf of the so-called mentally ill in commitment and foster care proceedings.
13. Abolishing the insanity defense.

References and Suggested Readings

Deutscher, G. *The Unfolding of Language.* New York: Henry Holt, 2005.

Deutscher, G. *Through the Language Glass: Why the World Looks Different in Other Languages.* New York: Henry Holt, 2010.

Drury, M. O'C. *The Danger of Words and writings on Wittgenstein.* Dulles, VA: Thoemmes Press, 1996.

Edelstien, M. G. *Symptom Analysis: A Method of Brief Therapy.* New York: W. W. Norton, 1990.

Hubble, M. A., Duncan, B. L., and Miller, S. D., Eds., *The Heart and Soul of Change: What Works in Therapy*. Washington, DC: American Psychological Association, 1999.

Moynihan, D. P. Defining Deviancy Down. *The American Scholar, 1993, 62 (1),* 17-30.

Murdoch, I. *Sartre*. London: Bowes and Bowes, 1953.

Ryle, G. *The Concept of Mind*. London: Hutchinson and Co., 1949.

Sarbin, T. R., and Mancuso, J. C. *Schizophrenia: Medical Diagnosis or Moral Verdict?* New York: Pergamon, 1980.

Skinner, B. F. *Science and Human Behavior*. New York: Macmillan, 1953

Szasz, T. S. *The Myth of Mental Illness: Foundations of a Theory of Personal Conduct*. New York: Hoeber-Harper, 1961.

Szasz, T. S. *Law, Liberty, and Psychiatry: An Inquiry into the Social Uses of Mental Health Practices*. New York: Macmillan, 1963.

Szasz, T. S. *The Manufacture of Madness: A Comparative Study of the Inquisition and the Mental Health Movement*. New York: Harper and Row, 1970.

Szasz, T. S. *Insanity: The Idea and Its Consequences*. New York: Wiley, 1987.

Szasz, T. S. *The Meaning of Mind: Language, Morality, and Neuroscience*. Westport, Ct., Praeger, 1996.

Szasz, T. S. *Pharmacracy: Medicine and Politics in America*. Westport, CT., Praeger, 2001.

Uttal, W. R. *The New Phrenology: The Limits of Localizing Cognitive Processes in the Brain*. Cambridge, MA: MIT Press, 2001.

Wynne, L., and Klintworth, C. S. *Warm Logic: The Art of the Intuitive Lifestyle*. El Paso, TX: Skidmore-Roth Publishing, 1990.

Wynne, L. The Missing Theory. *Ethical Human Psychology and Psychiatry,* 6 (2), Summer 2004, 135-146.

Wynne, L. Review of Szasz, T. S., *The Meaning of Mind: Language, Morality, and Neuroscience*. In *Ethical Human Psychology and Psychiatry,* 7 (2), Summer 2005, 167-171.

Wynne. L. *Healing the Hurting Soul: A Survival Manual for the Black Sheep in Every Family*. 2008.

Yoho, R. *Butchered by "Healthcare:" What to do about Doctors, Big Pharma, and Corrupt Government Ruining Your Health and Medical Care.* Pasadena, CA: Amazon, 2020.

Zmora, N. *Orphanages Reconsidered.* Philadelphia: Temple University Press, 1994.

The Evolution of Lifestyle Today: Prescribing Wellness Versus a DSM and ICD Diagnosis

Maria Malayter

Abstract: *The Industrial Revolution shifted into an information society which transformed how our economy operates. With the world of work changing, how has this impacted everyday living? It leads to the question about the scope of the Diagnostic and Statistical Manual of Mental Disorders (DSM) and International Classification of Disease (ICD) diagnosis process, and its evolution to meet the changes of the lives of individuals today. This chapter proposes an evolutionary assessment taken from a different academic discipline for a multiple dimension wellness view for living well. This perspective is taken from academic certificate programming for health and wellness promotion and sport kinesiology professional medical coaches. The chapter will explain the ten dimensions of wellness and include a couple of short vignettes where the core issue for the client was wellness, not a DSM diagnosis. It advocates for a more thoughtful investigation of wellness dimensions.*

"In life, the only constant is change" — this is a phrase often heard to help cope with changes. We live in a volatile, uncertain, complex, and ambiguous (VUCA) world. Yet, we have still not moved away from opening conversations with colleagues in other academic disciplines to discover how they view adaptations to changes that impact our wellness. This can often lead to discussions about various diagnoses in the *Diagnostic and Statistical Manual of Mental Disorders (DSM)* or *International Classification of Diseases (ICD)* when, instead, adaptations could be varying responses to the many dimensions of wellness.

The way we live and work has shifted as we moved from an agricultural society through four different industrial revolutions. We started with factory manufacturing, moved to technological manufacturing, and then to digital manufacturing. As of 2016, we are in Industry 4.0—artificial intelligence (AI) manufacturing. AI is quickly evolving and there are benefits, but also risks—the unknown—perhaps necessitating the need for policies or regulations. The truth is we have already embraced using AI almost every day as we determine how to travel via car with individual phone navigation systems. We are continuing to adapt to the changes of society.

In 1985, Warren Bennis and Bert Nannus, both management scholars teaching at the Army War College, created the acronym VUCA (which stands for volatile, uncertain, complex, and ambiguous) as a way of viewing the world. Maybe VUCA was not relevant on the assembly lines with the factory workers of the first Industrial Revolution in the Ford Motor plants as these were simpler, more predictable times. Yet, in 2020, VUCA was at the foreground as our way of working and living became disrupted by a major global pandemic.

Though the information society was prevalent before this time, the global society created a new economic way of being, communication pattern, and world of work. In December 2020, there were 350 million daily users of the Zoom technology platform for work, school, and basic communication. This is a world we are still learning about every moment as we are continuing to create and learn with video communication being a part of many individuals' daily lives. We are a true information and knowledge society, full of innovation which our lifestyles have been changing to adapt to.

This global VUCA event dramatically changed the way we live, work, and communicate. This chapter explores crossing the academic disciplines to share wisdom from the knowledge models of public health and sports kinesiology perspectives on approaches to living well. There are a variety of ways to live well. Together, we must create a multidimensional pathway to good living that is beyond a simple and narrow diagnosis.

After all, we are more than one narrow answer—we are complex beings with vast lives in a VUCA world that is ever-evolving. We need to look at how our lifestyles have evolved when we think about an individual's wellness and pursuit of good living in today's world.

Lifestyle Changes

In our developed country of the US, we have moved to a technological and information-based society that has greatly impacted our lifestyles. No longer are we working in the farmer's fields as laborers or on the factor's manufacturing line. Many jobs have greatly changed due to advances in technology which have also impacted on our education system. Children are introduced to technology before they even enter the traditional school system. The increased screen time impacts how they operate in the world. The variations of technological user knowledge can create disconnects across generations and lifespan development. This impacts every system in our society.

Since many workers have been able to alter their work location to be flexible—from a required in-office environment to the home—workers can be employed in any country yet live anywhere in the world. We have many variations of hybrid working models that impact the structure of the workplace. This globalization of the world of work has significantly shifted our lifestyles. One can no longer assume everyone is eating dinner at the same time as they may be still on their normal work shift or sleeping. We no longer have the psychological contract of the workplace being 8 am to 5 pm, we may or may not have a commute, and our adaptability to these changes is still occurring.

We have also emerged as a service economy. The quest for more in our culture has created more stress within everyday lives resulting in routine tasks, like grocery shopping, being automated. There was a time where it was vitally important for a family to make time to gather and sit down for dinner. Yet now, the restaurant service economy industry has expanded. It is easy for people to choose to have food delivered or they may go out to eat more frequently. This impacts all levels of our wellness dimensions, and where understanding the whole individual's lifestyle related to the various dimensions of wellness is very important.

The cell phone has significantly changed how we live. US culture is striving for the American Dream while working toward various achievements—they become more accessible with the global connections available through the tiny device in our hands. While technology speeds up many processes, it has also sped up our lives for achievement, evolving into a *doing* versus *being* society. The beverage market has come alongside to support the "go" culture with an increase of sold caffeinated beverages (with the global caffeinated beverage market expecting to reach $310.5 billion by 2025).

Where does wellness fit into these societal changes? How do these changes impact our wellness? We continue to experience a VUCA world and adapt—and so, our knowledge of wellness needs to increase.

Success and Being Well: The History of Wellness Dimensions

Being successful and being well has been taught in leadership development curriculums and community organizations for many years. As early as the 1900s and perhaps before, social and civic organizations connected their membership development programming to creeds of ways for well-being in life and living on purpose.

Individuals successful in life—like the founder of Ralston Purina Foods, William Danforth—wrote books about how to be the best leader with a strong sense of well-being through balanced living among mental, physical, emotional, and spiritual dimensions. Maintaining good health and well-being was one of the great measures of succeeding as a leader and in life. Nowadays, leaders cultivating environments of wellness for their employees is becoming more important as workers want a healthy working environment.

The multiple dimensions of wellness began from the studies of the medical doctor, Dr. Bill Hettler, in the 1970s and 1980s at the University of Wisconsin-Stevens Point. He had oversight of the health center, witnessed the various levels of wellness among university students, and wondered what areas of life students were thriving in.

This led to the creation of a multidimensional model for wellness with the following six dimensions: physical, intellectual, social, spiritual, occupational, and emotional.[1] Hettler continued his quest for the study of multi-dimensional wellness which led to its inclusion in academic studies of health promotion, public health, health sciences, sports, and kinesiology. It also led to the launch of a professional association named the National Wellness Institute aimed to further build up both the research and wellness profession.

Defining the Ten Dimensions of Wellness

There are many academic disciplines that define and study wellness, ranging from public health, psychology, IO psychology, social work, counseling, kinesiology, medicine, and even theology. How do you define wellness? Through years of extensive research studies on various populations and the compilation of various academic disciplines, wellness definitions have moved beyond the four and six dimensions. As such, the key to understanding is how wellness is *operationalized*.

When medical board-certified health and wellness coaches from the National Board Certification of Health and Wellness Coaches review an individual's state of wellness, they assess several dimensions. Through extensive empirical research across various populations, Dr. Francis Ardito, renown research scientist, sport physiologist, and creator of the Wellness Registry, expanded the definition of wellness to ten dimensions[2] to provide a wider range of an individual's wellness. The ten dimensions of wellness are:

1. Physical
2. Nutritional
3. Social
4. Emotional
5. Spiritual
6. Intellectual
7. Environmental
8. Occupational
9. Financial
10. Protectoral

---

[1] https://nationalwellness.org/resources/six-dimensions-of-wellness/
[2] https://hthu.net/wp-content/uploads/2018/05/cwa-and-pca-flyer.pdf

Physical Wellness

The physical aspect of wellness is related to an individual's state of their physical body and how it operates for daily living. Many people think of wellness and immediately think of the physical aspect—they think about the absence of disease.

There are many ways to consider the perspectives of physical wellness. Of course, the immediate baseline for physical wellness is the ability to care for oneself and their own daily personal activities. An individual needs to maintain a certain level of physical movement in their daily lives to remain well enough to continue their daily activities. While many people may relate physical wellness to extensive workouts, physical wellness can be as minimal as including ten- or fifteen-minute segments of movement throughout the day. The main key to physical wellness is to move.

Another aspect of physical wellness includes building a relationship with a primary care physician to maintain consistency in obtaining a yearly physical checkup. Creating a baseline of biometrics is vital to understanding when there might be changes occurring in one's own physical health. A basic physical with routine blood work is a good way to keep track of one's physical condition and to prevent chronic diseases.

Sleep is an important part of an individual's physical wellness. While it has been recommended for every person to get eight hours of sleep per night, it is important for each person to learn what their body specifically needs to function at their optional level. When a person does not get enough sleep, they will have challenges in understanding situations clearly, and emotions may have less regulation. The lack of sleep may create long-term health problems.

Nutritional Wellness

The nutritional aspect of wellness is related to how an individual consumes the right amount of food and water to sustain one's life. There are basic standards of water and food consumption each day that will be sufficient for a person to remain healthy. The nutritional needs will vary from person to person, making it challenging to provide one-size-fits-all dietary recommendations. The US Food and Drug Administration (FDA) recommends a diet of food and beverages that are nutrient dense and to monitor caloric intake.

The consumption of water is vital to our wellness. Civic Science[3] reports that almost half of Americans (47 %) consume far below (only three glasses of water per day) the recommended amount. This may create dehydration where the following symptoms could occur: headaches, extreme thirst, fatigue, dizziness, and confusion. Each person is different in the required adequate intake for water, and it may be different across the lifespan. Additionally, when people drink an excess of water, they may be flushing out nutrients in their body.

When a person is looking to lose weight, it is often encouraged to increase water to a significantly larger amount. There is a curbing of appetite by drinking more water as a person may think they are hungry but are in actuality thirsty. However, this can cause the person to accidentally drink too much water and flush out nutrients being consumed with food.

Social Wellness

The social aspect of wellness is related to the amount of time spent with family, friends, or engaging within the community. Engaging with others is an important part of wellness. We are naturally social beings, whether we are interacting in person or virtually. We like to interact and be socially engaged with others. The topic of belongingness is part of this aspect of wellness—individuals need to feel seen and heard as a part of their social wellness.

Therefore, social wellness is measured through actively engaging with others. It is natural to want to connect and converse with others and share life, whether it be the simple "hello" at a grocery store or a text via the phone. People need us and we need people. Social engagement can be achieved through many ways in our everyday local community or even through electronic communities, such as Twitch or Discord. Zoom

---

[3] https://civicscience.com/forty-seven-percent-of-americans-dont-drink-enough-water-plus-more-h2o-insights/

meetings can still connect us across the globe keeping us socially engaged on a large-scale level.

Emotional Wellness

The emotional aspect of wellness is related to an individual's understanding of their own emotions, expression of emotions, self-awareness, and self-regulation. There are many people who only understand basic emotions of happy, sad, and mad—and researchers of the 20th century have mainly focused on fear, sadness, anger, and joy. Yet, emotions are much wider than these few emotions. Studies are blending and mixing emotions to expand beyond the widely used Positive and Negative Affect Schedule (PANAS). Emotions are not that simplistic—and are an important part of our wellness.

Emotional wellness is knowing and understanding individual feelings. Learning how to work with personal emotions is also an aspect of emotional wellness. Some individuals may have varying levels of emotional wellness based upon how they have learned how to express or repress their emotions. There are also aspects of how an individual regulates their emotions in responding to situations that are also included in the dimension of emotional wellness.

Spiritual Wellness

The spiritual aspect of wellness is related to an individual's perception of having a sense of purpose in life, connecting with nature, or belonging to a spiritual group. The term spirituality is often connected to religiosity, though they can be different. Religiosity involves a belief in a God (or Gods) and participation in activities connected to these beliefs. The individual's belief in God may or may not be connected to organized religion.

Conversely, spirituality is a personal and unique experience for every individual. For some, connecting with their spiritual wellness can be found in natural settings. The individual may feel a spiritual connection to the earth and, specifically, within their experience of being away from larger urban areas. The individual might find peace by walking on a long path in the snow, on a sandy beach, or through a forest of evergreens. The individual might also feel like they are part of a greater aspect of life as they experience nature.

Spiritual wellness relates to understanding an individual's own values and how they connect them to their behavior in life. The identification of how an individual spends their time may indicate their values or purpose in life. Perhaps, the individual spends a lot of their time volunteering for nonprofit organizations or specific causes. They may feel like they have a great need or desire to solve a specific problem in the world as their life purpose.

Intellectual Wellness

When was the last time you learned something new? Was it a new and upgraded computer program or the history of a new place you visited? The intellectual aspect of wellness is related to an individual seeking new knowledge or staying up to date with topics of their own interest. We are wired to keep learning and growing just as our world continues to keep growing and changing.

The old paradigm that a person stops learning when they finish formal school is simply not true. An individual is always on a lifelong journey of learning. The intellectual component of wellness may be intimidating if an individual determines they may want to go back for additional training to upgrade their work skills. However, learning is always occurring as individuals may be updated to a new computer operating system on their computer or on their phone as technology continues to change. We need to keep learning to stay well.

Across the country, there are various learning programs that are thriving for the general love of learning. The lifelong learning institutes at many community colleges and universities are often filled with participants aged 55 and above, learning about topics from Shakespeare to music appreciation. The Road Scholar is an organization that creates travel learning experiences for those who enjoy detailed learning tours. Even some churches offer various learning experiences that are beyond faith or spirituality. All these types of opportunities are created and utilized based on the individual's desire for intellectual stimulation. Additionally, as society advances, many people will reinvent themselves for new careers or to start businesses as a part of the intellectual wellness aspect of life.

Environmental Wellness

Imagine you are looking to find out about the weather for tomorrow. You have a big day planned for a family reunion. The weather service states there is a major air quality alert due to smoke from the recent wildfires many miles away. This would be one example of environmental wellness — where an individual makes a choice about their wellness based upon the conditions of the external environment. Some individuals may choose to live in various parts of the world based on specific environmental conditions connected to the preservation of their own health.

Another way to consider environmental wellness is an individual's approach to the sustainability of the global environment. In various parts of the world, recycling and climate change are viewed very differently. An individual can respond within these various environmental dimensions such as reconsidering their carbon footprint by choosing to use public transportation instead of driving their own car or choosing to place solar panels on the roof of their home for the utilization solar power. Environmentally conscious wellness actions can also be demonstrated by always adhering to recycling as per the local standards of the community.

The way a person keeps their personal living space or workspace is another aspect of environmental wellness. Keeping an environment organized or unorganized can certainly have an impact on an individual's wellness. For example, an ultra-chaotic environment can be supportive of an individual's creativity or can create unrest, depending on the specific individual. This is how the environment may influence an individual's wellness.

Occupational Wellness

The occupational aspect of wellness relates to an individual's pursuit of a vocation, career, or job. A significant amount of time can be spent in a lifetime determining and pursuing occupational interests. There is the entry of an occupation through career planning, the shift after the end of a career, family-related caretaking roles, and other types of jobs. Others can view their work as a vocation instead of a career. Occupational wellness can also vary between gender and cultures.

An individual may pursue what they call their "life's work." This can be raising a family or working outside of the household. These types of work roles have changed as we have evolved through the industrial society to the information society of today. As a result, this can change our relationship with how we view our lifework and concomitant our occupational wellness. Relationships with organizations, companies, and co-workers—along with specific workloads and work schedules—can impact individual occupational wellness.

Our occupational wellness can begin as we are moving through our initial educational years preparing for our life's work. Individuals may already be predestined to work at a family business or continue as the next generation of a specific profession. These scenarios can determine whether an individual continues beyond a high school education and toward advanced education or not. As a result, these kinds of influences during this time can impact an individual's occupational wellness at a very early age.

Financial Wellness

The financial aspect of wellness relates to an individual's experience in their understanding of their personal finances, relationship with money, and financial goals. In the US, becoming successful can mean many things with regards to finances, all of which can vary between individuals and across subcultures within various states.

This will vary between individuals and their personal upbringing. The way an individual values money and how it is attained, spent, or saved can impact financial wellness. The relationship a person has with money can impact one's financial wellness. Based on an individual's upbringing, there can be an influence of abundance or scarcity that guides one's living condition. This attitude can influence all types of financial decision-making.

Money beliefs can also come from past generational experiences, member-ship in certain organizations, and general financial education. An individual with access to financial education will have more information to influence their financial wellness. Based on where and how a person has been raised, they may or may not have received financial education through school or from family members.

Protectoral Wellness

The protectoral aspect of wellness relates to an individual's general safety. This is being mindful of avoiding accidents, heeding caution toward potentially harmful life situations, or taking precautions like always using their seatbelt in a car. When considering the protectoral wellness dimension, an individual is concerned with, for example, how to care for their whole well-being in terms of levels of safety, avoidance of illness, and financial well-being.

If one were to take driving into consideration, the individual would first check to see if the vehicle had enough fuel in the car to travel to the destination. They would check to see if the tires had enough air and if the mirrors were in the right position. They would always fasten their seatbelt and make sure they had insurance to protect the car and its passengers.

Another aspect of protectoral wellness is the prevention of a health risk. This would be through individual choices a person makes, such as brushing their teeth to prevent cavities. Taking action to prevent the basic cold or general food safety through washing your hands is another example of protectoral wellness. The government also assists with protectoral wellness through the implementation of speed limits and changing traffic configurations to help reduce car accidents.

Practical Experiences of the Wellness Dimensions

Now that we have a better understanding of how lifestyles have changed over time, and an understanding of the many dimensions of wellness, let's review a couple of practical scenarios where exploring wellness dimensions can assist in improving a person's well-being.

Scenario 1: An individual arrives at a session feeling anxious and sad. After further assessing the individual across the ten wellness dimensions, the counselor discovers the following situations to have occurred in the past year: they lost their childhood best friend; they have endured a brand-new boss who is changing their work responsibilities; and they are having financial troubles because the new boss is reassigning their usual extra contract work to another employee, thus reducing their income.

There are several wellness dimensions to recommend for exploration and action within this scenario including, but not limited to, the emotional dimension to support possible grieving; the occupational dimension to navigate their new role at work or potentially plan to change jobs; and the financial dimension to review personal budgeting and possibly adjust to the pay decreases.

Recommended prescription for wellness: explore emotional, occupational, and financial wellness.

Wellness Dimension	Considerations	Your Recommendations or Questions
Emotional	What resources have you sought out for grieving from this important loss in your life?	
Occupational	In what ways are you working to develop the relationship with your new boss? If you are not getting along with your new boss, what other career options might you consider in this situation?	
Financial	How have you adjusted your budget with the decrease in pay? What resources might be available for working with a financial planner or guide in the community?	

Scenario 2: An individual enters the session with a sharp, almost angry tone of voice and seeming extremely defensive. While speaking, the individual describes a reorganization at the workplace and a new

manager overseeing their work team. They share that the manager appears to be taking a more critical notice of their work and is verbally discounting their work in public meetings. The stress of the situation clearly has an occupational wellness impact, yet it can (and is, for this individual) also impact other dimensions of wellness such as physical and nutritional wellness as this individual is not sleeping or eating well.

For others, these kinds of difficulties can impact social and emotional wellness as the experience of negative moods can make it difficult to relate to others. The fear of losing a job can create a lack of time to meet with others as work is more demanding, thus creating a sense of isolation. The issue of a bad boss can significantly impact an individual's level of wellness in many other dimensions.

Recommended prescription for wellness: explore environmental, physical, and nutritional wellness.

Wellness Dimension	Considerations	Your Recommendations or Questions
Environmental	In what ways might you more effectively engage with your co-workers and manager as the situations at work continue to be more stressful?	
Physical	How might you include more physical activity to balance out the pressure in life? In what ways can you focus on improving your sleep habits?	
Nutritional	How is your intake of water and eating habits during this time? What is your level of caffeine or alcohol intake?	

While there are many scenarios we can review as general life situations, by looking at the whole individual through the wellness dimensions we can find new ways to assist them in feeling better without necessitating the use of a *DSM* or *ICD* label. A core element of wellness that runs through most of the dimensions is being connected to others. Happiness researcher Sonya Lyubomirsky suggests that we find our greatest happiness through social connection. The truth is that we do not do life alone—we are a part of a connected society.

Prescribing wellness can build up an individual's sense of belonging. Many of the dimensions can challenge individuals to connect with others, whether to gain support or to access information. We are assisting in a way to help individuals feel as though they belong—that feeling we all deserve to feel. Wellness dimensions can help get us there—it builds bridges and not walls.

Practical Recommendations

Lifestyles of individuals—from work to home life—have greatly changed. Our global society has significantly changed and remains a VUCA (volatile, uncertain, complex, and ambiguous) world. We must look at all systems to review how to best serve individuals in helping them thrive. As such, we need a bigger perspective on how to be well and maintain wellness.

Fields of study train to view the world through the perspective of their models and theories. This is true when viewing the assessment of individuals by utilizing the *DSM* and *ICD* models of diagnostics. What if we took a larger view of people's lives and, instead, prescribed wellness?

Many in practice are already aware of the biopsychosocial model in working with clients. The model is a great starting point for expanding it even further on the multidimensions of wellness. Expanding this model to include the additional wellness dimensions can greatly help individuals improve their well-being and, ultimately, their lives.

We can use Dr. Francis Ardito's ten-dimension wellness model to understand an individual's overall well-being through these simple questions:

1. Physical – How are you Moving?
2. Spiritual – How are you Being?
3. Emotional – How are you Feeling?

4. Environmental – How are you Preserving?
5. Intellectual – How are you Learning?
6. Nutritional – How are you Eating?
7. Protectoral – How are you Safeguarding?
8. Social – How are you Relating?
9. Occupational – How are you Working?
10. Financial – How are you Spending?

Prescribing Wellness Now

Let's reflect on where we have been on this journey. We know that over time we have moved from an industrial society to an information society. With this, the *DSM* and *ICD* manuals have evolved with revised editions. However, have they evolved to meet our lifestyle changes and catch up with our monumental progressions in society? We need to evolve with the changing dynamics of society and further understand the dimensions of wellness to get a wider conceptualization of an individual's life.

It starts with understanding the wellness dimension models followed by educating and prescribing particular wellness dimension actions. This wider perspective can provide clients with better living, thriving, and a brighter overall wellness experience. We all strive for a good life each day — choose wellness.

Suggested Readings

Ardito, F. (2013). *The Consumer Wellness Advocate Certification Program.* Wellness Education. Agate Publishing.

Danforth, W. (1938). *I Dare You.* William H. Danforth, St. Louis, MO.

Hettler, B. (1980). Wellness promotion on a university campus. *Family & Community Health, 3*(1), 77–95. https://doi.org/10.1097/00003727-198005000-00008

Hettler, B. (1986). Strategies for wellness and recreation program development. *New Directions for Student Services, 1986*(34), 19–32. https://doi.org/10.1002/ss.37119863404

Global Caffeinated Beverage Market By Distribution Channel (Online and Offline) By Product (Carbonated soft drinks, Energy drinks, RTD Tea and coffee and Others) By Region, Industry Analysis and Forecast, 2019 – 2025 (2019). https://www.kbvresearch.com/caffeinated-beverage-market/

Lyubomirsky, S. (2010). *The how of happiness*. Piatkus Books.

Malayter, M. (2004). Boomers: Visions of the New Retirement. IUniverse.

Malayter, M. (2016). Navigating the RIDE of Change. Do What You Love Foundation.

Malayter, M. (2021). Investing the Time to Lead Well. Investing the Time to Lead Well. In book: *When Leadership Fails: Individual, Group and Organizational Lessons from the Worst Workplace Experiences* (pp. 17-27) DOI: 10.1108/978-1-80043-766-120211002

U.S. Department of Agriculture and U.S. Department of Health and Human Services. *Dietary Guidelines for Americans, 2020-2025*. 9th Edition. December 2020. Available at DietaryGuidelines.gov.

Watson, D., & Stanton, K. (2017). Emotion Blends and Mixed Emotions in the Hierarchical Structure of Affect. *Emotion Review, 9*(2), 99-104. https://doi.org/10.1177/1754073916639659

Watson, D. & Vaidya, J. G. (2013). Mood measurement: Current status and future directions. In J. A. Schinka & W. F. *Velicer (Eds.) Handbook of psychology. Volume 2: Research Method in Psychology (2nd Edition)* (pp. 369-394). Hoboken, NJ. John Wiley & Sons.

Releasing Addictions

Anna Yusim

Abstract: *This chapter delves into the multifaceted nature of addiction emphasizing its medical, psychological, and spiritual dimensions. Addiction is defined as compulsive engagement in a rewarding stimulus despite its harmful consequences. Addictions can be divided into three primary categories: substance addictions, behavioral addictions and psychological addictions. This chapter highlights the spiritual aspect of addiction, suggesting that it represents a disconnection from one's soul. It explores various cases—substance addictions, alcoholism, workaholism, and even addictions to certain emotional states like rage. Treatment approaches are discussed with an emphasis on spiritually-based methodologies. This approach is contrasted with traditional psychiatric methods that often prioritize medical and behavioral interventions. While the healing journey from addiction can be a long and complicated journey, true healing involves self-discovery, personal transformation, and a return to a state of wholeness transcending conventional treatment approaches.*

We often use the word "addiction" loosely leading to misconceptions about its meaning. Medically, an addiction is a compulsive engagement in a rewarding stimulus despite its harm. Psychologically, it is uncontrollable craving, seeking, and engaging in a certain behavior (including use of a substance) of which we have become dependent, and which results in impairment or distress.

In essence, engaging in an addiction is pursuing something that feels good despite it being bad for us. Spiritually, addiction signifies a disconnection with one's soul. [1]

Writing to the Alcoholics Anonymous founder Bill Wilson, the psychiatrist Carl Jung equated addiction with a spiritual thirst for wholeness. [2] People may resort to addictions to distract themselves from their inner turmoil or overwhelming feelings. In this context, we are going to consider addiction as an external thing we depend on for happiness and a sense of wholeness, even if it's harmful.

While an addiction is sometimes immediately destructive, other times—as in the case of smoking cigarettes—the detrimental effects can be more long-term. Having treated many cases of addiction as a psychiatrist for over 15 years, I see addictions as being divided into three primary categories: substance addictions, behavioral addictions, and psychological addictions.

- Substance addictions: nicotine, stimulants (cocaine, amphetamines, methamphetamines, caffeine, tobacco, etc.), depressants (alcohol, benzodiazepines, barbiturates, opiates, heroin), cannabis, inhalants, sugar,[3] chocolate.[4]
- Behavioral addictions: gambling, eating, sex, pornography, video games, work, watching TV, Internet, shopping, sleep, exercise, hoarding, and/or high-risk behavior.
- Psychological addictions: status, power, money, fame, achievement, attention, approval, chaos, drama, rage, and/or falling in love.

Addictions can dominate our lives by providing only fleeting satisfaction and leaving a void. Breaking the addiction often only treats the symptom, not the root cause. To truly overcome them, you have to address your core beliefs about yourself and the world, which are often rooted in the misconception that external sources can fill internal emptiness.

This belief creates the illusion that you will finally be happy and at peace if/when you can smoke a joint, have great sex, make more money, or create another specific outcome in your mind. This search for external solace is a misguided attempt to mask the pain of disconnection from our inner selves. We often seek out addictions to relieve our pain or remain in denial about what is missing in our lives. Addictions merely distance us from our inner truth.

The Root of Addiction

Numerous theories exist regarding the causes and origins of addiction. Classical psychiatry posits that addiction represents an effort to self-medicate underlying psychological concerns including unresolved conflicts, childhood traumas, social discomfort, and overall life dissatisfaction. From a biological perspective, individuals with a genetic predisposition exhibit a higher susceptibility to addiction.

Additionally, differing viewpoints on addiction's curability emerge with some advocating for recovery and others subscribing to the Alcoholics Anonymous (AA) philosophy that "once an addict, always an addict." Most would agree that addictions are influenced by complex physical, emotional, social, and genetic factors.[5]

For some, addictions may begin with prescription medication. That was the case with my patient, Luke. He was prescribed Valium, an anti-anxiety medication, to alleviate persistent gastrointestinal pain after other treatments failed. Initially, the Valium helped, but Luke soon required increasing doses for the same relief and experienced withdrawal symptoms that affected his work. Eventually, Luke and his doctor were at a loss as he became dependent on Valium.

Repeated exposure to any addictive drug changes the brain's pleasure pathway, the mesolimbic dopamine system (MDS). When that happens, the messages sent to the frontal lobes of the brain, where choices and decisions are made, cease to warn the person to stop doing something dangerous. Their impulse control diminishes, so the person feels like they can't stop. What once felt good and brought pleasure evolves into despair punctuated by temporary relief from the pain.

Addictions and Aloneness

In our society, we're often conditioned to feel isolated, perceiving ourselves as separate rather than part of a vast, interconnected web. Consequently, the primary root of addiction is the profound need to love and be loved.

Addiction psychologist Dr. Rosemary Brown views addiction as a form of emotional dependency. "Most of us never learn how to meet our own emotional needs," she says. We are conditioned to seek external validation, neglecting self-awareness and self-satisfaction.[6] Addictions frequently substitute our fundamental human desires for connection, attachment, and love.

Stream of Consciousness Writing Exercise: Identifying Your Addictions

A powerful way of accessing your inner truth is through the act of writing. For this purpose, I invite you to set aside a journal or notebook to chronicle your thoughts, insights, and inspirations. If you prefer to type, that's great too. The method we will use for much of our writing is the five-minute stream-of-consciousness writing method.

Stream-of-consciousness writing means that for five minutes straight. You will write from your heart and soul without lifting your pen from your journal or your fingers from your keyboard. Any and every thought that enters your mind will go down on the page. You will write for five full minutes without stopping, going back, editing, criticizing, judging, or becoming stuck on any one topic.

You just let the thoughts, feelings, sensations, and images come to you and then put them into words. There is no right or wrong. There is no good or bad. You just do your best to put your truth—what you feel in the depths of your heart and soul at the present moment—into words.

If you feel stuck, take a deep breath and just keep writing. If you can, set a stopwatch for yourself so that you can invest fully in your writing without having to monitor the clock. For the first topic, set your stopwatch to five minutes and write without stopping on the Questions for Reflection included below. These questions are included as mere guideposts. As with life, let your writing take you where it may. You may end up somewhere much better than you could have imagined or planned.

Questions for reflection

1. Can you concretely describe when in life you have felt empty and alone?
2. How do you fill that feeling of emptiness? Do you try to replace it with other feelings? Do you turn to a certain activity such as eating, drinking, smoking, exercising, or seeking out a friend or family member?
3. Do you turn to addictions of any sort? If so, which ones?

4. In what areas of your life do you look outside yourself for happiness?

Addiction to Drugs

Tamar's deepest longing was for love. But when she couldn't find it, she filled the void with heroin. No amount of heroin ever made her feel blissful for long and she quickly returned to a feeling of emptiness.

Tamar's mother, Rachel, met Tamar's father, Eli, while volunteering in Israel. He was a dynamic leader, and they quickly fell in love and married. When Rachel became pregnant with Tamar, the couple moved to New York to be near her parents. Eli never really fit in in the city. Back home he was a promising young leader. In New York, he was a foreigner who didn't understand the local ways of doing things. Rachel also found motherhood to be more of a strain than she expected.

As Eli and Rachel struggled, their marriage suffered which escalated when Eli started going to the pub every night and coming home drunk. He became unpredictable and volatile, creating an environment of fear for Rachel. There were instances when he became aggressive towards her and even shook baby Tamar. This continued for a year until Rachel packed up her things, took baby Tamar, and moved back in with her parents.

The subsequent divorce was fraught with emotional torment. Tamar's early life was overshadowed by conflict as Eli would angrily confront Rachel at her parents' house, either demanding to be let in or threatening suicide. A significant incident occurred shortly before Tamar turned two. Even with a restraining order, Eli came to Rachel's apartment, seemingly in a peace-keeping manner. He suggested that they all move to Israel for a fresh start. Rachel's refusal sent Eli into a fury, and in his anger, he picked Tamar up and walked out.

Frantic, Rachel called the police, leading them to Eli's house. Eli barricaded himself inside with Tamar and refused to respond to the SWAT team at the door. Then, he made a desperate move. He came out onto the balcony, holding Tamar in a baby blanket, and dangled her over the edge. "If you come any closer," Eli warned them, "I swear to God, I'll drop her." Tamar, of course, doesn't remember any of this; she was two years old. But our early years are the most formative years of our lives. We form our impressions of the world without yet being able to speak, ask questions, or clarify things. After the aforementioned event, Tamar was no longer a happy child.

At age twenty-one, Tamar was still looking for consolation and she thought that she'd found it in heroin. I first encountered Tamar during my early days as a psychiatry resident. She had battled with a heroin addiction since she was just thirteen years old. During our first session, she expressed her desire to turn her life around.

Tamar stopped the heroin use while in treatment. I assisted her during the withdrawal phase by prescribing buprenorphine, a medication which acts similarly to heroin but in a more controlled and less addicting manner. Instead of using substances to get a high, Tamar was taking this medication therapeutically. Once away from heroin, Tamar grappled with a profound emptiness. I could feel the intensity of her longing for connection.

The craving for love that had propelled her addiction was back. It was no surprise that she felt drawn to therapy sessions—they became her new "addiction." It's often beneficial during the early stages of treatment to transition from a harmful addiction to a healthy, constructive one (like therapy). I've always believed in the healing power of love. In Tamar's journey, a series of supportive and nurturing relationships—first with me, then with her family, then with a community at Narcotics Anonymous— enabled her to let go of her unsatisfying relationship to heroin. The next stage for her was to channel that love inwardly.

Over the next two years, Tamar stopped using heroin and received her high school equivalency degree. Five years later, she contacted me for treatment regarding deep-seated anxiety. During this period, she had abstained from heroin and had slowly stopped taking buprenorphine, a challenge even greater than quitting heroin. She eventually became a paramedic, and steadily rose in the ranks of her profession to be one of the top paramedics in New York City. Tamar finds her job fulfilling, having directly saved multiple individuals from suicide. Her own experiences give her a unique empathy for those struggling with drug dependency, and she's now adept at seeking love in healthy ways.

It is now fourteen years since Tamar stopped heroin and eleven years since she stopped buprenorphine. While she's made significant progress in various areas of her life, Tamar admits that she's still on a healing journey. She occasionally dreams about using heroin and experiences rare cravings. However, she's now equipped with the knowledge to replace the emptiness that drugs once occupied with positive alternatives.

A first step in addiction recovery is replacing a harmful addiction (like heroin) with a beneficial addiction (like therapy or a constructive relationship or meaningful work). However, it's essential to recognize that even the most positive habits can become detrimental if they dominate your life. Ultimately, the most effective remedy for addiction is nurturing self-love. Healing requires a deliberate shift from seeking external happiness to letting love fill your heart. The following exercises aim to guide you through this journey.

Exercise: Filling Your Heart with Love[7]

While we could go to all sorts of places to find love, these feelings are available to us simply by tapping into the intuitive intelligence of our hearts. You can find that beautiful place within yourself.

This exercise is designed to foster a deep connection with your heart. It is about immersing in feelings of love, appreciation, care, and compassion — and holding onto them. This is one of the most powerful ways of filling the inner emptiness that often leads to addiction.

By calming the mind and maintaining a solid connection with your heart for a minimum of five minutes daily, you harness the heart's power to heal. It's a gentle process — not something to be forced. When you are ready, sit in a comfortable position and ease into it.

1. Find a quiet place, close your eyes, and take several slow deep breaths:
   a. Inhale for two.

      b. Hold your breath for four.

      c. Exhale for eight.

      d. Repeat five times.

2. Now pretend that you are breathing through the heart. With each inhalation, imagine your heart expanding as it fills with love and light. As you hold your breath, focus on the love, appreciation, and compassion. With each exhalation, imagine your heart contracting as it releases negative energy and dark light. Repeat for a minimum of ten breaths, at least three times per day for one week.

Addiction to Rage

Rage, rather than substances, had become Marcella's addiction. Despite never indulging in illegal substances, Marcella, a successful coffee shop chain owner in Italy, had earned a notorious reputation for her explosive temper.

In the week of our first encounter, she had vociferously confronted three unsuspecting sales representatives, rejecting their unwanted products with a storm of emotions. Marcella's anger was no longer a fleeting emotional response; it had transformed into an addiction that seemed beyond her control. Much like any addiction, Marcella's rage provided a temporary high, swiftly followed by remorse and a profound sense of emptiness.

Her impulsive outbursts had become a way of life, and she experienced a growing internal tension when she hadn't "exploded" in a while, akin to withdrawal symptoms in a drug addict. This compelled her to actively seek opportunities for her next rage-fueled episode, often with a disproportionate reaction to the provocation. Her employees had a short tenure under her tutelage, and she had few friends who could endure her eruptions. Her devoted husband, viewed by some as either saintly or misguided, stood by her side through it all.

Marcella eventually sought treatment for her anger management, coming to the realization that her rage addiction was primarily harming herself. Her business suffered, her relationships were strained, and she was labeled as "toxic" by those around her. Marcella had become a slave to her impulses, compulsively discharging her anger at anyone in her vicinity.

Each rage episode temporarily filled an inner void and granted her a fleeting sense of power only to be followed by a profound emptiness, accompanied by feelings of shame, regret, and depression.

Therapeutic intervention aimed at helping Marcella redirect her frustrations into constructive outlets such as writing and communication, enabling her to express daily irritations and prevent larger explosions. Additionally, techniques like relaxation exercises, stress management, and the adoption of a daily meditation practice helped Marcella build her tolerance to frustration. Through these tools, she learned to communicate her grievances without losing control, ultimately conquering her rage addiction.

Surprisingly, as she embarked on this healing journey, Marcella discovered a newfound wellspring of energy during her days, previously depleted by her frequent rage episodes. This transformation allowed her to harness her productivity in ways she had not imagined when her rage remained unchecked.

Addiction to Work

Drugs were not Jay's addiction. At thirty-five, Jay was a business dynamo—a master of creating and selling start-ups, with four major successes and millions in earnings. However, Jay came to see me when his ninety-hour workweeks brought his marriage to a crisis point. While his wife, Amy, a busy Chief Operating Officer of a start-up, initially understood the demands of start-ups, the two grew distant over five years as she barely saw Jay and often competed with his phone for attention. Jay was a workaholic.

One morning, after a fleeting interaction, Amy told Jay that their current life was unsustainable, sending pangs of fear through Jay. This had happened before in a previous relationship, and he did not want to repeat that. Losing Amy would be devastating. When Jay came to me, he began to realize the truth: he was not just absent from Amy's life but also his own. Work was not as important to him as love. It was as if he were living someone else's life—someone who valued work more than love.

While exploring the root causes of Jay's addiction to work, we unraveled a critical insight. Jay's father had also been a workaholic. Growing up, Jay vowed never to tread that path, but he couldn't anticipate the persistent feeling of insufficiency that he would have regardless of his achievements. Paradoxically, the greater Jay's accomplishments and the wealthier he became, the emptier and more despondent he felt. He had believed that this path would bring him fulfilment, but his vision backfired and now his marriage was on the rocks.

In order to move past this addiction, Jay needed to recognize and confront his subconscious beliefs:

- Money equals happiness.
- I am lovable only if I am successful.
- If I get approval from the CEO, then I will know that I am worthy.

Jay was lucky because he had the financial means to step back and redesign his life. So, over the course of a year, I often asked Jay the question, "What do you most deeply want?" Eventually, Jay decided to leave the job at his start-up in order to save his marriage and reclaim his life. Shortly thereafter, he and Amy took their first vacation in five years.

Jay then entered "pre-retirement," a period in which he wouldn't work and instead would seek fulfilment by studying interesting things, taking up meditation, and thinking about his next life project. He hinted that this project might be starting a family with Amy. This, Jay told me, was his most authentic self. He no longer felt driven by fear of not being worthy or enough.

Addiction to Alcohol

Delving into one's true self can be a privilege that not everyone can afford. Steve struggled with introspection. He had built protective walls around himself that still left him feeling exposed. Whenever stress mounted, Steve's refuge was scotch. After exiting his fourth stint in rehab, Steve wanted to make permanent changes. He sought my counsel after a recommendation from a counselor at the rehab clinic.

Steve's prolonged absence had left his used car business in tatters. On the day we met, Steve discovered that his business partner had misappropriated ten thousand dollars from their dwindling funds to pay off a personal gambling debt. Steve vented to me about this. "This kind of thing always happens! [...] I need a partner to run this business, but every time I find one, I get ripped off, one way or another."

In therapy, it became evident that this pattern extended beyond his business. We found that Steve was not only drawing in dishonest business partners, but he also attracted dishonest friends and romantic partners. Steve's life illustrated a key spiritual principle: you don't draw into your life who you want; you draw in who you *are*. As you evolve, the people you draw into your life will change as well.

Throughout his therapeutic journey, Steve came to accept that he had not been honest with himself. In his previous relationships, showing vulnerability had been detrimental. Now he felt an increased comfort with the truth. This self-awareness led Steve to take small but meaningful steps toward greater honesty with the other people in his life. As he began to live more authentically and honestly, he began to attract more stable, honest, and trustworthy people into his life as well.

In essence, alcohol was the crutch that kept Steve stuck in maladaptive habits and behaviors associated with dishonesty toward himself and others. This thwarted his capacity to outgrow those parts of himself that no longer served him. By being able to see himself more accurately, Steve was able to take steps towards honesty and authenticity, and no longer needed the crutch of the alcohol that had once kept him stuck.

The Best Treatment

The underlying sentiment behind addiction is often a deeply ingrained belief that we are alone in a cruel, punishing world. We try to fill the void by seeking external solutions and validation. While addictions may fill this emptiness temporarily, true healing and contentment come from removing internal barriers that alienate us from love.

Addiction's underlying emotion is profound loneliness. Freeing oneself from addiction takes more than quitting drugs or a stressful job or giving up scotch for good. It's about learning to genuinely love yourself.

In the realm of medicine, addiction is one domain in which one of the most effective treatments is spiritually based involving twelve-step programs like Alcoholics Anonymous or Gamblers Anonymous among many other such programs. In the following exercise, I have adapted steps one through three of a twelve-step program. You're invited to use this exercise for any addiction that you are ready to release today.

Exercise: Surrendering Your Addictions

For this exercise, identify an addiction you would like to release. Reflect on your reasons for wanting to release this particular addiction and envision the transformations this could bring to your life. Ponder this addiction's origins and the initial purpose that it served for you. How has this addiction negatively impacted you? Do you feel ready to release it now?

If you're hesitant, I invite you to write down your feelings about why you're holding onto this addiction. Recognizing and understanding your resistance is crucial if we are not yet ready to release an addiction. Allow yourself the grace to reach a point of readiness, and consider seeking support from a friend, family member, or professional.

Step One: Be Honest with Yourself and Others

The first step is to admit to yourself and at least one person close to you that you have an addiction. In AA, this is the step that goes something like, "Hi. My name is Bill and I'm an alcoholic." For the sake of this exercise, you can use any language that resonates with you to communicate the following:

I, _____, admit on this date of _____ that I have an addiction to _____ that I would like to release, once and for all.

Confiding in someone you trust about your wish to release your addiction is beneficial in multiple ways. First, it shatters the secrecy and makes you be honest with yourself and others. Mustering the courage to open up fortifies your resolve to truly release this self-destructive habit. Second, it introduces a level of accountability beyond just yourself. Third, it guarantees that you have a support system, reminding you that you're not on this journey alone.

For those not comfortable with sharing with someone close to them, I recommend seeking out a nearby twelve-step group tailored to your specific addiction.

Step Two: Admit Limited Control over Addiction

For some people, sheer determination and self-awareness may suffice to stop smoking, abstain from alcohol or drugs, or stop a destructive habit or behavior. If you fall into this category, the first step above may be all that's required.

However, if the addiction returns or if, despite your best efforts, you find yourself relapsing, you will likely realize the extent of the grip of your addiction. When it comes to addiction, willpower is often not enough.

To execute step two, write or say the following affirmation:

> I, _____, having identified an addiction of _____ that I would like to release once and for all, admit my limited control over this addiction. My willpower alone is not enough to overcome this addiction. This addiction is greater than me, and I no longer want to overcome it alone.

Step Three: Surrender Addiction to your Higher Powe

If you have reached a point where battling the addiction alone seems insurmountable, it might be time to seek some help from above. You do not need to be religious or believe in God. Your Higher Power may be God, the Universe, Mother Nature, the essence of love, or any indefinable force that seems to guide people who are overcoming addiction.

Given that twelve-step programs are globally renowned and consistently found to be among the most effective treatments for addiction (with 1.3

million active members of AA in the United States alone, attending approximately fifty-seven thousand weekly meetings),[8] there's evidently a powerful entity aiding those who surrender their addictions to Him, Her or It and admit their struggles. Even if the concept of faith does not resonate with you, consider this approach as it is backed by empirical evidence.

If you are unsure about the existence of a Higher Power, lean into your doubts. This exercise can be a test rather than a definitive answer, and a Higher Power may reveal itself to you in time.

To execute step three, write or say the following affirmation:

> Given that I, _____, have admitted my powerlessness over my addiction to _____, I now open myself up to the possibility that Something greater than myself can restore me to a state of balance, peace, love and/or sobriety.

> On this date of _____, I surrender my addiction over to this Higher Power and ask for His, Her or Its help in ridding me of this addiction, once and for all.

Once you have requested assistance from a Higher Power, ask how this support and guidance might materialize in your life to aid in overcoming this addiction. Remain receptive to the ways the response may present itself in your journey.

This Approach to Addiction vs. Traditional Psychiatry

The approach to addiction outlined here diverges somewhat from the conventional methods typically employed in mainstream psychiatry. Mainstream approaches predominantly regard addiction through a medical or psychiatric lens, often emphasizing pharmaceutical interventions, counseling, and behavioral therapy as the primary tools for addressing addiction.

In contrast, this alternative perspective adopts a holistic and spiritually-oriented route, placing a strong emphasis on the idea that addiction entails more than just abstaining from substances or behaviors; it represents a profound journey of personal transformation, self-discovery, and healing.

Rather than focusing primarily on symptom management or harm reduction, this approach encourages individuals to delve deep into the root causes of their addiction. It underscores the importance of self-awareness, honesty, and a willingness to seek support, whether from trusted individuals or a Higher Power, irrespective of one's religious beliefs.

Ultimately, this alternative perspective views addiction as a doorway to inner exploration and a return to a state of wholeness, providing a unique and comprehensive pathway to recovery that extends beyond conventional methods.

Endnotes

[1] Yusim, A. *Fulfilled: How the Science of Spirituality Can Help You Live a Happier, More Meaningful Life.* Hachette Book Group, Grand Central Life & Style: New York City. June 2017.

[2] Letter from Dr. Carl Jung to Bill Wilson: Kusnacht-Zurich, Seestrasse 228, January 30, 1961. http://www.soberrecovery.com/recovery/the-famous-letter-from-carl-jung-to-bill-wilson-founder-of-alcoholics-anonymous/

[3] N. M. Avena, P. Rada, and B. G. Hoebel, "Evidence for Sugar Addiction: Behavioral and Neurochemical Effects of Intermittent, Excessive Sugar Intake," *Neuroscience & Biobehavioral Reviews* 32, no. 1 (2008): 20–39, e-pub 2007 May 18. Review.

[4] N. M. Hetherington and J. I. MacDiarmid, "'Chocolate addiction': A Preliminary Study of its Description and its Relationship to Problem Eating," *Appetite* 21, no. 3 (December1993): 233–46.

[5] N. D. Volkow, G. G. Koob, and A. T. McLellan, "Neurobiologic Advances from the Brain Disease Model of Addiction," *New England Journal of Medicine* 374, no. 4 (January 28, 2016): 363–71, doi: 10.1056/NEJMra1511480.

[6] Rosemary Brown with Laura MacKay, "Addiction Is the Symptom, Not the Problem," *The Fix*, Mar 20, 2016, https://www.thefix.com/addiction-symptom-not-problem.

[7] This exercise is adapted from the Heart Lock-In technique of HeartMath. See Doc Childre, Howard Martin, and Donna Beech, *The HeartMath Solution: The Institute of HeartMath's Revolutionary Program for Engaging the Power of the Heart's Intelligence* (New York: HarperCollins, 2011), 213–214.

[8] J. F. Kelly and M. C. Greene, "The Twelve Promises of Alcoholics Anonymous: Psychometric Measure Validation and Mediational Testing as a 12-Step Specific Mechanism of Behavior Change," *Drug and Alcohol Dependence* 133, no. 2 (December 1, 2013): 633–40, doi: 10.1016/j.drugalcdep.2013.08.006.

Soteria Houses: A Safe, Humane, Life-Enhancing Approach to Treating Psychosis

Al Galves and Susan Musante

Abstract: *This chapter describes the Soteria model of treatment for psychosis and its impact on the mental health system. The Soteria approach is described in detail including the physical, administrative, and staffing elements of the model and the mechanism of the treatment. A history of the model and evidence of its effectiveness is included. The impact of the model on the mental health system is described, including the following: the Soteria model is a demonstration of how to best help people who are experiencing the states of being, moods, thoughts, emotions and behaviors associated with diagnoses of mental illness; the Soteria model challenges the medical model of understanding and treating mental illness; the Soteria model challenges the belief that materialistic science and technology will be useful to the mental health of human beings.*

The Soteria Approach

Soteria is a Greek word that means deliverance or salvation. It was an interesting and apt choice for the name of a safe, humane, and life-enhancing approach to addressing what we call psychosis (also known as "madness" or "insanity").

Two brief stories demonstrate the difference between the conventional approach and the Soteria approach to addressing what most of the world deems "serious mental illness."

Time: 1970's. Place: admissions unit at a Connecticut state facility for mentally ill people.

Dee, an 18-year-old woman—still almost a girl—is brought in by her father and mother for commitment to the state facility to treat people exhibiting symptoms of mental illness. She has a bright and vibrant personality and attractive physical appearance. Her family complains of her "crazy talking" and her promiscuity. Father is conservative; mother is submissive and quiet.

Dee, who has recently become sexually active, is confused about this turn of events. In clinical terms, Dee would be described as "manic" with delusional thoughts. If you met her at a party, you would think she was a delight. Regardless, she is admitted for evaluation.

After a 72-hour hold, she is admitted for 30 days. This process for commitment is overseen by a "court" held at the hospital on the same unit where she was admitted and where most 30-day extensions for evaluation are rubber-stamped by a court-designated official. Dee is assigned a single bed in an open dorm that has at least 20 beds and is rarely quiet at night. What she really needs is a good night's sleep, which is almost impossible.

Bathrooms hold four toilets in stalls with no doors attached. Showers are open with no privacy. There is a day room with a TV that is on most of the day and often into the evening. Meals are served from a truck onto old brown plastic plates and consist primarily of carbohydrates (e.g., scalloped potatoes), meat (e.g., hamburger) and a canned vegetable (e.g. string beans).

Dee is allowed outside for recreation with staff supervision. They toss around a football. Dee becomes distraught and screams out at the staff as they toss the football, "Don't drop the baby!" Clearly, she is delusional, possibly hallucinating, and is diagnosed with schizophrenia.

She is prescribed Thorazine or Haldol (depending on the prescriber preference) and Cogentin to counter the other effects of the drugs that include parkinsonian-like tremors, agitation (often mistaken as a symptom), uncontrolled mouth movements and rigidity among other metabolic effects. Dee is discharged and readmitted on several occasions.

On her last admission known to this writer, she is given electroshock treatment (ECT) since the drugs are not doing what they are purported to do. The vibrant young woman leaves the facility with what could best be described as blunted or flat affect, shuffling and rigidity in her upper extremities, and weight gain, likely an effect of the prescribed drugs. She also leaves with memory loss which may or may not be permanent from the ECT.

Most notably, she does not leave with the vibrant personality with which she entered the facility. She is on the trajectory of being a chronic mental patient with little hope for a full life and valued role in society.

Time: 2000's. Place: Soteria-Alaska, Anchorage, AK.

Mimi, an 18-year-old woman—still very much a girl—is committed into the state-run facility for mentally ill adults from a youth residential facility on her 18th birthday with no advanced warning or preparation. *Happy birthday, Mimi!* Clearly, the world of mental health treatment and mental health commitments have not advanced very much from the 1970's.

However, there is limited availability of an alternative. A mental health family and youth advocate has gotten involved and told Mimi about a new program called Soteria House. It is a voluntary home-like environment with no locked doors, it has private bedrooms, and is situated in the community where residents can participate in community activities such as school, work, and recreation with support from staff. Mimi is skeptical, but a bit intrigued.

A visit is arranged to ensure informed choice. Mimi wants to move to Soteria House; the Soteria House staff are unsure if they can keep her safe given her history which included jumping off a roof. She has been in and out of youth residential treatment and taking medication on and off for some years. Mimi makes her own appeal to the director of Soteria. Her words: "If you let me in, you will never be sorry. I promise." The Soteria House director, impressed with Mimi's self-advocacy and desire to not be a chronic mental health patient, admits her into Soteria-Alaska.

At Soteria, there are no house requirements such as going to therapy or taking medication. There is, however, a culture where residents work alongside staff to upkeep the yard and the house. There are house meetings to address interpersonal issues and determine housekeeping tasks. There are educational opportunities within the house and within the greater community that are available to residents.

Mimi has not gotten an adequate high school education due to her problems and inability to fit into the school environment. At Soteria, she gets her GED, makes friends, and does volunteer service in the community to build self-reliance and work skills. She eliminates taking all of her prescribed medications with the support of staff and under the supervision of the consulting psychiatrist.

Mimi meets and develops a relationship with a young man in the military. Upon graduating from Soteria, she gets her own apartment. One night, a couple of months after she moves out of Soteria, she calls the executive director in the evening and say, "I know I am not supposed to call you at night, but I just wanted to tell you that I am soaking in my own bath in my own apartment, and nobody would have predicted this for me. I told you — you would not be sorry if you let me into Soteria."

In the supportive non-coercive environment of Soteria, Mimi left behind her trajectory of "chronic mental patient" and embraced her valued role in society as a student in a relationship with a hopeful future. Similar stories are told by other residents of homes using the Soteria approach.

A Brief History of Soteria

The first Soteria house operated in San Jose, California from 1971 to 1983. It was the brainchild of Dr. Loren Mosher, the psychiatrist who was Director of the Center for Schizophrenia Studies at the National Institute of Mental Health (NIMH). Dr. Mosher was disillusioned with the over-reliance on coercive, chaotic environments of mental hospital wards and the over-reliance on tranquilizing neuroleptic medications that had long-term debilitating effects.

He proposed and implemented an experimental program to see if people diagnosed with serious mental illnesses such as schizophrenia could recover better in a safe, friendly environment without the heavy use of the drugs. He dubbed his new environment, Soteria House. It was a house where people lived in the community without locked doors and where medication was used as a last resort rather than the first line of treatment.

The Soteria approach used a home-like environment that relied on relational support, role recovery, and community as the main treatment. The idea was to keep people safe and allow them space to go through the experience as one would support someone going through a bad psychedelic drug trip. It was based on the understanding that schizophrenia is a move by a wounded psyche towards survival, healing, and recovery. Early onset schizophrenia was considered an experience— not a lifelong debilitating disease. Soteria or *deliverance* was the goal.

Since it was a research project of the NIMH, a study was done to compare the outcomes of patients treated at Soteria with patients treated in the hospital. Patients were randomly assigned to Soteria or the hospital. Two years after treatment, investigators checked to see how the patients were doing. They found that the patients treated at Soteria were doing significantly better than the patients treated at the hospital in terms of social functioning, employment, reduced symptoms, and decreased rehospitalizations.[1]

The research demonstrated that the Soteria approach was more effective than treatment in a hospital using medication as the primary modality of treatment. People treated at Soteria House with no or minimal medication had far better outcomes in terms of role recovery (student, family member, worker, etc.), symptom reduction or symptom disappearance, and no or minimal use of medication. The daily cost was one-third the daily cost of hospital treatment. Nevertheless, instead of replicating it, studying variations of it and, if effective, expanding it, the NIMH shut it down, fired Dr. Mosher and buried the results in its archives.

We are referring to the Soteria model as an approach since Soteria Houses are fluid and reflect the culture of the community, its residents, its staff, and its place in time. Soteria Houses may all look different because of their

---

[1] Bola, J.R. & Mosher, L.R. (2003). Treatment of acute psychosis without neuroleptics: Two-year outcomes from the Soteria project. *The Journal of Nervous and Mental Disease,219*: 219-229

foundation in embracing the community and people they serve. What Soteria Houses have in common are shared values, beliefs, and approaches to addressing personal behaviors that can be challenging to individuals, families, neighbors, and communities.

To ensure that the effectiveness of the Soteria House was not an anomaly, Dr. Mosher and others developed replication programs. One was called Emanon House and was also in California in the 1970s.[2] Crossing Place, a crisis residential home in Washington, DC and McAuliffe House in Rockville, Maryland were founded by Dr. Mosher and had embedded Soteria principles.

Since then, there have been other Soteria houses. There has been one in Bern, Switzerland since 1978. There was one in Anchorage, Alaska from 2009 to 2015. There are four Soteria houses in Jerusalem with plans for many more. In Israel, the Ministry of Health and insurance companies are paying for treatment at Soteria houses. There is one in Burlington, Vermont that has been operating successfully with high rates of recovery for 8 years. There continues to be international interest in using the Soteria approach.

However, in the United States treatment for psychosis is based on the biopsychiatric model with patients being told they have a brain disorder, and that they'll have to take antipsychotic drugs for the rest of their lives. Neither Medicaid, Medicare nor insurance companies will pay for treatment at Soteria houses.

People who are afforded the opportunity of a Soteria House enter an environment that is safe—physically and psychologically—as they go through the psychotic experience. There is no pressure to get better, get back on track or stop having those thoughts or hallucinations. Rather, they are told that they can stay at Soteria until they recover, and the staff will be with them to help them go through the experience.

The treatment is based on relationships with the goal to help the person navigate the experience in a safe place where they are understood,

---

[2] Mosher, L. (1999) Soteria and other alternatives to acute psychiatric hospitalization. *Journal of Nervous and Mental Disease, 187.* pp. 142-149

supported, affirmed and can slowly and steadily recover. In their book *Soteria: Through Madness to Deliverance*, Loren Mosher and Voyce Hendrix, a long-time House Manager, describe the process through which relationships contribute to recovery.

- The first stage was the *Break*: when the patient took the initiative to make significant contact (beyond that necessary to survival) with some other member of the community.
- The second stage was *Friendship*: when the patient established an interpersonal relationship with another person in which the patient saw him or herself in a partnership with that person—in a symmetrical relationship that was honest, affectionate, caring and trusting.
- The third stage was *Communal Identification*: when the patient felt as a member of the Soteria family, not simply a member of the house.
- The fourth stage was *Extending*: when the patient began to establish relationships outside of the Soteria community.
- The fifth stage was *Network Balance*: when the patient's support system included persons from outside Soteria as well as within Soteria.[3]

With the Soteria approach, there is clinical oversight usually by a licensed counselor/psychologist and psychiatrist. However, most of the staff are people who have recovered from similar experiences and other non-licensed professionals who relate well with the residents—who help them make sense out of what is going on, understand what triggered it, and feel less agitated, upset, and alienated.

Some of the residents use psychotropic medication, but that is not the primary modality of treatment. Many residents do not rely on medication or use it intermittently. The primary modality of treatment is safety and affirming relationships.

---

[3] Mosher, L. R. & Hendrix, V. (2004). *Through Madness to Deliverance*. Bloomington, IN: Xlibris

Residents are involved in house upkeep and cooking as much as they are able. The typical resident becomes stabilized in about six weeks with an average stay of three to six months. Once they are stable, they are encouraged and helped to go out into the community. They participate in community activities, education, employment, recreation, therapy, and other forms of community involvement. There is an ongoing community of graduated residents who visit and/or volunteer after they have transitioned from living in the home.

The key principles of the Soteria approach are as follows:

- Home-like residence designed to treat persons who are experiencing their early psychotic breaks.
- There is psychological and physical safety through compassionate staffing relationships.
- There is no pressure to get back on track too quickly.
- Residents can stay until they have recovered and have a bridging plan into the community.
- Treatment is based on the relationship.
- The goal is to help the person navigate the experience in a safe place where they are understood, supported, affirmed, and can slowly and steadily recover.
- A resident may or may not use medication, but medication is voluntary and not the primary mode of treatment.

A key component of successful implementation of Soteria programs is staffing, both in terms of staff-to-resident ratio and staff characteristics. Staff characteristics include:

- Compassionate
- Similar experiences to residents
- Ability to provide safety and affirming relationships

Supervision and oversight are provided by a director who is a licensed clinician. There is a contract with a psychiatrist who provides psychiatric services as needed. There is no specific programming or model of treatment other than residents' and staff activities that can include:

- House upkeep, gardening, cooking, etc.
- Supported community activities: education, employment, recreation, family interactions
- Art
- Exercise
- Daily therapeutic house meetings (or more often, if needed) to develop relationships and manage the home environment.

Why Soteria Matters

The Soteria movement is an important step towards building a better mental health system. First, it is a demonstration that the way to help people—who are experiencing the states of being, moods, emotions, thoughts, and behavior that are associated with diagnoses of "mental illness"—are as follows:

> Help them realize that whatever is going on with them, no matter how painful, debilitating, impairing, or scary is understandable as well as somehow functional and potentially useful. Help them realize that the "symptoms" they are experiencing are a reaction to their life situation, life experience, and concerns they have about themselves and their lives.

> Help them experience the "symptoms" and use that experience to get to know themselves better—to become more aware of why they do, feel, and think as they do or don't. Thus, help them begin to develop a good relationship with themselves.

> Help them have experiences that will enable them to use their thoughts, emotions, intentions, perceptions, and behavior to live more the way they want to live.

This is very different from the medical model, on which the mainstream mental health system is based. The medical model tells people that their "symptoms" are indications of pathology—that they are sick; that the "symptoms" are alien; that they somehow came out of the blue; that they are caused by brain malfunction, chemical imbalances, and genetic anomalies; and that they have nothing to do with their lives and their reactions to it.

This is a very disempowering and cynical belief. If you carry it out to its logical conclusion, it is a belief that people don't have any control over the faculties they use to live their lives; that is, their thoughts, emotions, intentions, perceptions, behavior. It is a belief that people are at the whim of forces over which they have no control.

Allow me to elaborate. People don't have control over their brain function, biochemistry, or genetic processing. So, if you think your thoughts, emotions, intentions, perceptions, and behavior are controlled by those physiological dynamics, you believe that you don't have control over your thoughts, reactions to emotions, intentions, perceptions, and behavior. Again, that is disempowering and cynical. This belief has the benefit of taking people off the hook, of enabling them to not take responsibility for what is happening to them or what they are thinking, feeling, and doing.

That may be comforting in a way. Perhaps that is the reason people are attracted to the biopsychiatric belief system. It takes blame away: "It just happened to me," "I don't know why," "I am a victim," or "It was just random, came out of the blue." But wait—why should anyone feel blame about anything? People don't have control over choosing their parents or how their early lives played out. And what they experienced in their early lives can have a profound and major impact on what they do now—how they think and how they feel as adults. So, I suggest that we take blame out of the lexicon.

The Soteria movement is based on a very different understanding of human beings and how they operate. This is how John Weir Perry understood the psychotic experience.[4] Perry was a California psychologist in the 1950's who spent a lot of time with people diagnosed with schizophrenia. When a person who has been discounted, dishonored, put down, made to feel inadequate, abused physically, emotionally, or rejected approaches adulthood, he wrote that a change is initiated. The person's psychic energy is attracted to an exalted, powerful, capable but unreal, imaginary persona.

That change strips the rational part of the psyche of its usual energy and leaves it in a state of disorganization. They are understandably terrified of

---

[4] Perry, J.W. (1974), *Far Side of Madness*. Englewood, NJ: Prentice Hall

having to live in the adult world, having to take on the expectations and responsibilities of adulthood. Therefore, they may create a different reality for themselves—a reality that will make it possible for them to survive in a toxic world with toxic human beings. This is not a choice that is made by the rational part of the psyche. It is a choice or an intention that is driven by a deeper, healthier part of the psyche—a part that wants to survive and knows how to survive.

Based on this understanding of what is going on, the Soteria approach provides the person with safety, support, and affirmation as she goes through the psychotic experience. The person receives the message that, rather than being sick, she is moving towards healing and recovery. Although the experience can be scary, painful, troubling, and impairing, somehow, she is surviving. Thus, she is given the time and space needed to slowly become less afraid and, slowly at her own pace, begin to connect with other human beings who are going to treat her as a person on a path towards healing and recovery.

This is a challenge to the medical model. If it works, it is evidence that the medical model is not the best way to understand or treat mental illness. Does it work? The only study that compared patients treated at Soteria with patients treated at the hospital says that it does. This is the aforementioned study done by the National Institute of Mental Health (NIMH)—the one whose findings were buried. I know the results were buried because in 2010 I met with Sarah Morris, head of the NIMH's Schizophrenia Research Office. I asked her if she had ever heard of the Soteria house—she hadn't.

This was a watershed moment in the history of American psychiatry. Here you had a demonstration of an approach to treating first-episode psychosis that was more effective than the treatment in the hospital; that is, immediate prescribing of antipsychotics coupled with the message that "you have a brain disorder, a malfunctioning brain and you will have to take this medicine for the rest of your life." But instead of working at further developing the intervention, the NIMH decided otherwise.

Why did the NIMH do that? We can't know the answer to that, but we can infer why they did it. Psychiatry was clearly moving towards becoming a practice based on materialistic science—a practice that prioritizes things that can be measured, weighed, quantified, and seen on a brain scan. Psychiatry would no longer pay attention to the thoughts, emotions, intentions, perceptions of human beings.

You can't directly study those things under a microscope or see them on a brain scan. However, those are the faculties that people use to live their lives. So, in deciding to become a materialistic science, psychiatry turned its back on human nature and on human beings. The NIMH was in the process of becoming a laboratory for neuroscience, of focusing its efforts on the search for the biomarkers that could be used to diagnose mental illness and for the glitches in the neural circuits, neurotransmitters, glial cells and genetic anomalies that were the presumed causes of mental illnesses.

The result of that move can be summed up in this quote from Thomas Insel, the Executive Director of the NIMH from 2002 to 2015:

> I spent 13 years at NIMH really pushing on the neuroscience and genetics of mental disorders, and when I look back on that I realize that while I think I succeeded at getting lots of really cool papers published by cool scientists at fairly large costs—I think $20 billion— I don't think we moved the needle in reducing suicide, reducing hospitalizations, improving recovery for the tens of millions of people who have mental illness.[5]

One can readily see why the NIMH abandoned the Soteria experiment even though it was effective in treating first-episode psychosis. It is about as far from neuroscience or materialistic science as can be imagined. It is based on relationship. What makes it work is the ability of the staff and volunteers to be with patients in a supportive and affirming way and, in that way, help them go through the psychotic experience towards healing and recovery. One can imagine a neuroscientist or recently trained psychiatrist hearing

---

[5] Rogers, A. (2017, May 11). Star neuroscientist Tom Insel leaves the Google-spawned Verily for …a start up? Wired. https://www.wired.com/2017/05/star-neuroscientist-tom-insel-leaves-goolgle-spawned-verily-startup/

about the Soteria approach and saying, "I didn't go through four years of graduate school and four years of residency to do that."

The Soteria movement is a challenge to the idea that materialistic science and technology will be useful to the mental health of humans. As E.F. Schumacher says in his book *A Guide for the Perplexed*, you can study the brain with materialistic science, but you can't study consciousness or self-awareness and those are the faculties humans use to live their lives.[6] Humans don't use their brains to live their lives. They use their minds and emotions.

The mind is not the same thing as the brain. The brain is an organ, a piece of protoplasm. We have learned a lot about it. It is the seat of billions of neurons and trillions of neuronal connections. It uses neurotransmitters to facilitate the passage of neuronal transmission over synapses. We have learned something about the function of different parts of the brain. The mind, on the other hand, is a vastly powerful faculty. It is the faculty we use to understand the world, make decisions, solve problems, plan, build everything humans build, relate to each other, write books, engage in sports, and invent machines.

As William Uttal says in his book *Mind and Brain: A Critical Appraisal of Cognitive Neuroscience*, neuroscientists think they have a theory of how the brain creates the mind. However, they aren't even close to having such a theory, Uttal says, and it is unlikely that they ever will.[7] For example, neuroscientists have no idea about the difference in brain function when a person is planning a trip to Europe compared with when a person is solving a physics problem. They have no idea about how I can move my arm at the count of three.

Although they have been studying memory for years, they still have very little idea about how it works. They have no idea about what is happening in the brain when a person has the insight that the reason he needs approval from men is that he didn't get it from his father. They have no idea about

---

[6] Schumacher, E.F. (2015). *A Guide for the Perplexed*. New York: Harper Perennial
[7] Uttal, W. (2014). *Mind and Brain: A Critical Appraisal of Cognitive Neuroscience*. Cambridge, MA: MIT Press

how consciousness developed or how it operates. People use their minds to live their lives, not their brains. No matter how much neuroscientists learn about the brain, they are not likely to help people live their lives.

The Soteria approach helps people heal from psychosis by helping them use their minds and emotions to relate to other people. And once they are stabilized and less terrified of the world and humans, it helps them use their minds to get on with their lives—to find jobs and careers, go to school, marry, and build families. The Soteria approach facilitates the powerful self-healing properties of people. If you nurture those properties and give them an environment in which they can operate, they can help people survive and, eventually, thrive.

People heal with their minds, not their brains. They learn how to manage their thoughts, emotions, intentions, perceptions, and behavior to live the way they want to live. When people are living how they would like to, their symptoms disappear. Therefore, Soteria houses are not only effective treatments for psychosis—they are also demonstrations of how to effectively treat all mental illnesses. They challenge the idea that mental illnesses can be effectively treated primarily through the lens of the medical model. And they cast doubt on the idea that the mental health of humans can be helped primarily with materialistic science.

Soteria houses hold hope for a world in which most people who experience psychosis can recover fully. They are a low-tech, inexpensive, effective approach to treating psychosis. One can envision a United States in which every city with a population of 50,000 or more has a Soteria house available to people who experience psychosis. That is a future much to be hoped for and worked for.

How the Human Stress Response Explains Away "Bipolar Disorder"

Sarah Knutson

Abstract: *This chapter challenges the claim of mainstream psychiatry that "bipolar disorder" is the result of genetic defects or abnormal brain functioning. It posits that normal human stress and survival responses can produce and potentially explain the same phenomena. It draws on recent research showing that predators and prey use the same basic physiology to achieve their survival objectives, albeit for different purposes. Unlike prey motivation, where fear and defensive strategies predominate in order to escape threat, predator (appetitive) motivation creates intense states of emotional and physical arousal in pursuit of rewards. The latter has much in common with the DSM criteria for a "manic" episode. Each DSM criterion is then analyzed and explained through a stress/survival lens, demonstrating that the clinical (and allegedly pathological) criteria are virtually indistinguishable from responses that would be predicted by normal human stress and survival activation. Given the profound overlap, I suggest that ethical practitioners should be assessing for stress/survival reactivity, screening for biomarkers, and conducting a careful differential diagnosis to rule out possible stress/survival causality. I also discuss how stress/survival activation and the exhausted collapsed state that inevitably follows can be supported by learning to shift the underlying physiological baseline from sympathetic reactivity to parasympathetic well-being.*

Acknowledgement: A version of this chapter was first published by Mad in America on April 1, 2018.

My current diagnosis is "Bipolar I Disorder." In a few years, that likely won't exist. I might even be able to sue my clinician for not assessing — or ruling out — known biological markers of stress that overlap with conventional diagnostic features.

Here is how it works.

What we now know about the stress model

For a variety of complicated reasons, some of us develop an overactive stress baseline (sympathetic/fight-or-flight response) early on in life. Here's the down and dirty from Robert Sapolsky, world-renowned neurobiologist and primatologist at Stanford University:

> Across numerous species, major early-life stressors produce both kids and adults with elevated levels of glucocorticoids (along with CRH and ACTH, the hypothalamic and pituitary hormones that regulate glucocorticoid release) and hyperactivity of the sympathetic nervous system. Basal glucocorticoid levels are elevated—the stress response is always somewhat activated—and there is delayed recovery back to baseline after a stressor. Michael Meaney of McGill University has shown how early-life stress permanently blunts the ability of the brain to rein in glucocorticoid secretion. (Sapolsky, 2017, pp. 194-95)

A simple way of thinking about this is that a lot of us start our lives in 'high idle' mode. The engine is always a little too revved and runs a bit fast for its own good. Plus, it's harder than usual to calm it down. This puts added wear and tear onto the system and begins to show over the years.

There are a zillion ways the effects of a highly revved system can manifest. The stress response affects virtually every aspect of human functioning. Here are some that Sapolsky (2004) discusses in his best-seller, *Why Zebras Don't Get Ulcers: The Acclaimed Guide to Stress, Stress-Related Diseases, and Coping*:

- Functioning of glands, hormones, neurotransmitters
- Heart, blood pressure, cholesterol, breathing
- Metabolism, appetite, digestion, stomach and gut functioning
- Growth and development
- Sex and reproduction
- Immune system, vulnerability to disease
- Pain
- Memory
- Sleep

- Aging and Death
- Mental health and well-being
- "Depression," motivation, ability to experience pleasure
- Personality and temperament
- Vulnerability to addiction

In other words, there's practically nothing that happens in human minds and bodies that the stress response doesn't potentially affect.

How the stress response affects us individually is a different matter. Human beings are incredibly diverse in our life circumstances, experiences, interests, and gifts. There is no manual for life nor is there one right way of doing things. Rather, human development is more of a creative endeavor.

Each of us constructs a response to the challenges we face based on what we have to work with (personally, socially, environmentally) at the time. With time and repetition, some responses start to come more naturally than others. They start to feel like the essence of 'me.' In all likelihood, what I come up with — and what ends up feeling entirely natural to me — will end up being entirely different from what you come up with and what ends up feeling natural to you.

That's the beauty and diversity of life. It potentially gives us a lot to learn from each other.

So what's going on with 'mania'?

Well, here's a really interesting piece of information. As it turns out, the human stress response (sympathetic/fight-flight) is a real swinger. It plays for both teams. In other words, the stress response doesn't just get turned on by fear, like if I'm being chased by a bear (prey activation). It also turns on if I am the bear and chasing you (predator activation).

This was discovered by a bunch of researchers at the University of Florida (Bradley et al., 2001; Bradley & Lang, 2000; Lang & Bradley, 2010; Lang & Bradley, 2013; Löw et al., 2008; Schupp et al., 2004). They studied human beings in simulated predator-prey contexts and discovered that both frames of mind rely on essentially the same physiology. The major difference is in motivation and the emotional experience. Predator activation was motivated by obtaining rewards (appetitive motivation), leading to excited states of emotional arousal. Prey activation was motivated by escaping threats (defensive motivation), leading to fearful emotional arousal states.

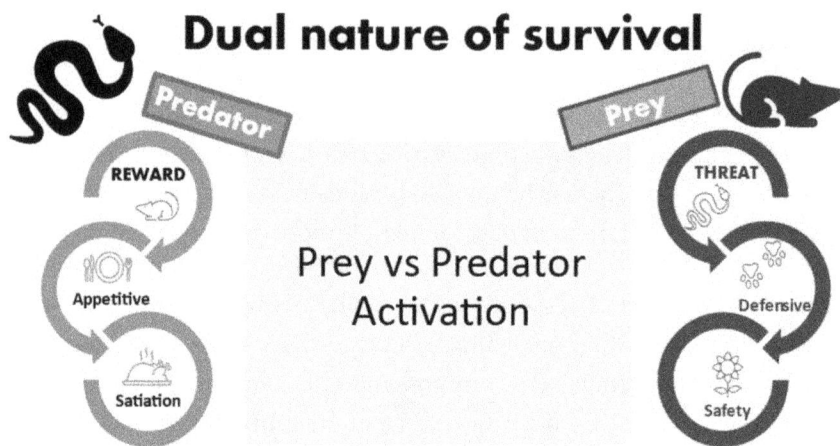

As you might guess, the upside of the stress response (appetitive motivation) has a lot of overlap with the exciting and pleasurable things that many of us tend to chase after when we're so-called 'manic' (see, e.g., Schupp et al., 2004, p. 598).

When you think about it, it makes sense. The human stress/survival response (sympathetic nervous system/fight-flight) developed to help us survive both as individuals and as a species. Our survival is not just about getting away from threats as fast as we can. Survival also requires us to be alert and on the ball for potential opportunities.

It's not enough to just know there's an opportunity. A lot of opportunities are only there for a moment. Like the classic cat and mouse, you have to gear up and go after it before it gets away.

Think of bargain shopping at Walmart on Black Friday. I have to be able to mobilize quickly if I'm going to snatch up that hot deal on a big screen TV. Fortunately, the survival response is there for me. It's all over the stuff that matters to human beings the most — thereby enabling me to out-hustle or out-wrestle the next guy who is all over the same Walmart bargain that I am.

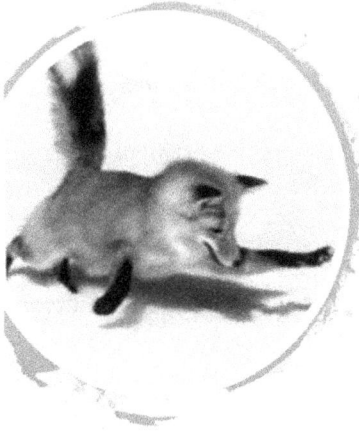

Nature of 'predator' survival motivation

Predator mindset	Adaptive responses
Rare opportunity	Eager, excited, expressive
High stakes	Agitated, high alert
Top fitness required	Preparatory activation
I must have this	Goal-directed, tunnel vision
Failure is not an option	Reckless, rationalizing
I made this happen	Self-importance

Physiology of "Mania": Symptom by symptom

Now that we have a basic outline of what's going on, let's take a look at so-called 'mania.' We'll go through the criteria for a 'manic episode' symptom by symptom so you can see how the stress response is potentially operating here.

DSM-5 Criteria for Manic Episode[1]

A) A distinct period of abnormally and persistently elevated, expansive, or irritable mood and abnormally and persistently increased goal-directed activity or energy, lasting at least 1 week and present most of the day, nearly every day (or any duration if hospitalization is necessary).

B) During the period of mood disturbance and increased energy or activity, three (or more) of the following symptoms (four if the mood is only irritable) are present to a significant degree and represent a noticeable change from usual behavior:

---

[1] The DSM-5-TR made some changes. I use this version because these were the criteria employed to diagnose me and those in effect when this piece was first written.

1. Inflated self-esteem or grandiosity.

2. Decreased need for sleep (e.g., feels rested after only 3 hours of sleep).

3. More talkative than usual or pressure to keep talking.

4. Flights of ideas or subjective experience that thoughts are racing.

5. Distractibility (i.e., attention too easily drawn to unimportant or irrelevant external stimuli), as reported or observed.

6. Increase in goal-directed activity (either socially, at work or school, or sexually) or psychomotor agitation (i.e., purposeless non-goal-directed activity).

7. Excessive involvement in activities that have a high potential for painful consequences (e.g., engaging in unrestrained buying sprees, sexual indiscretions, or foolish business investments).

Let's start with Criteria A first: elevated, expansive, or irritable mood, increased energy, increased goal-directed activity.

To really see what's going on, let's go back to that Walmart bargain and take a look at what is happening physically and mentally. First of all, an opportunity like this doesn't come every day. In all likelihood, I'm going to get something I desperately want at a price I can finally afford. But there's a catch: I get the bargain if and only if the item I want is still on the shelf, which requires me to activate like crazy to beat out the next guy.

So, is my mood expansive or elevated? You bet. It's the chance of a year and I might get it. Am I going to get potentially irritated? Well, if anything cuts me off or gets in my way, you bet. Is my energy increased? You bet. I have to make a dash for it. Am I goal-directed? You bet. That's the whole purpose.

Does it last a week? Probably not, because it's a one-day sale. But it could if I had to compete with the other customers in a survivor show for the chance to get the best deal and that competition went on for a week or a month. Then, if I really, really wanted that item and this was my one chance, I might well stay revved for as long as it took to give myself the best chance I could at landing the prize.

It's just the same as if I was in a war zone and had to stay in high alert. My body would likely rise to the occasion for as long as I needed it to in order to protect my interests as much as possible.

Okay, on to Criteria B.

Here's where you have to understand a bit more about the fight-or-flight response and how it actually affects us. When I'm chasing the opportunity of a lifetime, this is what my body does:

- Adrenaline surges. My heart pounds, lungs pump, and blood pressure amps. All of this is in the service of getting as much fuel and oxygen to my muscles as possible.
- My hair stands on end, my fists clench, and my legs get ready to run. Everything is primed and ready to pounce at the drop of a hat.
- My digestion shuts down. My stomach gets queasy and light. My bladder and bowels empty — just to make sure there's no needless surplus holding me back.
- Higher-order thinking (judgment) gets put on hold. That takes energy that my muscles need to move me. Thinking also takes way too long—this is a time for action! I can't afford to get bogged down in details. Once the cat is in the bag, there will be plenty of time for a more careful and reflective appraisal of whether I actually want or need it—or what I might do differently next time.
- With judgment out of the way, out come the fast reflexes and old habits. The autonomic system takes over behind the scenes and starts calling the plays. Whatever it is that I do and know best — whatever comes most naturally — is what that system goes with. After all, the stakes are high. This is the Super Bowl of my life. I'm not going to try out a new quarterback or a new play. I'm also not going to put in the second string. No way! It's the stuff I know by heart and have done a zillion times before that is going into my starting lineup, and going to get played again and again, in this frame of mind.

- Next come the tunnel vision and the tunnel hearing to shut out all the outside distractions. Attention rivets. This allows me to hyper-focus and totally zoom in on my vision of what I want to happen.
- I feel no pain. Literally. Endorphins, my body's natural opioids, are in full gear now, again making sure that nothing distracts me from the task at hand.
- It gets even better. The fact that I'm pursuing a highly meaningful personal goal is giving me massive hits of dopamine, which is essentially endogenous cocaine. In other words, I'm getting encouraged and reinforced by my body's own reward system to wholeheartedly pursue something I care about a lot.

Okay, now let's go back to Criteria B.

1. Inflated self-esteem or grandiosity.

Am I feeling pretty powerful here? You bet—an opportunity of a lifetime is within reach. Adrenaline is pumping up my muscles, creating a sense of strength and power I never knew I had. I'm feeling impervious to pain (thank you endorphins!).

I've got a personal cheerleading squad (dopamine) rewarding my efforts and boosting my spirits every step of the way: *You're doing great, keep going, don't stop now, you can do this, you'll get there. It's going to be so great, everyone will think you're totally amazing if you can just pull this off.*

Better yet, tunnel vision and hearing are shutting out any and all potentially discouraging outside feedback. In other words, thanks to the survival system, my sense of efficacy and personal power is being inflated to the max. But, far from being a disease, it's exactly the state of mind and body I need in order to take on and achieve the challenging task at hand.

2. Decreased need for sleep.

Let's be honest: is there any chance in hell my body is going to let me sleep in these circumstances? What predator worth their salt lets down their guard with potential prey so close at hand?

Equally important, this space I'm in is extraordinary and I know it. It's not just that I feel extraordinarily awesome. Clearly, I do. But when else in my life have I felt so capable and productive? Why risk losing it by going to sleep? Far better to keep up the momentum and milk this opportunity for all its worth.

3. More talkative than usual or pressure to keep talking.

Yep, for sure. If I care about you or you care about me, you bet I'm talking. This is the opportunity of a lifetime. I want you to know about it. I want you to get in on it. I want your support 100%. This is way, way, way too precious for either of us to miss out on—and I'm going to make sure you know that. I'm also going to make sure you have all the information you need to help this plan succeed. That way, you can assist as needed and carry on without me if I go down.

Plus, let's not forget that the mouth is a weapon. Jaws, teeth, and voice serve important survival functions. They are not just for pleasant conversation and consumption of food. If push comes to shove, I can bite, grip, growl, roar, scream, and yell for help among other things. Equally important, our talking apparatus is operated by muscles. Thus, the same adrenaline that is pumping up my arms and legs and priming them for action at the drop of a hat is also activating my jaws and speech apparatus. As a result, these muscles have an abundance of energy to fuel their operations and are more than happy to prattle on endlessly.

4. Flights of ideas, racing thoughts.

You bet. There's so much to figure out and so many angles to anticipate. All possibilities must be considered. All vulnerabilities must be anticipated and addressed.

5. Distractibility.

Frankly, I might never feel this good again. As already noted, I'm on a roll so I better take advantage of this energy while it's here. There's not a moment to lose. I need to make sure that I get to everything I can while the universe is being this generous to me and making me feel this amazingly great.

Yes, I know you might think you have important things to say to me, but that can wait. *We can talk anytime. You don't understand. This is a once in a lifetime opportunity.*

6. Goal-directed activity, psychomotor agitation.

Yep. This is here for sure, like we talked about above, for all the reasons above.

In particular, the goal-directed activity is supported by the cocaine-like effects of dopamine. As any good addict can tell you (me included), once that reward system kicks into gear, it can be hard to turn off. The natural desire to keep the 'high' going leads to looking for more goals to achieve in order to get more dopamine hits. It creates a vicious cycle that, all too often, only ends when I'm way past depleted and can no longer run on the fumes.

As to psychomotor agitation, thanks to adrenaline, muscles are loaded with energy and primed for some action. Think of kids on too much sugar. They are ready, raring to go, and a particle of dust can set them off.

7. Risky activities, high potential for painful consequences (unrestrained buying sprees, sexual indiscretions, or foolish business investments).

Exactly. This is where the survival response is both terrifyingly effective and mind-blowingly risky. Its whole purpose is to facilitate quick action and fast resolution.

To ensure that I'm on board, as soon as it notices the stakes are high the survival system intentionally pumps me full of chemicals that dull or deaden my awareness of risk:

- Adrenaline tells me everything is urgent and to go, go, go.
- Endorphins make me impervious to pain.
- Dopamine convinces me this is the opportunity of a lifetime: *not to be missed, must have now.* The rewards it promises for goal-

achievement ensure that I devote my energy and awareness exclusively to that. The resultant hyperfocus virtually assures that none of those lingering doubts or concerns about what could go wrong will make it past the firewall being patrolled by the associated sensory tunneling.

- The combination takes higher order thinking (judgment) offline and conspires to convince me I'm invincible.

In such circumstances, my better judgment really doesn't have a chance. It's under-resourced at the same time that my body is primed for action while my old habits are given a free reign. While this might sound crazy in a corporate environment, this is the response of choice in hunter-gatherer culture where buffalo, nomads or lions appear with nary a moment to waste. In such circumstances, one cannot respond too quickly: a moment's delay is likely death, or a precious opportunity missed.

When the stakes are this high, it is far better to err on the side of swift, decisive action. So, bag the prey or kill the foe right now. There will be plenty of time later on to think about what I did, how I did it, if I misunderstood or overreacted, how it might go better next time. "But" says the brain in a survival frame of mind, "this is not the time."

So that about does it

We have dispensed with all the symptoms of so-called genetic, chemically-imbalanced 'mania' armed only with the little ole garden-variety human stress response that happens for millions of Americans the day after every Thanksgiving.

If you've been following me so far, and relating it to your own experience, then you are quite possibly beginning to see how all of this might come together to create the 'perfect storm' that gets labeled a 'manic episode.'

About the crash

But what about that inevitable crash that comes after the so-called 'mania'? Where does that come from?

Piece of cake. The survival response runs on borrowed time and energy. It requires sacrifice from all sorts of other bodily systems. At the time, I have no idea that this is happening. The adrenaline, the power surge, the dopamine hits, the pain killers, the hyper-focus frame of mind all converge to keep me chasing short-term gains.

Once I come back to earth, however, it's payback time. There's a boatload of refueling, replenishing and damage repair that has to be done — at the very least in my own body, quite possibly in my life as well.

Let's talk biomarkers

Hopefully by now you can see how most — if not all — of the so-called 'bipolar' symptoms connect to the human stress (survival) response. The even better news is that there is a way to test to see if this is what's happening.

There are numerous biomarkers for these kinds of stress states: blood pressure, blood sugar and oxygen levels, blood and saliva tests for hormones (e.g., adrenaline, glucocorticoids), skin conductivity tests, muscle tension or twitching, frequency of movement, whether fine motor or large motor movements are more prevalent, pupil dilation, whether visual perception is biased toward detail or gross impressions, brain scans to see what neural pathways are 'hot' or 'cold'… the list goes on.

What about other DSM Disorders?

Yep, they all potentially have their stress response correlates with symptoms that match known 'stress signatures' as well. It's only a matter of time before we start to map them and do the real honest science that critical psychiatry circles have been calling for all along.

Why this matters

Let's suppose you tell me that the wreckage I create in a 'bipolar' state of mind is due to a genetic or disease condition that renders my brain structurally defective. If that's the case, then any hope I have of effective treatment is logically in the purview of brain scientists, doctors, and surgeons. My major role is to pray that they figure out a cure and soon.

On the other hand, suppose the problem isn't that at all. Suppose that what's really driving my so-called 'mania' is that my stress/survival response is firing wildly. Then the solution is a lot more within the realm of something I can work with.

Yes, I have some learning to do. I need to understand the basics of how the survival system operates. I need to learn what turns it on — and, even more importantly, what turns it off. But if I have that basic knowledge (which the average person can be taught in a few hours), then I have a tremendous amount I can work with through my own observation and trial and error.

Working with 'Mania'

Here are some basics that I've found useful for me.

What turns me on?

The survival response turns on for me any time the stakes are high. The activation it produces can be either predator (appetitive) or prey (defensive) in nature. Predator/appetitive activation and prey/defensive activation look and feel quite different. This is largely due to the effects of dopamine, which fires a lot more in predator mode due to the anticipation of reward.

In the simplest terms, here is how it works for me:

- Predator mode is activated by opportunities. I feel excited about capturing them and feel relieved (safe) when this happens. I fear and feel threatened at the prospect of losing them. I feel relieved (safe) if I can prevent this.
- Prey mode is activated by threats. I fear being overwhelmed by them and/or becoming someone else's opportunity. I get excited by the prospect of escaping such threats and feel relieved (safe) when able to do so.

What turns me off?

I used to think there was no way to shut this thing down. Survival activation had been a part of me — and basically running my life — for as long as I can remember. I couldn't imagine how I could work with it. I had tried so many things, none of which really seemed to work. The drugs shut me down but killed everything I enjoyed about myself along with it. I felt stuck.

Things started to change when I began to see my body as my ally rather than my enemy. The simple fact for me is this: my body basically hates being in survival mode. It's just not sustainable.

There are 37 trillion cells in the human body. The survival response oversupplies a few of them but leaves the vast majority high and dry. For the rest of these cells, life in survival mode is pretty dismal. The survival system burns up energy and resources like they're going out of style. As a result, the needs of my remaining body tissues are getting ignored and going unmet while the survival system is off and running. They are not happy about this. Nothing would make them happier than to exit survival mode and go back to the other option (content, sustainable, relaxed) that every human body has to offer.

This other option is the rest and refresh mode of the parasympathetic nervous system. Until recent years and with the advent of somatic experiencing and polyvagal theory, you didn't hear much about this system. It was considered boring compared to fight-or-flight. Instead of being the fighter pilot or star boxer, it is the mechanic/janitor that does all the clean-up, repair, and maintenance.

But, when you think about it, there is tremendous wisdom and potential in this restorative bodily system. The parasympathetic system is what lets us digest food, keep a steady heartbeat, not forget to breathe, replenish resources, and sleep at night. It's what allows us to grow, heal injuries, defend against infection, reproduce — and love and connect with ourselves, each other and whatever is beyond.

Better yet, this restorative (parasympathetic) part of us has been with us since the womb. It knows our needs and how to meet them better than anyone else could. No cell in the body is ever more than five cells away from the capillary network it manages. It literally does brain surgery on us every night while we sleep to heal the damage of the day.

Think about that for a minute because the implications are stunning. The 'dumbest' one of us on the planet has a parasympathetic nervous system that is smarter than any neuroscientist and more skilled than any neurosurgeon who ever lived. If that weren't the case, none of us would be alive right now.

Turning off 'mania' (and coming out of rebound depression)

If I want to function in this world, my body basically gives me two choices:

1. A survival activation system (sympathetic) that revs me up and keeps me running and chasing.
2. A restorative system (parasympathetic) that offers less excitement but the option of real serenity and sustainability (well-being).

My personal belief is this: I have to decide 'which wolf I want to feed.'

For me, that means actively choosing which bodily system I want to live in and use to relate to life as a human being. *Is it the body of trust and connection — of sustainability, restoration and well-being? Or is it the body of excitement, ambition and hot pursuit?*

There is more to it than that, however. In my experience, making the shift from survival reactivity to restorative well-being feels a bit intimidating. It calls to mind the addict who went to their sponsor and asked, "What do I have to change?" only to be told the answer is "Everything." What I mean by this is that cultivating parasympathetic well-being has required a totally different approach to life than I was used to. I have needed to develop a different mindset and way of being in the world. En route to making this transition, it helps me to keep the following ideas in mind:

- The survival activation (sympathetic) system goes on for a reason. It is signaling to me that something I care about feels unsafe or at risk. Once that risk is addressed, the system has no reason to stay on. It turns off naturally once I start to feel secure.

- As a result, I generally approach my activation with an eye to restore a sense of safety and well-being. I ask myself what I'm scared of (typically, FOMO-related) and try to listen honestly for the answer. Sometimes just doing this much — honestly owning that I'm scared of something and facing the truth of what that is — can help a lot.

- There's also a bit of a trick to making conscious contact with the body of well-being (restorative system). I can't access this part of me by trying harder or forcing myself to feel something. In fact, the harder I try, the more my survival activation system revs up—and that is as it should be. My survival system is all about trying and achieving. So, the moment I signal there's something I need to try hard for, this system comes online to help me make the grade.

- The restorative (well-being) system plays by entirely different rules. It shows up to help me relax and be with whatever is. Accordingly, this system turns on when I make a decision to trust, let go, and allow myself to be helped.

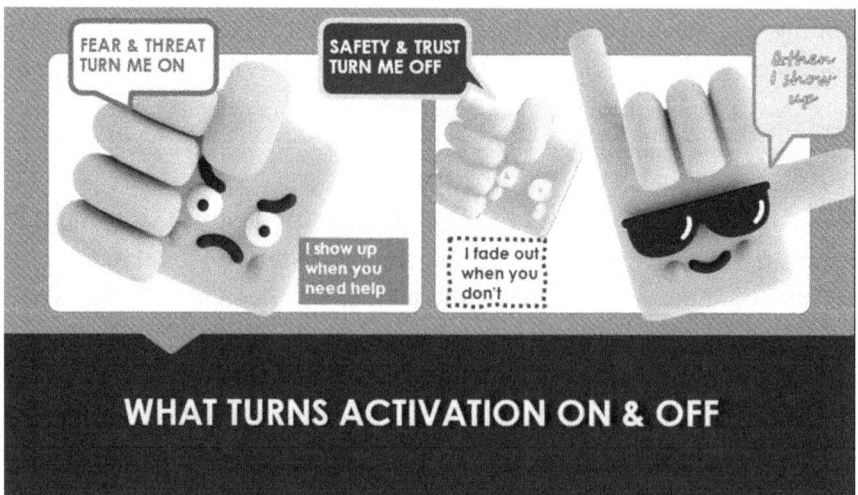

WHAT TURNS ACTIVATION ON & OFF

For me, this requires a conscious shift in focus from *trying to fix it* to actively cultivating my *capacity to trust and be cared for*. This parallels the wisdom of many religions (and Twelve Step programs). In my experience, a very different kind of Power emerges when I give up, stop trying so hard to control, and just let things unfold in the way that they will. The major difference is the Power is not somewhere "out there." It's an intuitive Presence that is very internal to me. And the capacities that make it possible are hardwired into my physiology and the body I was born with.

Below are some steps that I use to help me make the transition from activation to well-being. For me, they capture the essence of the principles I'm articulating here. It can help to practice them daily. The easiest way in times of stress has been just to:

1. Set a timer for a minute or two
2. Rest with a step until the timer dings
3. Reset the timer and move on to the next one.

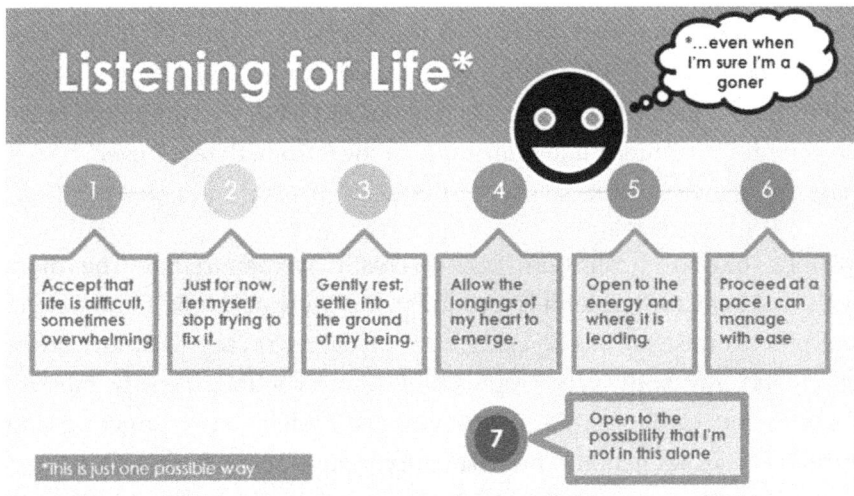

Usually, going through the process a couple of times will create enough space from stress for me to move on and start or restart my day.

Some other strategies

In trying to lessen the amount of time I spend in survival reactivity, it helps to learn to recognize the signs of amping up. I can then use that 'biofeedback' as a mindfulness bell to return to the body of well-being. Once back in that state of relative well-being, I can begin to gently inquire into what is scaring me and allow possibilities for addressing it to bubble up.

It can also help to do things that physically reassure my body and the tissues in me that we are not in crisis. I try to find ways to be with myself that are totally different from how my body would act if I were running from a bear. This includes moving slowly and intentionally, activating my curiosity about small things, doing stuff that takes fine motor coordination instead of large muscle groups, making tiny gentle touching movements one finger at a time, wiggling my toes one toe at a time, doing something familiar and easy like making my bed or washing a dish, playing my guitar... the possibilities are endless.

It's also important to be patient. As Sapolsky points out, the transition from survival activation (sympathetic) to restorative well-being (parasympathetic) is a delicate one. It's bad for the body to have both systems firing at the same time (like heart attack bad). Also, it takes a while to clear one set of hormones from the bloodstream and introduce new ones. Thus, my body needs time to make that shift safely. This takes a while — a minimum of 10-20 minutes and more likely an hour or two. Sometimes, I even find it happening over several days when I've been on a real emotional bender.

Waiting out this transition can feel really uncomfortable. The more activated I am, the harder it is to sit tight. But if I'm able to keep trusting in the process (instead of panicking and ratcheting myself back into stress reactivity), my body gets progressively more comfortable. My muscles relax as my cardiovascular and endocrine systems stop pumping and priming them for action. The circulatory system starts re-routing oxygen and glucose to my stomach, intestines, pancreas, kidneys and prefrontal cortex.

Queasiness, cravings, and gut discomfort dissolve as my digestive system reboots into a context of relative calm. Rational capacities return, and big picture perspective and judgment radically improve as my brain has increasingly more to work with. The end result is that I become progressively interested in — and capable of enjoying — rest, relaxation, sleep, healthy food, recreation, mundane social interactions, and life management tasks. My body repairs and restores. I feel like a human among humans again.

To sum up

As someone with a boatload of social trauma and a really bad relationship with my body historically, making this shift has not come easily. Nevertheless, I've found it possible with practice. The long and short of it is that there are a zillion ways to feel scared, but also a zillion resources for feeling safer. There are also a zillion options for finding something or someone I can potentially trust and let go with or let help me. That's where the diversity of life and experience on planet earth is a huge asset.

It works if I work at it -- and in a way that nothing else has for me. Over time, the internal motor has begun to slow down. Everything is not a crisis anymore. It doesn't always have to get fixed right away -- and sometimes not at all. There is a frame of mind that I can access where everything, really, is okay just the way it is.

References

American Psychiatric Association. (2013). *Diagnostic and statistical manual of mental disorders (5th ed.)*. Washington, DC: American psychiatric association.

Bradley, M. M., Codispoti, M., Cuthbert, B. N., & Lang, P. J. (2001). Emotion and motivation I: Defensive and appetitive reactions in picture processing. *Emotion*, 1(3), 276-298.

Bradley, M. M., & Lang, P. J. (2000). Emotion and motivation. *Handbook of psychophysiology*, 2, 602-642.

Lang, P. J., & Bradley, M. M. (2010). Emotion and the motivational brain. *Biological Psychology*, 84(3), 437–450.

Lang, P. J., & Bradley, M. M. (2013). Appetitive and Defensive Motivation: Goal-Directed or Goal-Determined? Emotion Review: *Journal of the International Society for Research on Emotion*, 5(3), 230–234.

Löw, A., Lang, P. J., Smith, J. C., & Bradley, M. M. (2008). Both predator and prey: Emotional arousal in threat and reward. *Psychological science, 19*(9), 865-873.

Sapolsky, R. M. (2004). *Why zebras don't get ulcers: The acclaimed guide to stress, stress-related diseases, and coping.* New York: Holt Paperbacks.

Sapolsky, R. M. (2017). *Behave: the biology of humans at our best and worst.* New York: Penguin Press.

Schupp, H., Cuthbert, B., Bradley, M., Hillman, C., Hamm, A., & Lang, P. (2004). Brain processes in emotional perception: Motivated attention. *Cognition and emotion, 18*(5), 593-611.

Contributors

Ron Bassman, as a 22-year-old, was involuntarily committed to a psychiatric institution for 6 months where he was diagnosed with paranoid schizophrenia and subjected to massive doses of medication along with a combined series of 40 insulin induced comas and electroshock. Three years later when he became stronger, he returned to Graduate school, earned his PhD in psychology and became a licensed psychologist. His written works include the book *A Fight to Be: Experiences from Both Sides of the Locked Door*. An article he wrote, *Never Give Up*, published in the peer reviewed journal *Psychosis* was voted by subscribers to be the best article of 2012. His current work centers on community inclusion and social justice.

Magdalena Biernat is a university accessibility expert for students with special educational needs and mental health crises, former coordinator of the Peer Support Centre at the Pedagogical University of Krakow, board member of the Human Foundation.

Mateusz Biernat is a special educational needs teacher, psychologist, therapist in the Open Dialogue approach and eCPR method, trainer of recovery assistants, president of the Human Foundation, member of the Mental Health Council of the Ministry of Health in Poland, speaker at international and national conferences, reviewer for Lancet Psychiatry and eClinical Medicine, expert on mental health, member of the Human Rights Committee of Mental Health Europe, with lived experience of schizophrenia, psychosis and multiple psychiatric hospital stays.

Ann Bracken worked in education for 22 years as a special educator, reading teacher, and a college instructor. Her writing credits include three volumes of poetry, a memoir, and several articles in *Mad in America* and the *Awakenings Review*. She serves as a contributing editor for *Little Patuxent Review*, and co-facilitates the Wilde Readings Poetry Series in Columbia, Maryland. In addition, she mentors several incarcerated people with their creative writing and works to advocate for a new paradigm of mental health care that is holistic, humane, and compassionate. Website: https://annbrackenauthor.com/

G. Kenneth Bradford, PhD is currently an independent scholar, Dharma teacher and contemplative yogin integrating Buddhist and Existential-Phenomenological thought and practice. Formerly, he was licensed as a clinical psychologist practicing psychotherapy in the San Francisco Bay Area, and Adjunct Professor at John F. Kennedy University and California Institute of Integral Studies. Publications include *Opening Yourself: The Psychology and Yoga of Self-liberation* (2021); *The I of the Other: Mindfulness-Based Diagnosis & the Question of Sanity* (2013); and *Listening from the Heart of Silence: Nondual Wisdom and Psychotherapy, Vol. 2* (2007, with John Prendergast); as well as numerous peer-reviewed articles intertwining psychology and spirituality, including on "Radical Authenticity," "Non-self Psychology" & "On the Essence of Freedom." He can be reached via his website: https://authenticpresence.net/

Phillipa Byers lives and works on Bundjalung country in Northern New South Wales, Australia. She has a PhD in philosophy and has taught moral philosophy and applied ethics at several Australian universities and to men living in prison. She has peer-reviewed publications in philosophy and ethics. She is also a social worker, most recently working within the New South Wales statutory out of home care (foster and kinship care) system assisting children and young people maintain and deepen connections with their families of origin from whom they are separated.

Natalie Campo, MD is an integrative psychiatrist practicing in Nashville, TN. She became interested in holistic treatment modalities in her first year of medical school at the University of Texas. After medical school, Campo trained in psychiatry at Yale and in medical acupuncture at Harvard. She obtained certifications from the American Board of Psychiatry and Neurology and the American Board of Integrative and Holistic Medicine. For many years, she taught alternative, holistic, and natural treatment options for anxiety and PTSD as a Yale faculty member. She serves as a Clinical Assistant Professor at Vanderbilt and provides consultation to the Osher Center of Integrative Medicine. She started her practice in Nashville called Mindful Medicine in 2011 to bring safe, effective treatments to people seeking relief from anxiety, depression, addiction, and the stress of a hectic lifestyle.

Arnoldo Cantú is a licensed clinical social worker with experience in school social work, community behavioral health, and currently working in private practice. His interests consist of working with children, adolescents, their families, and adults in a clinical capacity. Cantú was born in Mexico and considers Texas home, having grown up in the Rio Grande Valley. He is currently a doctoral student at Colorado State University with an interest in researching conceptual and practical alternatives to the DSM.

Professor Timothy Carey is the Chair, Country Health Research at Curtin University. Tim is a researcher-clinician with a PhD in Clinical Psychology, an MSc in Statistics, a Postgraduate Certificate in Biostatistics, and tertiary qualifications in primary, preschool, and special education. He is a senior Australian academic and Fulbright Scholar who has combined clinical practice with research and university teaching and training throughout his career. He has worked in rural and underserved communities in both Scotland and remote Australia and as an academic in Australia, the US, and Rwanda. He has over 175 publications and has presented his work at conferences and other scientific meetings both nationally and internationally. His In Control blog on Psychology Today has had over 1.48 million views. He is one of the world's leading scholars in the science of control and its application to wellbeing and harmonious social living.

Thomas E. Fink, PhD is a Pennsylvania-licensed psychologist with over 40 years of experience working in the mental health field with diverse clinical populations. He received his doctoral training in research and experimental approaches to learning and cognitive psychology at Temple University, Philadelphia, PA. and clinical training and supervision while working in settings that have included state mental hospitals and community mental health centers, as well as general and specialized outpatient settings. He is clinically credentialed with the National Register of Health Service Psychologists. He is interested in theoretical psychology and has presented workshops over the past 30 years critically reviewing the incorrect assumptions of a medicalized American mental health service delivery system. Current interests include understanding the misleading language used to talk about psychological and psychiatric problems and derivative models of therapeutic interventions. He lives and practices part-time in Camp Hill, PA, and can be contacted at drtomfink@gmail.com.

Dr. Daniel Fisher obtained a PhD, then worked at the National Institute of Mental Health, in the laboratory of Neurochemistry. While carrying out research, he was diagnosed with schizophrenia. To humanize the mental health system, he obtained an MD and carried out his residency in psychiatry at Harvard Medical School. He has worked for 44 years as a board-certified, community psychiatrist. Thirty years ago, he co-founded and is now President of Board of National Empowerment Center and is Vice Chair of the board of the National Coalition for Mental Health Recovery. Dr. Fisher was a member of the New Freedom Commission on Mental Health, and was a professor at U. Mass Dept. of Psychiatry. He is one of the developers and trainers of Emotional

CPR. He published a book about his journey of recovery and of the peer recovery movement called *Heartbeats of Hope*.

Al Galves is a psychologist in Las Cruces, New Mexico. He is President of MindFreedom International and a past Executive Director and long-time member of the International Society for Ethical Psychology and Psychiatry. He is a member of the International Society for Psychological and Social Approaches to Psychosis and the Psychotherapy Action Network. In 2007 he received the Distinguished Author and Humanitarian Award from the International Center for the Study of Psychiatry and Psychology. He is the author of Harness Your Dark Side: Mastering Jealousy, Rage, Frustration and Other Negative Emotions.

Kate Hammer is an existential therapist and coaching psychologist based in Central London (UK) with a thriving private practice online. Trained in existential analysis and logotherapy by Alfried Längle, the successor of Viktor Frankl, Kate also sees clients in-person for counselling and therapy. Client themes include anxiety, grief, stasis, worthlessness, non-belonging, racial trauma, gender questioning, uncoupling, cynicism and meaninglessness. Kate is a member of the Race Reflections community. Pro bono work has included Psychosis Therapy Project and piloting group coaching in the community with a local mental health agency.

David Healy has been a Professor of Psychiatry at McMaster University in Canada, at Bangor and Cardiff Universities in the U.K and is a former Secretary of the British Association for Psychopharmacology. He has authored 240 peer reviewed articles, 300 other pieces and 25 books, including *The Antidepressant Era, The Creation of Psychopharmacology, Let Them Eat Prozac, Mania, Pharmageddon, Children of the Cure* and *Shipwreck of the Singular*. He researches treatment adverse effects, the history of psychopharmacology, and the impact of clinical trials and psychotropic drugs on our culture. He is a founder of Data Based Medicine and RxISK.org.

J River Helms is an educator, writer, advocate, and psychiatric survivor. J has worked for Pathways Vermont since 2019. They began as a Service Coordinator on one of Pathways' Housing First ACT teams, supporting folks with experiences related to anxiety, sadness, extreme states, self-harm, suicide, and trauma. J is currently Director of Training & Advocacy, overseeing Pathways Vermont's Training Institute and facilitating various trainings for Vermont's Peer Workforce Development Initiative. They previously worked as a peer support advocate at a community mental health agency. J is neurodivergent, has navigated many experiences of intense emotional distress, and was suicidal for several years. J believes strongly that each person is the expert of their own experience, that people have a right to their own stories, insight, and meaning-making processes, and that all mental health services must be provided through a lens of cognitive liberty and epistemic justice.

Sarah Knutson is an ex-lawyer, ex-therapist, survivor-activist. Past experience includes work with Intentional Peer Support, Mad in America, and organizing (pre-COVID) online peer support for the psychiatric survivor community around a variety of realities that could not be safely named or discussed in mainstream clinical circles. Sarah is currently active with All Brains Belong in Montpelier, VT and working on a critical psychiatry book about the broader stress/survival/diversity paradigm.

Eric Maisel, Ph.D., is the author of 50+ books, among them *The Future of Mental Health, Rethinking Depression, Humane Helping, Redesign Your Mind,* and *The Van Gogh Blues.* He writes the "Rethinking Mental Health" blog for *Psychology Today,* with 3,000,000+ views, and is the developer of, and lead editor for, the Ethics International Press Critical Psychology and Critical Psychiatry series.

Maria Malayter, Ph.D. launched her career working alongside researchers from the University of Arizona Integrative Medicine and the U.S. Navy leading a health and wellness productivity program. She is an accomplished professor of applied behavioral science, leadership, and business psychology. Dr. Maria is the host of The Joy Chemistry podcast, author of several books, and has presented globally at academic conferences and leadership academies. She is a National Wellness Institute Certified Wellness Practitioner, Human Kinetics certified Coach, Intercultural Development Inventory Qualified Administrator, Positive Intelligence coach, affiliate member at the Institute of Coaching at McLean Hospital, and a Harvard Medical School affiliate. Dr. Malayter is a 2023 nominee for SUCCESS magazine's Women of Influence awards for her global impact in teaching, mentoring, and volunteerism.

Donald R. Marks is Associate Professor and Director of Clinical Training in the Department of Advanced Studies in Psychology at Kean University in Union, NJ. As a clinical health psychologist, Dr. Marks researches compassion-focused interventions for patients living with health anxiety, chronic pain, and life-limiting illness. He is Editor-in-Chief for *Ethical Human Psychology and Psychiatry,* the official publication of the International Society of Ethical and Human Psychology and Psychiatry (ISEPP). Dr. Marks is a past president of both the New York chapter of the Association for Contextual Behavioral Therapy and the Philadelphia Behavior Therapy Association.

Kathleen Martin is an Arrernte woman who has worked in Indigenous health for over 35 years and has a Bachelor of Applied Science in Indigenous Community Management and Development, with Curtin University. Kath worked as an Enrolled Nurse in 3 major hospitals in the Northern Territory and as a Senior Aboriginal Health Worker in Western Australia for several years on a Remote Aboriginal Community. She has developed and delivered training packages for Alcohol and Other Drug workers as well as Cross Cultural workshops and Aboriginal Health Worker Training. Kath has held numerous positions including the Coordinator of the Night Patrol and Sobering Up Services in Darwin, and the Senior Aboriginal Liaison Officer at Alice Springs Hospital. Kath has worked for Flinders University in Alice Springs and Darwin in a number of roles including a Topic Coordinator for Post Graduate studies and lecturing on Aboriginal Health in the Medical and Paramedicine Program.

Robert F. Morgan was born between the two world wars and is a Life Member of the American Psychological Association. He has been in the International Society for Ethical Psychology and Psychiatry (ISEPP) since 1999, is a former speech collaborator and project consultant for Dr. Martin Luther King Jr., the founder and editor of Cambridge University Press's *Journal of Tropical Psychology*, and founder of the Division of Applied Gerontology in the International Association of Applied Psychology (IAAP). He has supervised 126 psychology doctoral dissertations in California, Singapore, and Australia as well as has taught a contemporary trauma psychology seminar at the University of New Mexico (UNM). His publications include more than a hundred printed articles and 24 books on topics including lifespan psychology, trauma psychology in context, applied gerontology, and international psychology.

Susan Musante, MS, LPCC helped develop and was the founding director of Soteria-Alaska. As the first full-time director of CHOICES, a peer-led alternative to conventional outpatient treatment, she helped develop the peer workforce in Alaska. She is an educator and advocate for voluntary, informed, compassionate support that work. Her consulting activities focus on training and program development for recovery-directed, peer-provided alternatives. Susan has worked in universities, community-based centers, and consumer-run services. She has educated peer practitioners and masters-level practitioners. Her commitment is to respect the "lived experience" and support recovery.

David Newman lives and works on Gadigal country, Sydney, Australia. He is a faculty member of The Dulwich Centre and an honorary clinical fellow at the University of Melbourne School of Social Work. He has extensive experience in individual, couple and family therapy, primarily through his independent therapy practice Sydney Narrative Therapy, and currently works casually as a group therapist at a psychiatric unit for young people in Sydney. You can find out more about his work by visiting the following links:

https://sydneynarrativetherapy.com.au/#publications; https://dulwichcentre .com.au/holding-our-heads-up/; https://dulwichcentre.com.au/responding-to-suicidal-thoughts/

Michael O'Loughlin is Professor in the College of Education and Health Sciences and in the Ph.D. program in Clinical Psychology at Adelphi University, New York. He has authored or edited many books, Including, most recently, *Lives Interrupted: Psychiatric narratives of struggle and resilience (2019)*, and *Precarities of 21st century childhoods: Critical explorations of time(s), place(s), and identities* (2023). Since 2018 he has been coeditor of the journal *Psychoanalysis, Culture and Society*. He is also editor of the book series, *Psychoanalytic Interventions: Clinical Social, and Cultural Contexts*, and co-editor of the book series *Critical Childhood & Youth Studies: Theoretical Explorations and Practices in Clinical, Educational, Social, and Cultural Contexts*. He directs the Adelphi Asylum Project. He has a private practice for psychotherapy and psychoanalysis on Long Island, NY. (Personal website: http://michaelolough linphd.com/; faculty profile: https://www.adelphi.edu/faculty/profiles/ profile.php?PID=0064)

Wayne Ramsay, J.D. is a lawyer with the Law Project for Psychiatric Rights (https://psychrights.org/) and a retired airline pilot with captain ratings on the Boeing 737, 747, 757, 767 and Airbus 310.

Jonathan Shedler, PhD, an American psychologist, is known internationally as an author, consultant, researcher, and clinical educator. He is best known for his article "The Efficacy of Psychodynamic Psychotherapy," which won worldwide acclaim for firmly establishing psychoanalytic therapy as an evidence-based treatment. He is also known for his research and writing on personality styles and their treatment. Dr. Shedler is a Clinical Professor in the Department of Psychiatry and Behavioral Sciences at the University of

California, San Francisco (UCSF). Many of Dr. Shedler's publications are available for download from his website https://jonathanshedler.com.

Radosław Stupak holds a PhD in Psychology from Jagiellonian University. He is a Lecturer at the Institute of Psychology, Pedagogical University of Cracow. He has also studied at the Radboud University, University of Groningen and St. Petersburg State University. He is an Associate of the International Institute for Psychiatric Drug Withdrawal. He has written for media in Poland about the negative consequences of the dominance of the biomedical model in mental health care, and the harms associated with often unnecessary or avoidable prescription of psychiatric drugs.

Dr William Van Gordon is a Chartered Psychologist and Associate Professor of Contemplative Psychology at the University of Derby (UK), where he also Chairs the School of Psychology Research Committee. He is internationally recognised for advancing the Contemplative Psychology research agenda, to which he has contributed over 100 peer-reviewed papers. William writes a regular blog on Contemplative Psychology for Psychology Today (https://www.psychologytoday.com/gb/contributors/william-van-gordon-phd) and is author of *The Way of the Mindful Warrior* (https://a.co/d/aHdVnsf).

Harper West, MA, LLP is a psychotherapist at Great Lakes Psychology Group in Clarkston, Michigan. She is credentialed in Self-Compassion in Psychotherapy (SCIP), has completed training in Mindful Self-Compassion and Compassion-Focused Therapy, and was trained in transcendental meditation in 1978. Harper graduated from Michigan State University and the Michigan School of Professional Psychology. She is contributing author to the bestselling book *The Dangerous Case of Donald Trump: 27 Psychiatrists and Mental Health Experts Assess a President* and its second edition. Her self-help book *Pack Leader Psychology* won an IBPA Ben Franklin Award for Psychology. Harper serves on the Michigan Board of Psychology. (https://www.harperwest.co/)

Louis Wynne was born in Leeds, England, and received his early education there. He served in the Strategic Air Command during the Cuban Missile Crisis, later earned the PhD in Psychology at The Ohio State University, and then became an Adjunct Associate Professor of Psychiatry and Psychology at the University of New Mexico. He was later appointed Clinical Director of the New Mexico State Hospital. He was Co-editor-in-Chief of *Ethical Human Psychology and Psychiatry* and was the recipient of the Thomas Szasz Award in 2010. The American Board of Disability Analysis has inaugurated a scholarship in his name. He has been in solo clinical practice (adults only!) since 1988.

Dr. Anna Yusim is an internationally recognized, award-winning, Stanford- and Yale-educated Board Certified Psychiatrist and Executive Coach. With clients including Forbes 500 CEOs, Olympic athletes, A-list actors and actresses, and the Chairs of academic departments at top universities, Dr. Anna Yusim has helped over 3000 people in 70 countries achieve greater impact, purpose, and joy in their life and work. As a Clinical Assistant Professor at Yale Medical School, Dr. Yusim is Co-Founder of the Yale Mental Health and Spirituality Center. She is the best-selling author of *Fulfilled: How the Science of Spirituality Can Help You Live a Happier, More Meaningful Life.*

Margaret Zawisza, MA, has been working with the principles of eCPR as a trainer and facilitator since 2017. She works as a psychotherapist for the National Health Service (UK). She is also a practitioner of Open Dialogue. "What is important to me is the connection we make with others and the revitalization and strength we can experience through these human connections. Being present with another person experiencing crisis. I believe that listening with the heart begins the process of moving from crisis to safety. Being listened to, being heard and being seen are very powerful in recovery."

www.ingramcontent.com/pod-product-compliance
Lightning Source LLC
Chambersburg PA
CBHW021438180326
41458CB00001B/324